Dear Reader,

It's ten years to the day since *High Level Wellness* first came out, and its impact on the wellness movement has been so enormous that it has become a kind of classic (books that kick off movements get to become "classics" even if they aren't 100 years old). This anniversary issue showcases the original book, exactly as it was. We didn't want to tamper with the original flavor of wellness advocacy, circa mid-1970s, with all its wisdom, enthusiasm, fads, and goofs. We didn't want to rob you of the fun of finding out for yourself what this movement looked like way back when.

But ten years allow for a lot of hindsight, and Don Ardell has his own ideas about how he would redo things now. Thus he has inserted, around the "filling" of the original, the "bread" of his updated thinking. For those of you who already know *High Level Wellness*, his new material will explain itself. But for those who are reading this book for the first time, here are a few tools to help you out:

* This anniversary edition is formatted like a sandwich—the original material is in the middle, and the updates appear at the beginning and end.

* The updates are keyed to the original by title and by page numbers.

* Comments on the original material are introduced by the phrase, "Reflections on. . . ." Comments on material that never made it into the first edition are introduced by the phrase, "Lately I've Been Thinking About. . . ."

* The original included some very seminal tests—state of the art ways of finding out where you were on various wellness scales—in short, an important evolutionary step toward a wellness consciousness. Their historical importance requires that we include them here. But to find out Don's current recommendations for wellness tests, we suggest that you first read his updated chapters and take the new tests before looking over the old (and, in some cases, disavowed) ones.

* The original annotated bibliography still stands as one of the best in the field. To bring it up to date, Don has added a list of wellness books published since 1976 that he finds most valuable. This update appears at the end of the book.

* The original "five dimensions of wellness" in Part Two have been reorganized and somewhat changed. But essentially, the material is the same. The alteration is in emphasis and perspective, not content.

As for the rest of the book, it is self-explanatory. Don is a vitally concerned and funny guy. Enjoy his book—both the filling and the bread—in good health.

R

D1400984

Tenth Anniversary Edition

High Level
Wellness

An Alternative To Doctors, Drugs, and Disease

DONALD B. ARDELL

Ten Speed Press

1☯

Ten Speed Press
P.O. Box 7123
Berkeley, CA 94707

Cover Design by Brenton Beck

Library of Congress Cataloging in Publication Data
Ardell, Donald B.
  High level wellness.

  Includes bibliographical references and index.
  1. Health.   I. Title.
RA776.5.A73   613   77-10993

Previous edition published by Rodale Press in 1977
ISBN 0-87857-194-9

Ten Speed Press edition First Printing 1986
ISBN 0-89815-162-7

Printed in the United States of America

5   4   3   2   1   —   90   89   88   87   86

to Jeanne and Jon

ACKNOWLEDGMENTS
TO THE FIRST EDITION

Many people contributed to this book. I would credit them all if I had the space. Several, however, have to be recognized:

Bob Atkins of the Union Graduate School–West;

Don Gerrard, publisher of the Bookworks;

Carol Stoner, my editor at Rodale Press;

A. Kent Ballard, Executive Director of the American Health Planning Association;

John Travis, doctor of well-being in Mill Valley;

Debbie Eklof, my friend, who typed the manuscript; and

Mary and Roy Ardell, my parents, who got me started on a lifestyle of high level wellness.

ACKNOWLEDGMENTS
TO THE TENTH ANNIVERSARY EDITION

I want to thank all the people who helped me assess my first book, *High Level Wellness*, and prepare this ten-year retrospective commentary. It is not often an author gets to do something like this, and I am delighted to have had the opportunity.

There have been a lot of changes in the past ten years. I have changed a lot, too. But some things—including ideas, concepts, principles, facts, and so on—do not change. Many bear repeating, sometimes in a new context.

I cannot cover all the players, but the principal contributors to my labors at updating and critiquing this book who truly deserve my special thanks are David Randle, Barb Roths, Rosanna Allison, Jerry Gergley, Michelle Solon, John Travis, Mark Crookse, and John Langdon.

Thanks, also, to my editor, Naomi Steinfeld, and my "coach" and editor at Ten Speed Press, George Young.

Contents

Part 1

Getting Clear of Worseness 1
    Why Not Wellness? 3
    Exploring the Wellness Ethic 49
    Measuring Your Wellness 63

Part 2

The Five Dimensions of High Level Wellness................. 93
    Self-Responsibility 94
    Nutritional Awareness 113
    Stress Management 134
    Physical Fitness 145
    Environmental Sensitivity 162

Part 3

Toward a Healthier Nation...................................... 179
    Practicing the Artful Complaint 181
    Helping to Create A New Kind of Planning System..... 207

Part 4

A Wellness Resource Guide/The High Level Wellness
    Honor Roll of Books 215

Part 5

The New Part 295

Index.. 383

Foreword

I was really pleased when Don called and asked if I would write an introduction for the 10th anniversary edition of his book, *High Level Wellness: An Alternative to Doctors, Drugs, and Disease*. I view Don as the Ken Cooper of the wellness movement. Just as Ken Cooper has had a significant impact on aerobic fitness world wide, Don Ardell has had a similar impact in the field of wellness.

Even though Halbert Dunn and John Travis had written about wellness prior to the publication of Don's first book, it was the book, *High Level Wellness: An Alternative to Doctors, Drugs, and Disease* that had a massive impact on the American public. The book was read by professionals and lay persons alike. Ardell found himself being quoted by people from divergent backgrounds. The little yellow book with the smiling sun face could be found in corporate board rooms, classrooms, hospitals, and pulpits.

Don brings a fresh approach to the field of health. His lighthearted style is vastly different from the traditional health education presentation.

Don was misjudged, branded, and attacked by some of my physician colleagues. These detractors thought that Don was anti-doctor or anti-medicine. Don may occasionally exaggerate the relative value of a wellness approach. But when we compare his possible exaggeration with the millions of dollars spent each year by drug companies (claiming outrageous benefits from drugs that may actually cause more problems than they solve), how awful is Don's enthusiasm? It is exciting to observe that the recognition factor of the term "wellness" is far different today than it was ten years ago.

I recall a story a young woman told of an encounter in a Los Angeles bar. While on vacation from Stevens Point, Wisconsin, she was visiting relatives in a suburb of Los Angeles. During a visit to one of the local night spots, a young man approached and asked if he could buy her a beer. She indicated to him that she did not drink alcohol. He then offered her, in succession, marijuana, Quaaludes, and cocaine. After she declined all these offers, he said, "What do you *do*, anyway?" She proceeded to tell him that she was into wellness. The young man said, "*Walnuts!* What in the hell do you do with walnuts?" It is gratifying to note that today, people do not have to explain what it is to be into wellness. It is an accepted term. It is a term used to describe programs run by Fortune 500 companies. It is a term that has been used by the secretary of Health and Human Services and by leaders of the American Medical Association.

There are wellness programs in schools, churches, YMCAs, summer camps, hospitals, and businesses of all sizes. *High Level Wellness* has become a standard reference for all of these programs.

I am sure it is gratifying to Don and his publishers that so much of what he wrote ten years ago is still accurate and helpful today. It would be great if the field of medicine enjoyed that constancy. There are a number of surgical procedures that were done ten years ago that would be considered malpractice today.

The wellness movement is really based on the success model. In this book Don attempts to upgrade and revise the information that he provided ten years ago, as to how to live successfully. Orthobiosis is another term that could be used to describe successful living. Orthobiosis simply means correct living. The term *correct* is not used in a moralistic or dogmatic posture. It is used to indicate that there are ways of conducting one's life that are clearly more successful than others.

One of the beauties of Don's approach is to make it simple. The old KISS principle that we learned in school is evident in all of Don's writing—Keep *It* Simple, Stupid!

It is comforting to note that Don does not agree with everything he said ten years ago. What is even more comforting, though, is the ease with which he deals with controversy. He openly acknowledges that there may be differences of opinion concerning certain issues. Certainly, Don and I disagree at times;

but it never interferes with our mutual respect or our mutual goal of continued growth and development toward higher levels of wellness.

During the past ten years, Don has traveled extensively to promote the wellness concept. He has developed a breadth of knowledge and experience. Like a fine wine he has mellowed with the ten years of aging. The refinements and additions to this edition are valuable contributions to the growing resources in the wellness field.

Don is a voracious reader, a prolific writer, and a dedicated participant in this experiment called life. He moves with joy through his weekly activities. He tends to promote harmony rather than discord. He builds bonds rather than creating friction. His ideas are worthy of our attention.

BILL HETTLER, M.D.

Preface

High Level Wellness: An Alternative to Doctors, Drugs, and Disease marked a turning point in my life. I expect there will be other turning points to come, as there were before, but this book remains perhaps the most memorable of all. Its original publication by Rodale Press and the subsequent response to it affected my personal life and changed the direction of my career. The knowledge that it also was a major source of ideas and encouragement for others who would go on to shape and fuel the movement and expand the depth and range of the concept's application is more satisfying than anything else.

For these reasons, I embraced the opportunity to look back, reread, and comment on a book that I wrote ten years ago with a little anxiety and a lot of enthusiasm.

Actually, I never dared hope that *High Level Wellness* would be as influential as it was, but I surely am glad that it turned out that way. Not that it ushered in the millennium: For every person who has had any encounter with wellness, my book, or me, there are still about a million people who have never heard of any of these three. Furthermore, my wellness book was read by fewer than a tenth the number who read Fixx's so-called *Complete Book of Running* or even Miss Piggy's Diet Plan, neither of which dealt with matters remotely as consequential as wellness. (And I say that as a hard-core runner and an admirer of the mythical lady.)

But why be greedy? At least I'm still alive, and I did make my mark on the English language with the phrase "low level worseness," which is itself an (unfortunate but popular) alternative to Dr. Dunn's high level wellness. However, when Webster et al. finally acknowledge this phrase in their dictionaries, I hope that none of them prints my picture next to the term! How ironic and cruel a fate to be forever known—like Drs. Addison, Alzheimer, Hodgkin, and Hemorrhoid—as a disease. And the deadliest of all disorders, at that.

I hope you enjoy reading this edition as much as I enjoyed writing it.

Good wishes—and be well.

Introduction to the Tenth Anniversary Edition

"If only I knew then what I know now!" This kind of regret can make would-be time travelers of us all. Yet if I could return to 1976, to those long, halcyon afternoons on my balcony on Thoreau Circle in Mill Valley where I wrote *High Level Wellness* over the span of that year—knowing everything I know today of the growth/shape and discoveries in wellness that have occurred in the intervening decade—I would enthusiastically do again what I did before, with relatively few changes.

Well, this anniversary edition lets me go back and make those few changes. I welcome the chance to share with you my reflections on the original edition, based on the hindsight of ten years.

This book is my favorite of all those I have written since, for several reasons. The obvious ones are that it launched my career and helped advance a health movement; but my other, more personal reasons are my fond recollections of the wonderful days I spent writing it, and the fact that the basic principles have clearly stood the test of a decade, if not of time. (The jury will be out for quite a spell on the latter.)

"High level wellness is an alternative to doctors, drugs, and disease." "Modern medicine is a wonderful thing, but there are two problems: people expect too much of it and too little of themselves." These and other assertions of the early edition are still evident, more dramatically than ever—only now is the public beginning to act according to the book's iconoclastic perspectives. Similarly, most of the original assertions about wellness as a lifestyle of zest, purpose, and serenity seem more valid today than ever.

Nevertheless, there have been changes, and I know a lot more about some subjects now than I did then. After all, there has been a rich if brief wellness history these last ten years, manifested in hundreds of conferences, books, video and audio tapes, articles, and more. In short, because of the tens of thousands of people who have participated in and helped to shape the wellness movement in America, there are data, facts, insights, and initiatives to draw from today that were unavailable ten years ago.

Thus, this ten-year anniversary issue is itself a form of time travel, especially if you are new to the subject or unacquainted with the first edition of *High Level Wellness*. When you read the original pages you are the time traveler. You get to see what wellness was like back then, both in concept and as interpreted by the (then) few who were exploring ways to promote it in the medical, corporate, and other sectors, as well as how it seemed to apply in five key wellness dimensions.

I received an enormous amount of positive reinforcement from the publication of *High Level Wellness*, including fame, fortune, and offers of marriage. But I also received a few brickbats. These always concerned me, especially when I suspected or knew that the complainant had a telling point. Much as I enjoyed the compliments, I learned more from the suggestions for reforms, whether they were communicated as tactful hints or as gruesome scoldings. I have taken these letters, book reviews, and comments about the book into account in writing the material for this edition of the book. To all my friends and everyone else who took the time to tell me what seemed true and what deserved more (or less) attention in future efforts, I extend my grateful appreciation. What follows is stronger for all this feedback—and, of course, much improved, owing to the opportunity provided by the good folks at Ten Speed Press to time-trip back and forth between 1976 and 1986!

All in all, my sense is that 85 percent of what I wrote in 1976 has stood the test of ten years time, and I am very pleased that I feel that way. I hope most if not all of my colleagues in the field agree with me on this. I'll readily grant that about 14 percent of the parent edition is, understandably enough, either dated, inaccurate, misleading, incomplete, or irrelevant. And the really good news is that only 1 percent of the original 1976 version is out-and-out dangerous nonsense! That's not bad, in my opinion. If those percentages held for the production of American automobiles, we would have fewer recalls and a lower trade deficit; if medical care itself were so managed, medical malpractice claims would decline precipitously, life expectancy would improve by a decade, and the costs of treatment would be several billion a year less than they are now.

Maybe I should have been a doctor, or chairman of the board of the Chrysler Corporation. After all, I'm more sincere than Marcus Welby and cuter than Lee Iacocca. Such is fate.

Garrison Keillor, whose new book was on the top of many best-seller lists, was asked by a *USA Today* reporter (October 4, 1985) whether the book might make him famous. Keillor talked about enjoying the fame, then added, "There are things I would change, though it's a good book. I feel good about it. I think you avoid a lot of problems if you become semi-famous for something that's pretty good to begin with, rather than, say, becoming famous for embezzlement." That's pretty much how I feel about *High Level Wellness* and becoming famous or semi-famous.

This ten-year evaluation assesses and updates each section of the original outline, beginning with the front cover and continuing through the four major parts and headings therein. Enjoy—and remember: "The future lies ahead." Your comments on the current version are warmly solicited, and may be used in the next decade's edition. Just know that, other things being equal, the author prefers warmly phrased compliments (if not marital proposals) to gruesome scoldings.

Part 1

Getting Clear
of Worseness

Imagine that you live in a dictatorship. The leader is a tyrant and a bizarre character, even by authoritarian standards. While you and most other citizens are reasonably prosperous, educated, and secure, you are required to pursue a certain kind of lifestyle. Specifically, you must refrain from all vigorous exercise, eat a high-fat diet laced with refined white sugars and flours, and take plenty of additives, preservatives, and stabilizers in your food each day. You are expected to weigh at least 20 pounds more than the optimal range for your age, sex, height, and bone frame. In addition, there are certain quotas expected of you: you must consume large quantities of coffee, cigarettes, alcohol, aspirin, and other drugs. Computers are set up to monitor your adherence to these regimens; deviations are treated harshly. Naturally, no meditation or other forms of relaxation are allowed. Once a year, however, on the tyrant's birthday, you are permitted to enjoy natural foods, refrain from caffeine, smoking, and the drinking of intoxicants. You can pursue the exercise of your choice on this day, and any form of stress management is similarly looked upon as a permissible endeavor on this particular occasion.

Isn't it amazing how many of us act as if there really *were* a tyrant programming us to self-destruct before our time? Imagine what would happen on the tyrant's birthday when a 24-hour period of health-enhancing behavior was possible. How many folks do you suppose would pass up the single chance to get out and run, play, and feel alive on this special day? How many would choose the health-robbing diet when a nutritious alternative was possible? And wouldn't this occasion be a time of experimenting

1

with some form of stress management to allay anxiety, tension, and upsets?

You have such a day—every day. The only tyrant you face is your own inertia and absence of will—your belief that you are too busy to take your own well-being into your own hands and that the pursuit of self-health through a wellness-promotive lifestyle is too hard, complicated, or inconvenient.

Good news! You can depose this inner tyrant and set up a new government of you—to preside over a different kind of lifestyle for a fuller kind of life. The difference can be greater than night and day. The difference can be high level wellness— as opposed to low level worseness.

I wrote this book for people who feel controlled by sickness-inducing habits and who are dependent upon others for their health and well-being. I wrote it for *you* if you feel hooked by doctors, drugs, or disease. My basic goal is to show that a healthy lifestyle can provide more joy, satisfaction, and zest in living than you could ever obtain from the predominant behavior patterns in contemporary America (smoking, eating junk food, not exercising, living with uncontrolled stress, refusing accountability for your own health, etc).

You won't find any cures, remedies, or prescriptions in this book; no one approach to inner peace, outer riches, or complete and bionic superhealth; no gurus to believe or promises to take on faith. Instead, I urge you throughout to chart your own life course, guided and aided by an awareness of some rather fundamental health principles, five key dimensions, and a wide range of alternative approaches, strategies, and techniques. All these elements are part of a lifestyle philosophy called high level wellness. Maybe you are at a place in your life where this philosophy will work for you. I hope this is the case. Enjoy.

Why Not Wellness?

Modern medicine is a wonderful thing, but there are two problems: people expect too much of it, and too little of themselves.

I have long been a Mozart fan. I especially love "Eine Kleine Nachtmusik," "Serenata Notturna," and the piano concertos; at one time in my life I tried to read everything I could find about this ill-fated genius whom many credit with bringing more beauty into the world than anyone before or since. (That is quite a claim, even for a Mozart.) One of the Mozart books I discovered contained an anecdote which I think applies to modern medicine. As a young man, Wolfgang Amadeus was a court composer in Vienna at the palace of Emperor Joseph II. Required to produce what he considered slight and unchallenging works for the limited tastes of the nobility, he is said to have been asked how he felt about the compensation he received. His alleged reply has stayed with me these many years: "It is too much for what I do, and too little for what I could do."[1]

Modern medicine costs Americans over $140 billion annually, about 8½ percent of the value of all goods and services produced in a year. What we get is called the health system. In many ways, modern medicine is good, invaluable, and worthy of our highest regard.

But modern medicine is not the same as health. If we could purchase health for $140 billion a year, we would be getting a good buy. The cost would, in fact (to paraphrase Mozart), be too little for what health is worth. But we are not buying health with these great investments of the national treasure. Health cannot be bought—at any price.

---

1. Benson Wheeler, and Claire Lee Purdy, *My Brother Was Mozart* (New York: Henry Holt and Co., 1937), p. 126.

Yet, Americans spend vast sums of money for the treatment of diseases that could have been prevented free. They undergo god-awful suffering and give up years of life because health and well-being seem too much trouble to think about—until it is too late. The most crippling iatrogenesis (doctor-caused illness) inflicted by the medical establishment is benign in relation to the illness which individuals foist upon themselves through destructive lifestyles.

But you can join the ranks of thousands who have started to look to themselves for health—and who use modern medicine (and what is misleadingly called the health system) only when they have already done what they can for themselves. What you can do for yourself is a great deal; what medicine can do for you is rather limited. My emphasis is on what is within *your* power and my concern centers around self-responsibility for rip-roaring good health and well-being. This approach is known as high level wellness. I call it an alternative to doctors, drugs, and disease because a lifestyle that's consistent with wellness principles and that integrates wellness dimensions will help you avoid disease and need doctors and drugs far less than you probably do right now.

My "Roots" in Wellness

My background is in health planning. For the past 10 or so years, I have worked in the medical system as a health researcher, consultant, administrator, and teacher. I wrote this book after I "dropped out" of the health-planning system. I left because I finally came to accept what I suspected for several years, namely, that health planning has almost no effect upon the health system—and that the health system in turn has little effect upon the health of the people.

As a health planner, I worked for and later directed agencies in Minnesota and California in attempts to make the medical system more efficient. Our concerns were excess hospital beds, plans for new technologies, doctor services, medical costs, and review of proposals for federal and state grants for new facilities and equipment. We were not expected to ask if all this had a positive impact on the health of the people, though some people did voice misgivings, on occasion. What really got me going in this direction was encountering the work of two physicians, Halbert L. Dunn and John W. Travis.

In 1961, Halbert L. Dunn published a little book about the interrelated and interdependent whole human being composed of body, mind, and spirit. The individual, wrote Dunn, must find personal satisfactions and a sense of purpose in life: to do so, he/she needs opportunities for the expression of uniqueness and a place of dignity amongst others. Dr. Dunn went on to describe health as so much more than the absence of illness. He talked about a state wherein you actually glow with well-being, a state, in his words, wherein you are "alive clear to the tips of your fingers. You have energy to burn. You tingle with vitality. At times like these, the world is a glorious place." Dr. Dunn gave a special name to this state of well-being, the same name that he gave to his wonderful book: high level wellness.[2]

I came upon *High Level Wellness* when Dr. Henrik Blum, head of the health-planning department at the University of California at Berkeley, handed me this worn little 5-by 7-inch book and said, "You can't afford not to read this!" He was right; reading Dr. Dunn's book in early 1975 was something akin to being hit with a bolt of "benevolent" lightning. "This is what we health planners should be attempting," I thought to myself. I began reading all the health books I could find, visiting "holistic"[3] health centers, talking to and exchanging letters with other people throughout the country interested in similar notions, and beginning to explore and experience on a personal level some of the techniques (e.g. biofeedback, meditation, etc.) of the "new medicine."

---

2. (Arlington, Va.: R. W. Beatty, 1961). See review in the Wellness Resource Guide.

3. *Holistic* means "viewing a person and his/her wellness from every possible perspective, taking into account every available concept and skill for the person's growth toward harmony and balance. It means treating the person, not the disease. It means using mild, natural methods whenever possible. For the person, it means engaging in a healthier lifestyle to enjoy a higher level of wellness. The holistic approach promotes the interrelationship and unity of body, mind, and spirit. It encourages healthy, enjoyable activity on all these levels of existence. A holistic approach differs from simply following an "alternative" therapy. It is not an alternative to conventional medical practice. Rather, it includes judicious use of the best of modern western medicine combined with the best health practices from East and West, old and new."

Dr. Halbert Dunn died at age 80 in late 1975. I never did have the opportunity to meet him; I suppose I'll always regret not having had the chance to thank him for being such an influence on my development, and for his courage in speaking and writing about wellness at a time when some colleagues and medical experts thought the idea unrealistic and impractical. I have had the good fortune, however, to come to know another of my wellness mentors.

While attending a lecture at the Wholistic Health and Nutrition Institute (WHN) in Mill Valley one evening, I met John Travis, M.D. Dr. Travis had a two-projector slide show, which he employed to explain the nature and purposes of his Wellness Resource Center. This encounter was the second "benevolent lightning bolt" in my early evolution into wellness. I'll tell you a lot more about Dr. Travis and the Wellness Resource Center in just a moment—for now, I'll just mention a few of my earliest conclusions about wellness:

- Attention to lifestyle and environment offers the most rewarding paths to improved levels of health. It is the only way to reduce the staggering cost burden of American medicine, and the best way for you to reduce your chances of premature aging and unnecessary suffering from degenerative disease.
- Wellness initiatives in one area of your life will reinforce health-enhancing behaviors in other areas. If you take up jogging and stay with it for a week, or if you develop a meditation technique or other relaxation skill, or if you do any one of hundreds of possible things appropriate to your unique pace and preferences that makes you feel more alive and vigorous, this effort will carry over, sustain, and motivate you to pursue other dimensions of high level wellness. And the more positive things you do *for* your body, the fewer negative things (e.g. smoking) you will want to do *against* it.
- It is even possible to be "well" in the midst of illness and dying. You can learn to interpret illness as a message from within—a signal that some aspect of your life de-

serves attention and reform. Similarly, you can learn to accept the eventuality of your own mortality—and experience the dying process as another aspect of human reality. If you do this, neither illness nor the acceptance of eventual death will inhibit your acceptance of life—and the treasuring of optimal good health that will enable you to achieve the fullest existence within your potential. For there is always illness and death in wellness and life and, in the last analysis, the ratio between birth and death will be one-to-one.

• A state of high level wellness is within the reach of all. A wellness lifestyle will not only drastically reduce your risks of illness or disease; it will provide for you a life of greater satisfactions, increased serenity, and an expanded interest in the future.

These were among the ideas that got me going in my first years of active study and pursuit of wellness. I know there were many influences on me in addition to Drs. Dunn and Travis—their impact just seems especially dramatic, in retrospect. I do not believe there is a single *cause* of wellness, or any one thing you can do to get into it, or a course or book that alone will motivate you and point the way. No part of the brain can be localized and stimulated to turn you on to wellness, so please stop looking right now for a button to be pushed or, as I figuratively noted, a benevolent lightning bolt or two waiting to fall. What I have come to realize, and what I have used as a unifying theme in this book, is that wellness consists of many wonderful possibilities, and that you can come at it from whatever direction you choose.

One approach that some have found useful is to spend time at holistic health centers or even at a wellness center. This might be a good time to tell you about these interesting places, where the idea of self-responsibility for health and wellness is expressed in a variety of creative ways. You might want to go to one of these centers someday; more likely, you will probably just want to think about some of the approaches being taken and perhaps try some of them on your own.

7

Welcome to the
Wellness Resource Center

As I've already told you, one of the major influences on my thinking about health as something quite different from medicine was John Travis, founder of the Wellness Resource Center in Mill Valley, California. A physician with all the credentials of the medical order (Tufts M.D., residency in Preventive Medicine and Master's in Public Health from Johns Hopkins), Travis seems to have realized the forecast made in 1957 by Dr. D. C. Jarvis in his famous book, *Folk Medicine*. Jarvis predicted that "the doctor of the future will be a teacher as well as physician, whose real job will be assisting people to learn how to be healthy." Following this pattern, the staff of the Wellness Resource Center uses no drugs, gives no prescriptions, does no lab work, conducts no physical examinations, and sees no patients. People who show up at the center with physical symptoms or illnesses requiring treatment are referred to other physicians. So you might wonder, what does it do? A great deal, it turns out.

Travis, whom I think of as a doctor of well-being, has organized the Wellness Resource Center, its staff, and its programs to support his contention that self-responsibility is the key to high level wellness. Programs at the center take several forms, although the basic approach takes one direction. In the first place, people are acknowledged as clients rather than patients; the distinction is important in underscoring the importance of the commitment to self-responsibility. At the center, emphasis is on coming to know yourself, and learning to recognize and effectively express your emotions and feeling states.

If you are beginning to suspect that John Travis and the Wellness Resource Center are different from your friendly neighborhood medical clinic, you are on the right track. That any similarities are both coincidental and unlikely is demonstrated by the skills which clients develop in the course of a four- to eight-month program. If you joined such a program, you would learn to:

- Relax—regularly reach deep relaxation of body tension at will.
- Experience Yourself—experience rather than intellectualize physical and emotional feelings to become more aware of the body-mind connection.
- Remove Barriers—clear away self-imposed barriers by examining "forgotten" or suppressed experiences and by releasing an emotional charge.
- Improve Communication Skills—develop better communication skills to effectively express (rather than repress) emotions such as sadness, fear, anger, and enthusiasm and to learn how to ask for what you want.
- Enhance Creativity—express talents and creative abilities which often manifest themselves as stress and symptoms if not allowed full expression.
- Envision Desired Outcomes—use creative energy to visualize actual results you would like to manifest in your world.
- Take Full Responsibility for Yourself—see exactly how you are contributing to your problems and how to take charge of your own life in order to create what you want.
- Love Yourself—gain a greater sense of self-worth and self-acceptance which enables you to see yourself as a Wonderful Person, love yourself, and thereby be able to love others.

Now I do not know what your experience with physicians has been, but my own encounters have been quite a bit different from this. I recall asking Dr. Travis what, in a few words, the staff was trying to impart at the Wellness Resource Center. He told me the aim was to assist clients to become experts in themselves—a goal which deserves the commitment and status usually associated with pursuing an advanced graduate degree. At one point, Dr. Travis said that going through the center is akin to earning a master's degree in yourself. According to him, "There are as many degrees of wellness as there are degrees of illness. The idea of measuring wellness and helping people attain higher levels of wellness is relatively new."

Travis recognizes the historical neglect of health measures due to the association of the term with the absence of illness, and he has devised a model to facilitate a reorientation from health as nonsickness to health as a positive state of well-being. The model is a continuum which Travis uses to give equal time to wellness. Here it is.

As Travis describes the continuum, "Moving from the

WELL MEDICINE

disability symptoms signs

PREMATURE DEATH

HIGH LEVEL WELLNESS

education growth self-actualization

TRADITIONAL MEDICINE

Neutral point no discernible illness or wellness

center to the left shows a progressively worsening state of health. Moving to the right of center shows increasing levels of health and well-being. Traditional medicine is oriented towards curing evidence of disease, but usually stops at the midpoint. Well medicine begins at any point on the scale with the goal of helping a person move as far to the right as he is willing to go."[4]

Travis believes that wellness begins when an individual sees himself or herself as a growing, changing person. High level wellness means giving care to the physical self, using the mind constructively, channeling stress energies positively, expressing emotions effectively, becoming creatively involved with others, and staying in touch with the environment.

In contrast to this ideal, the center believes that many people who may lack obvious physical symptoms of illness are in fact bored, depressed, tense, anxious, or generally unhappy with their lives. These emotional states often lead to physical disease through the lowering of the body's resistance. The same feelings can also lead to abuse of the body through smoking, drinking, and overeating. Usually, these behaviors are substitutes for other, more basic human needs, such as recognition from others, a stimulating environment, caring and affection from friends, and growth towards a higher degree of self-awareness.

---

4. See my article entitled "Meet John Travis, Doctor of Well-Being," *Prevention*®, (April 1975), pp. 62–69; also, see the brochure entitled *Well-Medicine: Client Information.*

The Wellness Resource Center staff works to help clients learn how to take charge of their own lives and to feel good about themselves. What happens is not medicine, as most of us think of medical services; it is an alternative approach wherein Travis and staff are facilitators and assistants to clients moving toward high level wellness.

Usually a potential client telephones, then agrees to proceed, and an appointment is made. The center then mails to the new client a battery of questionnaires, one of which is the Wellness Inventory (a Travis creation) containing 120 questions. The client checks those which apply to him or her. He or she is also given a booklet,[5] which also contains extensive footnotes explaining the health implications of selected items, and is divided into 10 categories. The categories, along with sample questions, are as follows:

Productivity, Relaxation, Sleep
04 ☐ If awakened, it is usually easy for me to go to sleep again.
09 ☐ I meditate or center myself for 15 to 20 minutes at least once a day.

Personal Care and Home Safety
12 ☐ I regularly use dental floss and a soft toothbrush.
17 ☐ I minimize my exposure to sprays, chemical fumes, or exhaust gases.

Nutritional Awareness
20 ☐ I eat at least one uncooked fruit or vegetable each day.
29 ☐ I have a good appetite and maintain a weight within 15 percent of my ideal.

Environmental Awareness
30 ☐ I use public transportation or car pools when possible.
33 ☐ I set my thermostat at 68° or lower in winter.

Physical Activity
43 ☐ I jog at least one mile twice a week (or equivalent aerobic exercise).
48 ☐ I do yoga or some form of stretching-limbering exercise for 15 to 20 minutes at least twice per week.

---

5.   The Wellness Resource Center offers a wellness self-evaluation in the form of a wellness workbook. Available from the center, 42 Miller Avenue, Mill Valley CA 94941, at a cost of $25 (at the time of this writing), the 100-page workbook contains all the questionnaires used at the center as well as specific guidelines for how to increase one's wellness.

Emotional Maturity and Expression of Feelings
51 ☐ I think it is OK to feel angry, afraid, joyful, or sad.
53 ☐ I am able to say "no" to people without feeling guilty.

Community Involvement
65 ☐ I would at least call the police if I saw a crime being committed.
68 ☐ If I saw a car with faulty lights, leaking gasoline, or another dangerous condition, I would attempt to inform the driver.

Creativity, Self Expression
77 ☐ I like myself and look forward to the future.
79 ☐ I find it easy to express concern, love, and warmth to those I care about.

Automobile Safety (optional)
81 ☐ I wear a lap safety belt at least 90 percent of the time that I ride in a car.
84 ☐ I frequently inspect my automobile tires, lights, etc., and have my car serviced regularly.

Parenting (optional)
94 ☐ I do not store cleaning products under the sink or in unlocked cabinets where a child could reach them.
98 ☐ I frequently touch or hold my children.

In addition to the Wellness Inventory, clients complete the Health Hazard Appraisal, a medical history questionnaire, a life-change index and a purpose-in-life test, a computerized dietary inventory, a vision questionnaire, and a nutrition/health/activity profile. Clients are asked to write a paragraph on each of four dimensions of wellness, and to use the sample questions under each dimension as guides to their response, which should be brief. The dimensions and sample guide questions are:

1. Stress Control
   Do you meditate? If so, how often and in what way? Do you often feel tense or have cold hands or feet? What do you do for fun? Do you let yourself have massages? How often? What are your creative outlets? Are you satisfied with your abilities to relax?

2. Self-Responsibility
   Do you believe you are responsible for the quality of

your life? What, if anything, would you like to be different in your life? Please mention any counseling or growth-related processes you have been involved in. Are you satisfied in this area?

3. Nutrition
   How much attention do you pay to the content of the foods you eat? Do you use supplements or vitamins? Do you eat home-cooked meals or eat in restaurants? Are you satisfied with your nutrition?

4. Physical Fitness
   What kind of vigorous exercise do you get, if any? Have you had positive or negative experiences with athletics in the past? Do you do any stretching (yoga) exercises? Are you satisfied with your physical condition?

In addition, each person responds to four open-ended questions leading to a client/center "contract":

1. The major things I want to accomplish by being in the WRC program: (example: Be able to dance, sing, cry, yell, say "no," and love myself instead of giving myself high blood pressure.)
2. How I plan to accomplish them: (example: Go dancing, read *Born To Win*, learn how to fight effectively with my spouse, ask for strokes and learn to feel comfortable getting them.)[6]
3. What I might do to sabotage myself to keep from getting them: (example: "Make others wrong" for expressing themselves openly, act sullen, and provoke negative strokes from spouse.)
4. How I will know when I have met my contract: (example: I'll be dancing and singing at least once a week, having normal blood pressure, and enjoying getting strokes and having free time without feeling guilty about it.)

All of this is designed to help the client get the most from the Wellness Evaluation visit. Travis emphasizes that the questions are designed to stimulate the client's thinking about the state of her or his wellness as well as to serve as a guide in initial discussions.

---

6. As defined in transactional analysis, a *stroke* is "any act implying recognition of another's presence." See Muriel James and Dorothy Jongeward, *Born to Win* (Menlo Park, Calif: Addison-Wesley, 1973), p. 44.

After evaluation, many clients enroll in the one-to-one sessions with a counselor and join a "lifestyle evolution" group to explore the basics of wellness. At the Wellness Resource Center, these are the basic areas (in order of emphasis) and the general approach taken.

Stress Control

From the inventory data, the staff knows whether and to what extent the client meditates; frequency and type of stress experienced; ability to have fun and stay loose; creative outlets favored; and other information about the client's ability to relax.

The staff then employs various techniques—some through group methods—to strengthen the client's ability to use a stress-reduction approach. Though Travis believes biofeedback is sometimes built up into a panacea by excessive claims, he does employ it as the major stress control and energy-channeling device. Biofeedback, in case you aren't familiar with it, measures very subtle changes in the body, such as muscular tension, and displays the information back in a way that enables the person to achieve unusually deep states of relaxation. In concert with techniques such as meditation, guided fantasy, massage, sauna and hot tub baths, the staff has had success using biofeedback for such stress symptoms as headaches, back problems, insomnia, and an inability to concentrate.

An important part of the center's approach to stress control is managed by two staff members who specialize in clearing, visual stress reduction, and the process of visualization. They assist clients in specific areas of concern, such as personal effectiveness, persisting conditions and problems, defense mechanisms, and automatic behavior. By clearing mental blocks and emotional charges, the client can experience freedom from compulsions, and an increased ability to communicate freely, attain goals, and overcome personal limitations. One center staffer works with clients' vision. Through Bates Method exercises, clients with normal vision and with refractive error learn to relax strained eyes. Clients also learn the skills of visualization, which help them to attain specific desired states or conditions, such as deep relaxation, new personal attributes, changed relationships, and new commitments in life.

While some of this may begin to sound far out, Travis told me that these approaches really work, particularly in evoking creativity. When clients learn to visualize themselves relaxing, for example, their tension levels dissipate and their bodies begin to feel better. The clients then are ready to learn how to apply visualization to imagine states of well-being, which in fact helps them realize desires for well-being.

Books on the center's reading list for this dimension include Walter McQuade and Ann Aikman's *Stress*, Barbara B. Brown's *New Mind/New Body*, Hans Selye's *Stress Without Distress*, and Herbert Benson's *The Relaxation Response* (several of which I review in the Wellness Resource Guide).

Self-Responsibility

The center believes that having an aim in life or a sense of purpose is crucial to one's ability to prevent illness, avoid damaging stress, and achieve a high level of wellness. Clients are therefore encouraged to find the means of self-expression most appropriate to their lives, and to chart a path to personal balance and self-esteem.

At the center, an effort is made to aid clients in understanding how they are responsible for the pressures and tensions in their lives. The favorite approach to this objective combines transactional analysis (TA) and psychosynthesis, which are described elsewhere in this book.

Clients are encouraged to keep a journal or self-evaluation log, and share it weekly with the center staff and, if they choose, with the group in which they participate. The journal contains information about significant self-observations, emotional responses to events, new insights based on readings, experiences, and similar recordings. Ten topics the center staff suggests for weekly journal coverage are:

1. My predominant internal themes this week.
2. Feelings (glad, mad, sad, scared, or other) I was particularly aware of this week.

3. Some inner quality of myself that I've become aware of and really like.
4. A behavior of mine I'd like to change.
5. Bracing or internal tension I became aware of this week.
6. How I handled a time of intense stress.
7. What I learned from reading this week.
8. Amount of exercise.
9. Number of meditation or relaxation periods.
10. Amount of time spent nurturing myself.

The center's reading list on self-responsibility features Thaddens Golas's *The Lazy Man's Guide to Enlightenment,* Muriel James's and Dorothy Jongeward's *Born to Win,* and Ram Dass's *The Only Dance There Is.* (See the Wellness Resource Guide for a review of *Born to Win.*)

Nutritional Awareness

Rather than urging a particular diet, specific foods, or favorite vitamins and minerals on clients, the center staff simply encourages and aids them to become better informed about basic nutritional requirements. A counselor begins by describing the multiple threats to a balanced diet created by American culture and the food industry. Then, working with the results of the client's personal computer-processed nutritional report, he helps the person grasp the significance of whatever gap there may be between that person's actual consumption of nutrients and the recommended requirements of protein, fiber, vitamins, and minerals.

Travis, who admits to vegetarian leanings and seldom eats red meat, believes this nation will experience a slow evolution in its diet toward more basic foods for both economic and health reasons. While believing that it's important for people to find their own way, he does urge such basics as adding bran to the diet for bulk, reducing sugar intake and eating more raw vegetables, fresh fruits, unprocessed foods, and taking vitamins B, C, and E, plus minerals, especially from natural sources (e.g., yeast and liver).

As part of the wellness education program, a reading list is made available which includes books, audiovisuals, catalogs, and brochures describing wellness activities in the community. Some of the books on the Wellness Resource Center reading list in the dietary category are Paavo Airola's *Are You Confused?*, Roger Williams's *Nutrition Against Disease*, and Frances Moore Lappé's *Diet for a Small Planet*, all of which I review in the Wellness Resource Guide.

One of the basic principles at the Wellness Resource Center, which is emphasized in connection with the nutritional awareness dimension, is avoidance of an overemphasis on one approach. The staff feels that too many advisors think the way to well-being lies only in their special area. Nutrition enthusiasts too often ignore stress control, while some stress-control "gurus" dismiss physical awareness, and so on. If there is one principle about which the center is adamant, it is the value of integrating the different dimensions in a balanced approach to well-being.

Physical Fitness

The center does not conduct any fitness activities, but does encourage clients to consider initiating and/or supplementing fitness regimens. Particular encouragement is given to those efforts which enhance endurance, flexibility, and strength. The staff especially emphasizes aerobic exercises for cardiovascular benefits and yoga for body toning. The reading list features Ian Jackson's *Yoga and the Athlete*, George Leonard's *The Ultimate Athlete* (reviewed in the Wellness Resource Guide), Kenneth Cooper's *Aerobics*, and George Downing's *The Massage Book*.

Naturally, a client does not move sequentially from one dimension to another; all four areas are integrated and tailored to suit a particular client or group.

One client who has worked with the center, Peter Sorgin, a 41-year-old salesman living in San Francisco, said that he went to the Wellness Resource Center one year ago with a chronic headache problem. Working principally with biofeedback and transactional analysis approaches, Peter claims he soon learned the basis of these pains (emotional conflicts) and how to control and effectively deal with conditions which precipitated his

17

symptoms. He seldom has headaches now, but more important, he has come to view his health as a matter of more than just not being sick. He is currently attending the center on Tuesday evenings, working with a group of eight persons on relaxation exercises and problem-solving discussions related to each of the four wellness dimensions.

Peter emphasizes that it takes hard work and a commitment to realize positive health. "One has to take a firm stand to say I'm not going to go with donuts and coffee and smoking and the commuter crush and pollution in the air and all the rest."

Finally, Peter stresses that wellness is even more than taking responsibility for one's own health—that it implies a concern for the larger society as well in the sense of doing what one can to help others. He would like to see programs like that at the Wellness Resource Center conducted in schools, union halls, work places, churches, and throughout the community.

Another client of the center, David Isaacs, 39, also gave high marks to the biofeedback aspects of the program, but seemed most enthusiastic about the processes employed. He said that the staff "makes available alternate pathways by which people can experience what's going on within themselves." David likes the way Travis avoids a parental role, emphasizing instead the options available as people work to find autonomy within themselves. As he said, "It's a subtle thing, but very effective."

Travis thinks the 400 percent increase in malpractice premiums is one symptom of public dissatisfaction with the traditional physician role. He thinks many doctors have been too willing to assume a demigod posture, raising impossible expectations, with the resultant legal backlash when unrealistic hopes are unmet. Naturally, his own malpractice insurance premiums have been unaffected—mainly because he does not carry any insurance. This is hardly a great risk for a physician who makes no promises to *do* anything *for* anybody, but rather acts as a facilitator to those who choose freely to do for themselves. Few M.D.'s are as unlikely as Travis to violate the abused medical maxim, "First, do no harm." In the Wellness Resource Center context, a disgruntled client would have to sue himself.

18

As you can sense from the above description, Travis has organized a team approach involving professionals with varied skills. People come from near and far; several clients commute nearly 100 miles weekly to attend sessions.

Lasting approximately eight months and encompassing weekly visits for individual and group sessions, the center program costs approximately $1,500—though the expense is less if the client chooses to "graduate himself" earlier. Twenty people were enrolled at the center when I made my visit; Travis estimates that twice this number can be accommodated, which means that 80 clients can attend the center's program annually.

In addition to the ongoing individual and group-oriented program, the center conducts workshops, provides 10-day intensive wellness programs for persons traveling to Mill Valley from distant places, and trains physicians and other health professionals in the organization and approaches of a wellness center. Over 5,000 copies of the Wellness Inventory have been sold, and Dr. Travis has personally given a wellness slide presentation and lecture to approximately 100 groups throughout the country within the past year.

Neither the center nor Dr. Travis himself practices medicine. Travis believes strongly in the separation of wellness programs from treatment or care-giving of any kind. But a number of health centers exist that *do* combine modern medicine and wellness, and it might be a good idea at this point to highlight a few of these interesting places. There are four such centers I would like you to know about: Meadowlark in Hemet, California; the New England Center in Leverett, Massachusetts; the Wholistic Health and Nutrition Institute in Mill Valley, California; and the San Andreas Health Council in Palo Alto, California. Each has an unmistakable commitment to encouraging self-responsibility, to working with the *whole* client as an interconnected being of mind/body/spirit, to using appropriate nontraditional approaches similar to those employed at the Wellness Resource Center (e.g. wellness assessments, relaxation techniques, nutritional counseling, fitness routines, etc.), and to facilitating the client's efforts to comprehend root causes of problems in order to move ahead to a wellness lifestyle.

Let's begin with a visit to Meadowlark, and by meeting Evarts G. Loomis, M.D., another physician as remarkable as Drs. Dunn and Travis—in his own special way.

Healing the Whole Person at Meadowlark

Located about 100 miles southeast of Los Angeles on a 20-acre wooded estate, Meadowlark is the oldest of the wellness resource centers noted in this book. Established in 1958 and nurtured through the years by Dr. Loomis, Meadowlark provides "an atmosphere for self-healing, self-exploration, and personal development." There are two basic beliefs which color and shape the activities at Meadowlark: the first is that mental and emotional tensions coupled with toxins in the body lie at the root of illness; the second is that the human body has an innate, root wisdom with which it maintains or recovers its own perfection when it is allowed to function unhindered. These twin beliefs are expressed in varied ways in Meadowlark programs. A brochure on the institution as a "health and growth center" provides further insight into the environment which Loomis has fashioned in carrying through his concept of treating the whole person's body/mind/spirit.

At Meadowlark we are a *family*, interacting with each other, learning and applying the ways of wholeness, health, and peace. Meadowlark is not a hospital nor a rest home. It might be described as a community where one may learn to help himself to health and high level wellness by practicing, under guidance, tested techniques for living.

Meadowlark is a place to awaken one's awareness of oneself, within and without, in relationship to people, the world, and the universe.

Meadowlark offers its services and programs to all those who are active and healthy but desire a greater understanding of life; successful people who have a sense of unfulfillment; vital people who feel a loss of meaning creeping into their chosen field.

The Meadowlark program in part reflects Dr. Loomis's Quaker background, his study of the healing principles of Hippocrates, Plato, Pythagoras, and Hahnemann, and his visits to eight of Europe's leading health spas. The result is a composite of medicine and religion, art, psychology, homeopathy, and nutrition. All have been brought together in a unique Meadowlark blend. The major forms which express this blend are meditation, nutritional awareness, music, body movement, and art workshops. Loomis believes that within this philosophy there are many paths available at Meadowlark on which guests can approach their highest potentials, their own beings, and special journeys in this life. His role, and that of the center's staff, is to indirectly assist people "to live in awareness of a responsibility for their own process."

So, what should you expect if you were to be a guest at Meadowlark? To begin, you would complete a series of medical forms and attitude inventories and spend at least an hour with a staff counselor. You would be given at least two major programs per day (e.g., biofeedback, yoga, polarity therapy, art and color workshops) and encouraged to take up some form of physical exercise, mental stimulation, and spiritual refreshment. The meals may be different than what you would expect, given the Meadowlark approach to nutritional well-being. This is one of the most important dimensions of the program. Loomis thinks of nutrition as inseparable from absorption and elimination; he told me that "although nutrition is not the only factor in high level wellness, sustained good health without good nutrition is impossible." You could expect a lot of whole grain foods, with a high percentage (50 percent) of meals consisting of fresh raw vegetables/vegetable juices and fruit. (Such foods would make up 100 percent of your diet at times when you were physically ill.) You would also eat plenty of fresh raw seeds, nuts, wheat germ, and brewer's yeast. Most meals begin with a salad and/or fresh vegetable juice or fruit; certified raw milk, buttermilk, yogurt, cottage cheese, and natural cheese are also available, as are vitamin supplements. What you would decidedly not find at the table would be processed or canned goods containing white sugar or flour, fried foods, anything treated with preservatives or sprays, artificial sweeteners, coffee, tea, chocolate, or carbonated beverages. The day, incidentally, begins at 7:00 A.M.! No guest has to do anything, though people are encouraged to participate in the daytime programs and the evening group discussions and interactions. As you might expect, alcohol and smoking are not socially acceptable forms of expression at Meadowlark.

The statistics on the center may interest you. About 20 guests per week are in residence; counting volunteers and part-time people, the staff numbers about 30. The annual budget is approximately $250,000; guests pay a basic rate of $177 to $270 weekly, which includes board, lodging, and the regular retreat-type program experience. There are extra charges for special programs (e.g., fasting, polarity therapy, extended counseling). Guests desiring any kind of medical treatment are requested to stay at least two weeks. Last year, around 500 people stayed at Meadowlark, and 1,400 received a quarterly newsletter. In addition to the regular program, the center is sponsoring workshops for former guests on varied subjects, including personal journal-keeping and an introduction to psychosynthesis. A fund drive has been initiated to raise money for a Loomis Research Clinic to be built on the grounds at Meadowlark. This will contain teaching and laboratory facilities, extra housing, holistic services for nonguests, lecture accommodations, and a chapel dedicated to Loomis's mother who, incidentally, is still active in developing and taping meditations in her home nearby.

Some people are initially drawn to Meadowlark by the personal charisma of Dr. Loomis, as was a 48-year-old California lawyer I talked with recently who specializes in real estate development. This person, who asked to remain anonymous, told me that his interest in Meadowlark was sparked by hearing Dr. Loomis give a talk at a holistic health conference and by his own general interest in alternative approaches to well-being, scientific curiosity, powers of the mind, and "coping with the world." The lawyer visited for a week, and has been back twice since. An articulate person, this man talked about the characteristics, skills, and roles of each staff member at Meadowlark, and also described to me at some length the basis for his high estimation of Dr. Loomis and his 97-year-old mother, Amy. When I asked him to summarize just what happens at Meadowlark to account for such enthusiasm, he told me about a variety of specific activities (water fasts, dream work, expressive drawing, journal-keeping, inner dialogues, and varied processes for discarding excess passions, such as writing them down—and then throwing the paper in the fireplace), but emphasized that Meadowlark is a many-faceted experience. For him, it has been a "marvelous" process, and he says he is healthier emotionally, mentally, and physically as a consequence of having been a part of Meadowlark. As to the experience's staying power or impact on his life when he is not in Hemet, his reply was that through Meadowlark he strengthened his own resources and gained a "perspective" that he now finds invaluable in business and life.

Flo Ray Harmon, a 42-year-old woman from Belmont, California, went to Meadowlark in 1976 after trying unsuccessfully to resolve a complex of problems using surgery, psychiatric treatments, and drugs. She was at "the end of my rope, hooked on doctors, and totally dependent on having someone else take care of my problems and give me 'the cure'." Then Flo read about Meadowlark in a magazine and decided to give it a try. She stayed two and one-half months. The staff of Meadowlark worked with her as a whole person. "It was the first time I was encouraged to think of myself as a mind and spirit as well as a body. I'm convinced it was the integrated approach that got me well." Flo said she started out with homeopathic remedies and a 14-day water fast, then went to juices, and then to a diet that revolutionized her consciousness about food. The exposure to the other dimensions of healthy living; exercise, stress management, and taking accountability for her own health, led this woman to the conclusion that "Meadowlark saved my life. The staff does not do anything *for* you, they give you the tools to work with. I have been back for brief visits on several occasions—I think of myself as part of the Meadowlark family."

The theme of Meadowlark as a way station for spiritual journeys was also expressed by Louise Gates, a 59-year-old resident of San Leandro, California. Louise went to Meadowlark around Christmas season, 1975; though she stayed but two weeks, in some ways she never left. While this client had some physical symptoms, her motivation in traveling to Meadowlark was more related to "a need to discover me." Louise said, "I knew from my friendship with Dr. Loomis and from the philosophy of his center that if there was anyplace where I could find out who I was, it would be there. There is no way I can explain it or put a value on it, Meadowlark was an inner experience. How can I describe that? They just love you and you know this. They don't have to say this, and they never did, they just do it. The vibrations are tremendous. It is a special place in my life, it turned me around."

Much of what Meadowlark represents is attributable to the influence and energies of Evarts Loomis. He, like Travis, tries to deemphasize his role and direct all public credits to the talents and commitments of those who work at the center. This acknowledgment is certainly valid in the sense that people who gravitate to the centers as staff do so for reasons of ideological and personal fulfillment, are highly qualified and capable, and invariably earn less than they would command elsewhere. Yet, the presence of a Loomis at Meadowlark and a Travis at the Wellness Resource Center makes these places special, and different from what they will be in the future when the guiding innovators move on. Of course, that is exactly what these physicians expect and desire. It was of some interest to me that Loomis, at 66, seemed to have such detailed plans for the Meadowlark of the future. He may or may not be around in the year 2000, but I'm pretty sure Meadowlark will be.[7]

Like every other center, Meadowlark is not for everybody. Some may feel uneasy about the spiritual, meditative quality of the place; others may find the "atmosphere of love" that Loomis believes "a prerequisite for a successful healing retreat" to be uncomfortable. That is another reason I am so pleased with the variety of holistic health centers that already exist and are, in my opinion, certain to become the predominant pattern for the delivery of medical care in the years to come. You will get a good sense of this variety by considering at this point the philosophy and methods of the New England Center.

---

7. For information about Meadowlark programs, write to Dr. Loomis at the Friendly Hills Fellowship, 26126 Fairview Avenue, Hemet CA 92343.

Personal and Organizational Wellness
at the New England Center

The New England Center is located on 11 acres of undeveloped land bordering the State Forest of Mt. Toby in Leverett, Massachusetts. In existence since 1971, it is a nonprofit adult educational and training institute. The center has a professional staff that works as a team to provide clients with "education and treatment in the various therapies in the humanistic movement."

Having been there recently, I can attest that the center provides clients with an auspicious setting for its far-ranging services. These include personal counseling (using transactional analysis, Gestalt therapy, body integration, bioenergetics, and psychodrama), massage, corrective body integration, consulting for social service agencies and industries, and sponsoring a journal and workshop series on humanistic and transpersonal education. All of these strands are tied together, according to Katie Baker, the center's executive director, by the belief that an individual client must have available "a range of options in searching for his or her own meanings and values."

One of the principal efforts of the center is an internship/work/study program which, depending upon comprehensiveness desired, can be for one-, two-, or three-month periods, or an intensive nine-month program. Workshops are an important part of this residential program, and are designed to assist the client explore his or her energies and develop skills in group leadership, counseling, and educational techniques. In addition to the approaches already noted, the center emphasizes the methods of humanistic psychology, psychosynthesis, Feldenkrais, body integration, movement awareness, meditation, and yoga. The intention is to offer experimental learning methods not available in more traditional settings.

The heart of the New England Center's program, however, is in the workshop offerings which provide intensive sessions led by well-known facilitators (scheduled in the current year to visit the center were Alexander Lowen, George Bach, Albert Pesso,

Jeanne Houston, Jack Canfield, and Leonard Orr, among many others).

Baker said the approach of the New England Center is holistic in attempting to facilitate the client's basic and natural human potential through mind-body processes of sensory perception, effect, cognition-intuition, and body movement. These processes are expected to generate awareness, understanding, learning, and feeling well. The goals are self-actualization and wholeness.

Ron Dorson, 32, writer and former Greyhound bus driver, visited the New England Center at a time when his life was in disarray, to put it mildly. In response to my request for a commentary on why he chose the New England Center, what was happening in his life when he went there, and what he got out of the experience, Ron offered the following account:

> In the spring of 1976, I dropped out of a creative writing program at the University of Massachusetts in Amherst to go through the Greyhound training academy in Los Angeles. After graduation, I logged 10,000 miles as a "hound-jockey" out of Salt Lake City.
>
> I am a literary adventurer. But the aftershock of the Greyhound odyssey left me in a severe state of depression. When I was furloughed from Greyhound, in the fall of '76, I returned to Amherst to do some writing and tie up some loose ends. I planned to stay for two weeks. But the magazine editor who had assigned me to do a full-length feature on the Greyhound experience quit his gig and the new man gave me a kill fee and told me to get out of his face. My lady, who had pledged eternal love, decided to shine on our relationship, and my writing instructor at U-Mass thought the Greyhound piece was only worth a B, and my talents minimal.
>
> It had been three years since I was published. I was beginning to feel like a one-book phenomenon. The depression I experienced was crippling. I could hardly get out of bed in the morning or find the energy to walk down the street. My body felt like I had a fever of 110 degrees. I felt suicidal. I went to see a psychiatrist and he looked at me out of the corner of his eye like I was a leper. After our first session he told me that maybe he could turn me around in five years; three times a week, at $40 an hour.

A friend of mine had a pamphlet on the New England Center, a personal-growth community. I envisioned group tongue sucks and zipped-out gurus. But I needed immediate relief and was willing to try anything. I drove out there and talked to the director of the center, Katie Baker. "Fire your shrink," she said, "and come live with us." I did just that and even though it took a few weeks to feel at home, the New England Center experience changed my life. It was great to be a part of a supportive community and to receive some warmth and positive reinforcement rather than the hostility and negative input I was used to. I learned some invaluable survival tools at the center and my self-concept improved tremendously.

What we desperately need, in my humble opinion, in this country at least, are communities like the New England Center where people can go periodically to get their self-concept batteries recharged and feel some warmth and compassion. Because too often it is easy to sink into the cesspool of despair, and believe there is no way out.

Last year, the center conducted nearly 100 workshops and involved from 2,500 to 3,000 people, earned $152,000 in income, and distributed 35,000 copies of the program brochure.[8]

Baker remarked that the greatest strength of the center is that it has survived for five years; her long-term goal as reported to the Board of Directors was "to be in business next year."

The Wellness Resource Center, Meadowlark, and the New England Center, though unique unto themselves, all share the wellness notion that you are in charge of your life, that you can choose health instead of illness, and that learning who you are and how you want to be is fundamental to your health.

Seizing the "Teachable Moment" At WHN

Yet another approach to high level wellness is available just a few miles from the Wellness Resource Center at the Wholistic Health and Nutrition Institute, better known as WHN.

WHN offers "multidisciplinary therapies" in what it calls *holistic* or *whole person*, humanistic health care "dedicated to

8. For more information about the New England Center, write to Katie Baker at Box 575, Amherst MA 01002.

high level wellness and unity of body/mind/spirit." In the WHN context, therapy takes the form of guidance, with physician and client becoming coworkers toward optimal well-being. One reason WHN incorporates treatment medicine with wellness or health promotion is the institute's belief that a crisis (i.e., illness) often enables and motivates an interest in the lifestyle changes required for personal growth and better health. WHN provides another style of guidance in a person's self-exploration and assumption of responsibility for his own well-being. It offers adult education, certification in holistic health studies, medical services, health evaluations, and research and special programs for professional health workers, such as internships, residencies, and continuing education for nursing credits.

Although it has become a medical clinic and research center, WHN is best known in the San Francisco Bay Area for the wealth of diversified wellness and holistic health classes which are conducted at the institute at least three nights weekly and every weekend. In January of 1977, for example, 18 different subject areas were offered to the public; several of these were single evening lectures, others were part of a package of classes lasting several weeks.

At the core of the WHN approach is the health evaluation, which is performed in three phases. The purpose is to help the client assess and understand his or her overall health status as a first step toward increased vitality and well-being. The focus is on areas of health potentials, health hazards, stress levels, and what the client considers "imbalances" in aspects of his or her life. Rather than just a search for illness, the health evaluation is billed as a source of data leading to a healthier awareness of oneself. The tests, like the overall program, reflect a blend of medicine and health promotion: many of the questionnaires, indexes, surveys, and so forth used at the Wellness Resource Center are included, but so are such physical checks as blood and urine lab tests, biometric readings (blood pressure, pulse, vital capacity and skin fold, etc.), and consultation with a physician. For those interested in a little "experimental" medicine, WHN has a supplemental (optional) evaluation which includes spiritual consultation, an iridology reading, and a hand reading.

WHN has a staff of seven, supplemented by local "healers" or practitioners of varied health-related arts. Insight into this unusual approach to both medicine and wellness can be gained from a listing of WHN's clinical services.

MEDICAL SERVICES—Provides both preventive counseling as well as expanded general practice with a focus on causal factors. This approach employs medical therapy, physical therapies, hypnosis, nutrition, and herbs.

NUTRITIONAL SERVICES—An in-depth analysis of key factors within diet and lifestyles as it pertains to one's health. In-depth questionnaires, diet diary, and computerized nutrient-health-activity profile which is returned to the client are included within the substance of the consultation. One's restoration of their [sic] nutrition utilizes specific herbs, natural supplements, and diet therapy. Special counseling is available concerning pregnancy and lactation, infant and toddler feeding, and prenatal care.

PSYCHOLOGICAL SERVICES—An wholistic approach to clinical psychology including psycho-diagnostics, therapy, hypnosis, biofeedback, sexuality counseling, meditation, with an emphasis on the human "soma" toward increasing mind-body integration.

ACUPUNCTURE—The health care of a large portion of the world's population is based on the principles of Oriental medicine. Acupuncture is one of the oldest forms of medicine, having been used in China for over 5,000 years. It has withstood the test of time and is a complete system of healing governed by specific laws, offering good results in a wide range of health situations.

PODIATRY—An approach emphasizing the alternatives to conventional means of treating foot disorders. Special emphasis is placed on preventive foot care, rehabilitation, and treatment of chronic pain syndromes, utilizing acupuncture, manipulation, and nutrition.

SPIRITUAL CONSULTATION—A clairvoyant has access to the energy field which surrounds living matter, and to information not ordinarily considered accessible, such as energy patterns, thought patterns, and specific causes for the individual's present state of physical, emotional, and spiritual affairs.

ADJUNCT CLINICAL SERVICES—include herbal consultation, homeopathic consultation, and physical fitness consultation.

As you can sense from this unusual interdisciplinary mix, WHN is indeed an expanded form of medical clinic. According to its founder and medical director Richard Shames, the focus is on helping the client discover which of many possible avenues is most fruitful for him or her. Or, to quote Dr. Shames, which combination of approaches is most appropriate for "the triad of well-being—healing, maintenance, and growth." Shames believes that illness represents an auspicious "teachable moment," and the WHN program is set up to reflect and build upon that conviction. The point is that WHN and other helping agents are most effective when they can assist the client to "seize that teachable moment as a turning point" in his or her life.

Dr. Shames told me a holistic center should incorporate a wide variety of activities, as illustrated in the following range of programs available at WHN:

- *a clinic* where licensed professionals in the fields of nutrition, physical fitness, psychotherapy, medical treatment, biofeedback, spiritual consultation, hypnosis, massage, and many others are available for individual advice or therapy.

- *a public educational program* of classes and workshops in a wide selection of wellness-related topics. The focus is on personal health and on learning tools to have greater control over it. It is a basic tenet of the holistic view that the power and responsibility for health lies more with the individual than with any healer or therapy.

- *an overall health evaluation* of strengths and weaknesses in body, mind, and spirit, including an analysis of food intake, movement output, health hazards, stress levels, life goals, as well as medical history, physical measurements, and lab tests.

- *a variety of special interest groups*, such as weight management programs wherein group process and dynamic leadership combine to foster extra motivation. Each program employs a multidimensional approach to the issue at hand.

- *a professional training department*, for exposing present and future health workers to this new field.

- *a research wing* to investigate the validity of holistic concepts and efficacy of specific alternative methods.

What kind of people go to WHN and other health centers? How do they come upon such places, and what do they get out of the experience? The motivations for visiting a WHN or a Meadowlark are as varied as the centers.

Dianne Duchesne, a 31-year-old nurse from New York City now living in Fairfax, California, learned about WHN through its quarterly program catalogs while working in a local hospital. Dianne went to an evening lecture out of curiosity, and got "hooked" on holistic health. In the year that followed, she attended a great many lectures, read extensively on the subject of holistic health, and took the comprehensive WHN wellness evaluation. At the conclusion of the evaluation, she set a number of goals for herself, and found in two months that most of them had been realized. More important were the changes taking place in her life, in good measure due to the WHN experience, including quitting her job at the hospital, which she said was making her sick, and getting much more in touch with the person she was and wanted to become. About WHN, Dianne remarked: "It has been a 'far out' experience—the communication processes there are beautiful. Also, all my test results have improved (blood pressure, skin fold, pulmonary function), I feel better about my life, and I am truly enjoying my work. My work? I'm making carrot juice for a local health food store, and spreading vitamin A throughout the county."

Barbara Eversole, 32, of Larkspur, California, has bronchial asthma, which she believes is caused and aggravated by a chain-smoking habit and nervousness. She has been to a variety of traditional physicians, all of whom put her on drugs which, if anything, seemed only to make matters worse. Friends and a local medical doctor trained in homeopathy asked her to give WHN a try. At WHN, the approach was to focus on Barbara, and to deal primarily with her sense of self-esteem, life purposes, and other dimensions of the whole person who also happened to have certain unwanted symptoms. Barbara is now working with a staff counselor on a weekly basis; most of her time to date has been spent in general counseling, and on breathing exercises and others that promote body harmony and relieve tensions. Though she does not expect any quick results, Barbara is confident that WHN's nonmedically focused approach to the larger aspects of her life is going to do more for her well-being than past attempts that centered upon her illness.

The value of a holistic approach is as often founded in the process of caring as it is in the product of healing. A nine-year-old boy named Reed Fromer from Mill Valley, for years has had an unusual problem of periodic seizures. According to his mother, Jacki, at least 20 different physician-specialists were unable to diagnose these seizures as other than an emotional problem. No physical basis could be found. Furthermore, Jacki told me that never, in her opinion, did the physicians take a genuine interest in the child himself, or show much compassion for his illness. After talking with friends and listening to general information about WHN circulating in Mill Valley, she decided to give the institute a try.

Jacki told me that the approach and the degree of concern for her child at WHN have been quite different from what she had come to expect from the medical system. In addition to a sense of genuine caring and attention to Reed and not just Reed's problem, the WHN staff has employed a variety of alternative techniques (homeopathy, biofeedback, iridology, psychic readings) in conjunction with certain standard medical tests and analyses. By looking at Reed during a seizure (something not done before), the staff has also isolated a physical manifestation associated with the difficulties.

At the time of my visit, Reed remained a client at WHN, so the impact of the program upon the boy is still to be seen. But, his mother is high in her praise of the *process* of WHN. The humanistic orientation, the fact that there are no drugs or medications being used, the willingness of the staff to incorporate new disciplines *with* existing medical practice have all, said Jacki, given *her* a lot of support and Reed a better chance for a normal life.

Last year WHN saw nearly 2,000 clients; the mailing list for the seasonal free catalogs of holistic medical services and educational activities now has over 11,000 names.[9]

About 50 miles to the south of WHN, near Stanford University, there exists an education center with yet another perspective on ways to promote high level wellness. It's called the San Andreas Health Council.

An Educational Medical Council

The primary purpose of the San Andreas Health Council, located in downtown Palo Alto, is to help people discover how they can play a greater role in their own health care. Begun in 1973, the center has a staff of 20; 44 others are also listed in the council catalogs (published each season) as "people involved" in the general programs. The San Andreas folks sponsor a "Passage" program for people over 60, a counseling center, biofeedback clinic, blood pressure screening, and a "Lite" program for clients with life-threatening illnesses. The council also conducts "Friday night lectures" and approximately 175 courses a year. These last from three to eight weeks. A sampling of class descriptions from a recent catalog should give you a sense of the council's commitment to getting people to play a greater role in their own health care. I think it also shows a belief that health care "involves maintenance of an optimal state of health," not just the treatment of a disease. Though the council has not organized its programs this way, I have arranged a sampling of the San Andreas Health Council class descriptions under the five wellness dimensions used in this book.

---

9. For more information about WHN, write to: Wholistic Health and Nutrition Institute, 150 Shoreline Highway, Mill Valley CA 94941.

Self-Responsibility

• PAIN-IN-THE-NECK WORKSHOP AND PICNIC—
The neck is an artful system of ropes and pulleys which
pivots our head, attaches the arms, holds the shoulders in
place, and anchors the air-bellows system. It also houses an
air hose, a food conveyor, a sound-producing apparatus, a
number of valves, and several small chemical manufacturing centers. The whole complex is arranged around a
column of hollow tubes through which passes the wiring
which connects the brain to the rest of the body. Small
wonder many people have neck problems. The workshop
will discuss the where and whys of neck pains, cramped
muscles, and headaches, and what to do about them. Mind
and body exercises as well as massage and pressure-point
techniques will be taught. This outdoor class will include a
picnic lunch. Bring a jug of juice . . . .

• A PSYCHOLOGICAL APPROACH TO PHYSICAL
ILLNESS—"Each symptom, mental or physical, is a clue
to the resolution of the conflict behind it, and contains
within it the seeds of its own healing"—Seth. This will be
an experiential group for those with physical problems of
either a chronic or acute nature, who want to explore their
responsibility in the onset and maintenance of the disease.
With the assumption of the presence of underlying conflicts
we will work towards their resolution to allow a natural
healing process . . . .

• TOUCH FOR HEALTH—This class will offer a layman's
approach to the techniques developed by Dr. George
Goodheart, the father of Applied Kinesiology. The course
will instruct the participants in kinesiological muscle testing
and give methods whereby the weak muscle can be
strengthened with neurovascular, neurolymphatic, and
acupressure techniques. The overall view of the course is to
bring the class member into a realistic appraisal of his/her
health and provide techniques to correct minor health problems . . . .

• CENTERING—This is a group to learn how to center
ourselves. Centering is the free harmonious interplay of
both hemispheres of our brain. The form of consciousness
controlled by the left hemisphere appears to be sequential,
logical, and verbal. The other, controlled by the right

hemisphere, timeless, intuitive, and sensual. Our society has massively specialized in the development of left-brain functions to the neglect of the right brain. This will be a course to acquire techniques to use altered states that involve right-brain functions—dreams, meditative techniques, trance and imagery states.

Throughout the course we shall emphasize the use of these techniques to function more competently and efficiently . . . .

● HOW TO QUIT SMOKING WORKSHOP—This is a self-directed program for people who want to quit smoking. Participants will be instructed in aversion and behavioral techniques and will experience relaxation, role playing, and group support. Many of the methods were developed through the Heart Disease Prevention Program at Stanford . . . .

Nutritional Awareness

● NUTRITION IS A WAY OF LIFE—"You are what you eat."—There is much truth to that statement, and researchers have found that the standard American diet can actually lead to disease. Principles of body function and pathways of digestion will be explained, with attention to the way eating habits can affect conditions like nervousness, muscle cramps, skin blemishes, tiredness, and even ill temper. Part of each session will be devoted to preparation of simple, tasty, nourishing, natural dishes which we will share . . . .

● BREAKING THE OVERWEIGHT HABIT—The reasons for overeating are many, and the difficulty of achieving permanent weight loss has filled many shelves with dieting manuals. Yet the main problem seems rather simple: lack of knowledge, and therefore lack of active participation by the dieter.

Emotional and nutritional aspects of the food habits of each group member will be initially assessed and evaluated by means of a personal interview, a one-week food log, and a second personal session in which individualized nutritional approaches will be discussed. Group sessions consist of short topical lectures, discussions, light exercises and games, after which we will share a simple but tasty low-calorie meal. With active involvement, group support in times of crisis, and constant guidance, we will work toward the goals of improved health and appearance, emotional relief and permanent weight loss.

This is an ongoing group which may be joined at any time after the initial individual sessions.

• GROUP FASTING—Food is a drug that many of us are addicted to. By fasting, we can gain a sense of freedom and release when we realize, by experience, that we do not suffer dire consequences if we miss food for a few days. One may even experience some rejuvenating effects or a pleasant lightness of spirit, surprising alertness, improvement of vision, or swiftness of thought.

The three course leaders will help individuals choose an appropriate fast and will be available by telephone throughout the fast for support and consultation. The group will meet together three times for support and interaction, and to share experiences of the same adventure . . . .

• NUTRITION AND THE HOLISTIC APPROACH TO PSYCHOLOGICAL WELL-BEING—This workshop will focus on learning how to use nutrition and other modalities (acupressure, integrated movement, respiration) to the promotion of a more balanced body ecology and psychological health. Participants will learn how to determine their personal nutrition patterns. These patterns are suggested through applied kinesiology muscle testing (determination of change or imbalance in muscle tone) and by a careful diary. The role of megavitamins, hair analysis, and food allergies in promoting psychological health will be presented through research and sharing of clinical experience . . . .

Physical Fitness

• JOGGING AND YOGA—This course is a way of developing total fitness. Through recapturing the playful spirit we've lost to the claims of adult responsibilities, we will regain the vitality and resilience of youth. The course includes elements of yoga, dance, jogging, and aerobic play.

• TAICHICUAN FOR MENTAL AND PHYSICAL FITNESS—This form of the classical Yang-style exercise has been officially adopted by the Chinese government and is practiced daily by millions of people as a lifetime health conditioner. It consists of relaxed, continuous, smooth movements, with the primary motivating strength in the legs and waist. Palo Alto students of this instructor have reported improved balance; disappearance of some chest pains, backaches, muscle cramps, and allergy symptoms; a reduction of stress; and a greater sense of calmness and well-being. Individual attention is given.

Stress Management

• UNSTRESSING—Many of us hold tensions which block or deplete our energy. The focus of this class will be to develop those skills of awareness and quieting which allow us to grow toward more optimal health—physical, emotional, and spiritual. Techniques to be included are meditation, autogenic training, systematic desensitization, Jacobsen's progressive relaxation, and biofeedback.

• SELF-DIRECTED COUNSELING—Self-directed counseling is the process of recovering one's ability to release emotion. It is a unique technique, not only for working out accumulated distress from the past, but for dealing with new stress situations and present events. Participants are taught to use special counseling methods and to be a counseling partner to others. Through counseling partnerships, class members help each other to release the effects of past and current hurtful experiences.

Environmental Sensitivity

• SENOI DREAMWORK—We all dream much of the night. Frequently we forget our dreams and then we forget that we forgot, so it's as if we haven't dreamed at all. Forgetting and ignoring our dreaming is thus severing ourselves from half of our creative mental life.

In this class we will apply techniques to our own dreams derived from the Senoi, the dream people of the Central Malay Peninsula, techniques to remember our dreams with some vividness, to lucidly dream (be aware we are dreaming while dreaming) and thus exercise some control of what occurs in the dream state, techniques to continue specific dreams, complete dreams, and establish continuity between what happens in the dream states and what happens in waking perception states.

This will be an experiential class emphasizing the practical day-to-day use of dream states. The idea will be to gain skills.

• CLAIMING WOMAN: THE QUESTIONS OF POWER —For women who wish to explore their sources of personal power and renewal. We will not focus on force or aggression in the traditional sense, but will use the direct awareness and experience that movement work provides to explore the connection between power, strength, survival (standing on your own two feet), and sexuality. Pictures, instruments, and art materials will be used along with movement experiences in centering, being effective, recognizing our own uniqueness, and other topics.

• ASSERTIVENESS THROUGH MOVEMENT—The body is a powerful tool for discovering feelings and gaining awareness of interaction patterns. The body often communicates better than words. To be convincingly assertive, affectionate, or angry, we must learn to use our bodies to say what we mean to say. Workshop participants will move, dance, role-play, and Gestalt their way toward spontaneous and full expression of warmth, anger, and desires.

• HOW TO FIND WORK YOU ENJOY . . . AND GET PAID FOR IT—The work you do has a tremendous impact on your total well-being. Since it is impossible to separate your work situation from the rest of your life, a dissatisfying, unrewarding job can take its toll on your bodily health and energy level, self-concept, relationships, and enthusiasm for living.

This workshop will explore your career from a holistic standpoint, helping you discover how to enrich your life by finding work in harmony with the "real you." Time will be spent pinpointing your strongest skills, interests, and talents and showing how you can apply them in new areas of work. At the end of the workshop, you will be prepared to make a safe transition to a satisfying job.

The council advocates an holistic approach to health care, which the staff believes integrates aspects of a person's life, enables him or her to work toward optimal health, and to be in a better position to benefit from diagnosis and treatment when physician care is needed. A festival is held each quarter to acquaint people with the council and its programs. The annual budget is now around $130,000; part of this helps to defray the costs of distributing 10,000 copies of the quarterly program listings and other health-education pamphlets and brochures.[10]

Again, a few personal vignettes of clients who went to San Andreas and what they got out of it may lend some perspective.

David Minor, a 49-year-old mathematics professor living in Fremont, California, went to the San Andreas Health Council for three months in connection with headache and other pains caused by an auto accident. Though the council seemed a rather unusual health establishment compared to those he was used to, David had heard good things about it from his wife and several of her friends. He said, "I was willing to try something different, I was open, and I needed a new kind of atmosphere." I asked David how the San Andreas approach was different and what effect it had upon him. "The total atmosphere was different," he reported, "so very positive and supportive. I did not get any 'treatment,' just training sessions on autogenics and relaxation exercises. The staff explained things; they made it clear that progress was up to me. This was quite a contrast from the physical therapy and other 'treatments' to which I had grown accustomed. In the past, getting information about the procedures and alternatives was like pulling teeth. I'm a firm believer in the holistic philosophy I experienced at San Andreas." David also noted that he recommended the council to his sister, who traveled from Southern California to attend for related difficulties.

Alston Rigter, a professor in the Health Sciences Program at San Jose State University, incurred a lot of trauma (no physical injuries) in a 1975 auto accident caused by failed brakes. Shortly thereafter, she developed a tremor, which several physicians diagnosed as a benign essential tremor for which they could do little. Having a predisposition for self-help, a back-

---

10. For more information, write to the San Andreas Health Council at 531 Cowper Street, Palo Alto CA 94301.

ground in and a solid understanding of the holistic concept that symptoms can be a manifestation of inner imbalance and unresolved tensions, she suspected all along that something could be done if the underlying tension could be resolved. As the professor put it: "If something is eating you and you only get rid of the symptoms, it will get you somewhere else." She said she was impatient with physicians placing so much emphasis upon pathenogenicity, and having so little interest in learning what needs to be known about healthy people, and how they stay that way.

Alston went to the San Andreas Council and worked on breathing, stretching, and relaxation exercises, bringing her energy into better distribution and learning to feel muscles that had been forgotten for years. "I found it was hard for me to relax, to let go—I think because I have led such a disciplined life. But it was the Hatha Yoga taught by an O.T. [occupational therapist] that did it for me," she said. The professor continues to visit and participate in occasional council programs, though her tremor disappeared about ten days after she started going there. Her activities today include Hatha Yoga, Rolfing, various relaxations, and occasional participation in the Passage group which, she was happy to report, is "definitely not one of those coffee and cookies affairs."

The founder and director of the San Andreas Health Council, Susan Harman Stuart, believes that such wellness-oriented medical centers will become quite popular in the years ahead. They meet a growing public demand for knowledge about health enhancement, and the fact that physicians are integrated into such centers rather than dominate in them, is an attraction for both clients and staff. In this egalitarian atmosphere, clients have a better chance to recognize that their well-being is more dependent upon what they do for themselves than is the case in a doctor-dominated and "care"-oriented non-wellness clinic.

If he had in mind "self-responsibility" in using the term "prudence," then Euripides had its merits in mind some time ago when he wrote, "While our lives may be chains of chances, chance fights ever on the side of the prudent."

Oneness of Mind/Body/Spirit at the East West Academy

One other approach to high level wellness has been pioneered by the East West Academy of Healing Arts (EWAHA), located in San Francisco. Unlike the other wellness centers, EWAHA is almost entirely a volunteer operation, save for its founder and head, Dr. Effie Poy Yew Chow, and one administrative assistant. EWAHA has managed to organize and conduct four major conferences in the past year. The subjects were (1) holistic approaches to health care; (2) holistic health and healing energies; (3) the rituals and practices of other cultural healing systems; and (4) stress and tension in connection with cancer, death, and dying. All together, about 2,500 people have participated in these events.

EWAHA does more than sponsor conferences, however. The academy uses the systems approach to encourage those involved in Western medicine to consider both ancient and other contemporary cultural healing systems and to investigate the validity of preventive practices, lifestyle modification, and humanistic approaches to health. The concept of health is given a broad focus, and attention is concentrated on the effects of nutrition, environment, the social and health sciences, and other factors upon the individual's "optimal survival."

In a recent newsletter, Dr. Chow offered a summary of EWAHA programs and purposes, saying they are:

> . . .designed to allow all levels of health professionals, personnel, and consumers to investigate, study, and train in holistic and cultural health care with a view toward actually integrating concepts, skills, and practices learned into modern Western health care settings. The ultimate goal is the creation of expanded health service systems which will actively assist all classes and cultures of our American population in developing and maintaining our individual health, well-being, and self-dignity.

In addition to conducting major conferences, the academy has developed holistic health curricula for interdisciplinary health education, organized short-term training programs for health workers and consumers, and established an extensive network of wellness advocates and interested parties. The academy maintains a membership directory, distributes periodic newsletters, and, in cooperation with another organization, produces video and audio tapes of holistic presentations for sale to the public. About 50,000 people are currently receiving information from the academy regarding holistic health practices, seminars, and directions.[11]

One other effort underway has wide implications for raising the wellness consciousness of professional health workers (a benefit that thereby will eventually be relayed to the rest of us). It involves the formation of a Council of Nurse-Healers, intended to "foster the reemergence of caring (humanism) and healing as fundamental aspects of nursing and health care. To heal (from 'haelen', to make whole) is to promote health and to mobilize the client's recuperative powers." This endeavor is being organized on a national and international basis "to enhance the treatment and prevention of disease by encouraging methods which take the total dimension and well-being of the individual into account."

Esalen—A Rustic Pleasure Spa for Self-Responsibility

Located 300 miles north of Los Angeles on the rugged coast at Big Sur, the Esalen Institute is an educational laboratory and personal growth center. Founded in the early 1960s, Esalen quickly became internationally known as the trend setter for the human potential movement. The tools and techniques developed as part of this movement are still available at Esalen "for individuals to use to realize their own healing and growth through self-responsibility." One purpose, according to the latest catalog, is to promote health through an emphasis on the "potentialities and values of human existence." The basic pur-

---

11. For further information about the East West Academy of Healing Arts, write to Dr. Chow at 33 Ora Way, San Francisco CA 94131.

pose and guiding principle is best explained by the cover page used on each of the Institute's quarterly catalogs. This is entitled "Who's Responsible at Esalen?"

> In our position as educators, we invite people to take responsibility for their whole life situation while at Esalen. This includes taking responsibility for who they select as their teachers, their leaders, their gurus, their authority figures . . . and so on—and to be aware, whenever possible, what effect this has on them. We, of necessity, are setting up a situation for our seminarians to learn the practice of self-responsibility from the time they consider selecting a workshop, not just during the workshop. In effect, we are asking that this self-responsibility attitude be present in the initial contact with Esalen. Ideally, the same attitude will pervade after a workshop when our seminarians go back to the community and seek out others—physicians, teachers, counselors, mental health professionals, etc.
>
> As we have become more thoughtful and self-critical about the overall direction of Esalen we have begun to concentrate on enhancing our basic commodity—the Esalen environment and lifestyle. Our primary emphasis is not on teaching particular truths or personal and interpersonal techniques for daily life; rather our primary concern is with a particular consciousness and developing an environment to support the evolution of that consciousness—the consciousness of self-awareness/self-responsibility.

What Esalen has become is a residential center for workshops and seminars on a dazzling variety of human potential topics, with the added attractions of a splendid natural setting, hot baths from sulphur springs that overlook the ocean, and a reasonable assurance that other registrants attending Esalen will be interesting discussants and active participants in the programs and activities. Unlike the other holistic resource centers, Esalen is quite well known and draws from across the nation, and around the world.

Nearly everyone who has started a movement or written a book in the field of human potential and the transformation of human consciousness has appeared at Esalen at one time or another. Workshop and seminar leaders have included Gerald Heard, Alan Watts, Arnold Toynbee, Frederic Spiegelberg,

Ken Kesey, S. I. Hayakawa, Linus Pauling, Paul Tillich, Gary Snyder, Norman Brown, Rollo May, Bishop James Pike, Carl Rogers, B. F. Skinner, Abraham Maslow, William Schutz, Ida Rolf, Stuart Miller, and Fritz Perls, to name a few.

Activities range from weekends to week- and month-long seminars. Esalen attempts to encourage, synthesize, and evaluate various kinds of holistic approaches to well-being. Fields of interest include education, religion, philosophy, and the physical and behavioral sciences. Special emphasis is given to body awareness, massage, and personal integration. The focus at Esalen is on experimentation; nothing of a "cure" or treatment nature is attempted or encouraged.

I asked Dick Price, cofounder of Esalen and cochairman of the Board, whether the leadership thinks of Esalen as a health-oriented center, and was not surprised to learn that the managers do not so interpret the Esalen experience. The individual coming to Esalen might go through three stages, according to Price. The first is an introductory time, a period of getting the "feel" of being in the natural environment, being exposed to a multitude of ideas, and being affected by conversations and varied influences of other people at Esalen. The second is a miscellaneous phase, wherein the guest picks up a few ideas here, concepts there, and so forth, by attending Gestalt, massage, or other single-focus programs (often, people can sit in on other groups besides the one for which they registered). The third phase, according to Price, is a directive phase, a watershed time when individuals decide to make a personal commitment to their own health and well-being when they leave Esalen. In the past year, there have been several workshop offerings which appear to foster this last phase, as the following excerpts from recent catalogs suggest:

> Inner Road to Health—This is a workshop for staying well and helping others to stay well. The subjects covered include many of the health approaches taught at Esalen. . . . Throughout the five-week program the main emphasis will be on discovering and awakening inner resources. In this connection, regular meditation, yoga, tai chi, massage, and other quieting practices will help still the

mind and relax the body, permitting new awareness and sensitivity to emerge. Our eventual goal is to integrate and make whole all the diverse aspects of our being: physical, mental, social, emotional, energetic, and spiritual. This result may not come for many years, but the process leading towards wholeness can be well on the way by the end of the workshop . . . .

A Practicum in Preventive Medicine—This seven-day workshop is designed as an intensive practicum for physicians and other health care professionals. We will look at the nature of health and how to maintain optimum levels of well-being. The areas of focus are: acupuncture, stress, body work, biofeedback, yoga and meditative techniques, psychosocial factors of disease, preventive medicine, dietary considerations.

Body Awareness, Moving, Relaxation, and Vitality—Fixed patterns of movement create tension in the body and rigidity in the mind. We will experience new ways to move which are functional with constant focus on breath and directed awareness of body sensation. Massage with directed energy will heighten our sensation of ourselves and others, allowing for dissolution of stress and increased vitality. We will use Feldenkrais movement, sensing, meridian awareness, touch, and visualization with music.

Mind As Healer, Mind As Slayer—This weekend explores the neurophysiology of stress and human consciousness; the interaction between states of mind and physical health or illness; psychological factors in cancer and hypertension; and applications of biofeedback and meditation in self-healing. Participants will engage in meditative practices, visualization techniques, and use biofeedback instruments with emphasis on health maintenance.

The meals are vegetarian (with occasional meat alternatives), with herbal teas, whole grain breads, and nonrefined fresh fruits and vegetables from the Esalen garden plentifully available. Unfortunately, smoking is permitted in the dining room, which interferes with the pleasant atmosphere. Price told me this is a matter of dispute among the current directors, with the predominant view at this time being to underscore individual choice and responsibility by keeping the matter open for personal discretion.

Esalen is big business, relative to the other centers. About 70 people live on the grounds as guests, along with 50 paid staff and as many as 20 "work-scholars." Esalen is not cheap: a week costs $270, which includes room, board, and all program costs. The annual budget is now over $1 million; 35,000 catalogs are distributed quarterly.

Bette Fuller, a humanist counselor who has been involved with Esalen as a seminarian, resident fellow, and leader of groups since 1966, told me that Esalen is, more than anything else, " . . . a platform. It is a context for people on the cutting edge of new learning in sociology, religion, health, and a myriad of other areas. The support and recognition it provides have nurtured many people over the years, and from Esalen's unique atmosphere have come important concepts and methods that today are part of established institutions. One example is in the field of education—Esalen was the place where early experiments and study in affective learning (involving working with children at the emotional level) took place." Betty described other instances wherein leaders of creative movements (e.g. Ida Rolf, Fritz Perls, Moshe Feldenkrais, Lawrence Le Shan, Jack Worsley) were able to explore their ideas in a safe, high energy environment. The results, said Betty, have been "a string of important contributions to public well-being and human consciousness."

I asked Betty to tell me about the meaning of Esalen to her, personally. "Its impact on my life has been tremendous: I left my job (theatre) and studies (psychology) to develop my own area of life work. I now combine mind/body/spirit possibilities using Gestalt, encounter, psychosynthesis combined with Feldenkrais body work, massage, meditation, song, dance, and laughter. I have learned to dare, to come from my experience, to value my judgment, and to trust myself. I have great respect for the potential of human beings. Esalen has been a very important source in my evolution."

One of my neighbors in Mill Valley is George Leonard, a well-known author (*Education and Ecstasy, The Transforma-*

tion, and *The Ultimate Athlete),* student of holistic health, holder of the black belt in Aikido, and leader of periodic workshops at the Esalen Institute. I called George and asked him if he considers Esalen a health-promotion center. "Indeed I do," was his reply: "It emphasizes the rejoining of mind, body, and spirit and the interconnectedness of these aspects of our being, it promotes alternatives to the traditional medical model, and it fosters self-responsibility." George then quoted a physician friend of his who said "the Esalen catalog alone is better preventative medicine than anything you will find in most doctors' offices." Since Esalen has been doing health promotion from its beginning, George termed it "the granddaddy of holistic health."

If your interest in wellness tends to emphasize pleasuring, natural beauty, a range of programs from which to choose, and a nonideological program, Esalen might be the kind of place that could be of value in your own evolution.[12]

As you have no doubt realized by now, however great their diversity, the Wellness Resource Center, Meadowlark, the New England Center, WHN, the San Andreas Health Council, the East West Academy, and Esalen have much in common. Each promotes self-responsibility by actively involving the client in his or her own well-being. Each works with the whole person, and focuses on the roots of the symptoms that are the surface barriers to self-realization. Each promotes positive health through education in the basic dimensions of well-being. Each places an emphasis on lifestyle strategies for the highest levels of health achievable, and all utilize a wide range of facilitators instead of relying primarily upon doctors.

Despite the sometimes impressive results which I have reported in the vignettes, none of the centers' personnel offer or believe in fast cures. They have no new technologies or secret theories. The clients I met may or may not be representative,

---

12. For more information, write the Esalen Institute, Big Sur CA 93920. To receive the Esalen catalog and occasional mailings, send a check or money order for $2 to the Institute.

for I made no effort to do a scientific survey with double blind/cross-over controls or other rigorous studies. I just talked to a random sample of interesting people, and I was surprised at their willingness to share with me—and now with you—intimate aspects of their lives. I know these individuals did so because they have come to believe so strongly in the value system of wellness, as expressed in various ways by these different centers for health and well-being. They wanted to share their experiences with you through this book in the hope that you might find some encouragement and support to pursue wellness in your own fashion.

I suspect there are other wellness-oriented centers in this country, many just beginning to emerge from once-traditional medical practices, former neighborhood health centers, human potential or consciousness-raising organizations, free clinics, and other starting points.[13] The highlights of the few just presented are just that: highlights. All this is suggestive, not definitive. I wanted to show you through real world cases and events that high level wellness is not just a theory, a fad, or an impractical approach to better health. It is a practical reality—an option that you can choose—and which you can carry out for yourself. The centers are fine places and, if you have the time, money, and interest, you would probably enjoy the experience of being at one for a short period of time. But you do not *need* a center. On your own you can learn all you need to know about how to take charge of your own life; and singlehandedly you can shape your lifestyle and environment to the extent necessary to experience the personal and health rewards of a high level wellness way of living.

A good way to start is to consider what I believe is the basic credo of high level wellness.

---

13.   In fact, I know there are such places, including holistic health centers in West Newton (Mass.), Berkeley, Los Angeles, Santa Monica (Calif.), and Hinsdale and Woodridge (Ill.). In the years to come, as I have suggested already, I believe it will be easier to list the cities and towns *without* such centers.

Exploring the
Wellness Ethic

If you are less healthy than you want to be, if you are tired of spending so much of your money on drugs and medicines, if you question the wisdom of reliance upon a medical system, if, in short, you are sick of being marginally well, you are probably ready for high level wellness.

There are many roads that will take you there; you will want to choose your own maps and ways, tailoring specific activities to your unique background, current needs, and future expectations. However, we all share a great deal, and I'd like to set out a number of guidelines you might find useful.

The Principles of High Level Wellness

1. You Are the Chairperson of Your Own Well-Being. You can carry the key to your own physical, emotional, and mental well-being in the way you choose to live. Doctors and others can help you, can give you advice, can save your life in certain instances, and can usually make things easier, but in the overall analysis, you have the responsibility for whatever goes well or poorly; for your own health and well-being.

2. Forget About Magic Bullets or Instant Solutions. So many of your fellow citizens are sick and dying from the diseases of civilization, the debilitating pathologies of premature aging brought on by aberrant lifestyles. Despite this fact, the not-so-subtle message from the medical media is that somewhere there is a medical solution to these problems, that no challenge is too great for medical technology, and that health can be purchased by greater investments in medical research facilities, procedures, and techniques. Unfortunately, there is no pill or

49

other magic bullet that will cure cardiovascular disease, cancers, cirrhosis of the liver, and all the other infirmities caused by years of high-risk behaviors. The nation as a whole, in my opinion, would be better served if we spent less on the search for biomedical cures and more on ways to motivate ourselves to avoid known disease-causing behaviors.[1] You will be better off not depending on easy or effortless answers to the terrible problems brought on by health-denying lifestyles.

3.   Heed   Not   the   Counsel   of   the   Adipose   Physician.

Examine your doctor before you let him examine you. Improvements in our health status would come about much faster if physicians, the most respected and esteemed of all health-care providers, could take it upon themselves to teach us how to maintain and improve our health and choose better for ourselves. Instead, the medical profession as a whole, and 98 percent of its members' energies, are devoted to the treatment of illness symptoms, diseases, injuries, and the unending struggle against death. It seems to me that physicians who themselves pay little regard to the importance of nutrition, exercise, stress management, and self-responsibility are highly unlikely to promote lifestyle reform to you and me. Fortunately for us, if not for the doctor, this kind of attitude will be apparent in the appearance of treatment-centered providers, as well as in their manner and philosophy. By all means discount not just the counsel of such doctors, but also your relationship with them. After all, their ambitions for *your* health are unlikely to be much greater than the commitment they evidence for their own.

---

1.   A large-scale health survey based on a study of 7,000 adults in California over a period of time demonstrated an 11.5-year greater life expectancy for people whose lifestyle incorporated six or seven basic health habits versus those who only followed three or fewer of them. The life-giving patterns? (1) no smoking; (2) moderate drinking; (3) seven or eight hours sleep per night; (4) regular meals with no snacks in between; (5) breakfast every day; (6) normal weight; and (7) moderate, regular exercise. These results were duplicated in a Wisconsin study of 2,000 persons, with added findings that connected such personality traits as moderation, serenity, optimism, interest in others and the future, with good health and long life. See Nedra B. Belloc, *"The Relationship of Health Practices and Mortality," Preventive Medicine* 2 (1973):67–81; also George Leonard, "The Holistic Health Revolution," *New West,* 10 May 1976, p. 42.

4. Your Body Is the World's Greatest Healer—Let Nature Do Its Thing.   Your body is a marvelous creation. It is designed to work well; it is equipped with self-generating antibodies which mend damaged tissue, regenerate dying cells, and otherwise keep you healthy. These "self-regulatory" processes include your body's ability to maintain optimum temperature, heart, and respiration rates; blood flow and blood pressure; acid-base balance; and electromagnetic properties. But marvelous though it is, your body cannot, over the long haul of the years, resist and survive the punishment occasioned by disuse, misuse, neglect, and denial. So, don't fight nature's remedy. Develop an understanding and appreciation of your body, consider natural laws of healing, and avoid behaviors, ingestions, and inhalations which block nature's processes. Your body is beautiful just as nature designed it—please don't do anything to void the warranty.

5. God Makes It Her Business to Stay out of Ours.   A wellness philosophy, as I see it, holds that you are on your own in this world, neither favored by nor discriminated against by a higher power or powers. When you are ill, it is to your advantage to accept responsibility and work as you can with the condition; when you are well, give yourself some credit for your good fortune. William Nolen, M.D., wrote something I think makes a lot of sense:

> . . . The more all of us know about the healing process the more likely we are to pursue life and health along channels that are apt to be productive. I spent the better part of two years looking for quick, magical, miraculous answers to problems of life and death, only to find that those answers do not exist. I'd like to spare others that pursuit.[2]

George Bernard Shaw once hinted, tongue in cheek, that people who believe in miracles are blaspheming the Almighty, explaining that "you go to Lourdes and you see piles of crutches and piles of wheel chairs, but you don't see any glass eyes, or

---

2. William A. Nolen, *Healing, A Doctor in Search of a Miracle* (Greenwich, Conn.: Fawcett Crest, 1974), p. 238. See review in the Wellness Resource Guide.

toupees, or wooden legs. Therefore, Lourdes implies a limitation on the power of God, and that makes it blasphemous."[3] Shaw's comment was made in the same spirit of good-natured irreverence that I intend in referring to "the higher power" in the feminine gender, which I thought would help you remember the principle.

6. Neither Rome nor a Wellness Lifestyle Can Be Made in a Day. It is hard work to live well. It is easier to eat junk food, ignore exercise, disregard tension, and "let-someone-else-do-it" than it is to develop an individualized wellness program in each of the five dimensions. Each wellness area is a complex field having many disciplines and numerous approaches; it will take time for you to experiment and discover what you like in each dimension. But, there is no hurry, Rome was not built in a day and neither can or should a lifestyle schemed in wellness be designed or implemented in an abbreviated time frame.

7. Don't Sacrifice, Deny Yourself, or Give Up Destructive Life Habits—Until You're Ready to Do So. Joan Gomez has observed that "a moral veto is no good against an instinctual drive."[4] This means that it is fruitless and inappropriate for me or anyone else to tell you that you shouldn't smoke, or that alcohol is bad for you, or that porno food is poison, etc. However true such imprecations may be, they will be ineffective in motivating you to change your behavior. If you *do* attempt lifestyle reforms due to external pressures or guilt, you might experience so much trauma and generalized distress that you will soon go back to cigarettes, whiskey, and your wild, wild ways. However, if you are presented with information about health enhancement in an interesting, nonthreatening, low-key manner which emphasizes the positive aspects of lifestyle reforms—well, then I think you will take note. And you may eventually make changes, when you are ready. It seems to me that when people themselves decide they can do nicely without the cigarettes and

---

3. Quoted by Dr. Jerome Frank, author of *Persuasion and Healing* (New York: Shocken; 1963) at the Conference on Future Directions in Health Care held in New York City, 10, 11 December 1975.

4. *How Not to Die Young* (New York: Pocket Books, 1973), p. 212.

whiskey (wellness is not puritanical), they can make that choice without leaving a gap in their lives which might be filled with an activity as dysfunctional as that foregone. When you know it is right, when you understand why you are doing (or avoiding) something, and when you anticipate the benefits of a new health-promoting behavior, then the change in activity brings a satisfaction that reinforces while it pleases. Not smoking, for example, will produce a sense of satisfaction, not feelings of self-denial or agonizing sacrifice usually associated with medieval torture.

8. No Medicine Is Good Medicine—As a Bendable Rule.
Americans are pill freaks. We consume 20,000 pounds of aspirin annually. That's 225 tablets for every man, woman, and child. Valium and Librium are the staple of U.S. medicine: 75 percent of all doctor visits end with a prescription for one medication or another. Spend an hour before the tube and you will be assaulted by the pharmaceutical industry with offers of pills or other nostrums for improved sleep, excretion, energy, youthfulness, smell, and, naturally, overall health. Mood elevators, amphetamines, tranquilizers, narcotic pain pills, and antihistamines seem more American than apple pie, which is bad enough! There are occasions when medicine is warranted, but the general attitude of the wellness adherent is that natural remedies, time, will, and an integrated lifestyle are quite sufficient, thank you, for most of what does or could ail you. A high level wellness lifestyle is, in itself, a state of being that affords high resistance to disease.

9. It's Better to Be a Client than a Patient.   The term *patient* connotes a subservient quality in the nature of your relationship with a physician; as a client, on the other hand, you are the responsible party in transactions with the provider. (That's because in the wellness framework, the provider is a facilitator of learning, an ally, and a guide in the healing process—not an authority figure.) The distinction is more than a rhetorical gesture: the ethic of active self-responsibility for your well-being is the foundation of a wellness philosophy, and the idea that you are the sovereign of your own well-being is simply easier to recognize when you are respectfully treated as a client than it is when you are condescendingly managed as a patient. The patient takes the doctor's orders; the client considers his or her advice.[5]

10. High Level Wellness Is More Rewarding than Low Level Worseness.　　As an ever-changing state of feeling good about your body and purpose, high level wellness is such a positive, "turned-on" way to live that after you experience it the alternatives will become totally unattractive. As Dr. William Glasser, who studied thousands of dedicated runners and meditators, has shown in *Positive Addiction* (New York: Harper and Row, 1976), you can actually become "addicted" to positive behavior which develops your character and your body and leads to documented increases in mental alertness, self-awareness, confidence, and personal esteem. High level wellness is, quite simply, more fun than "low level worseness." It is more powerful than illness and, once started, more infectious than disease. It is a richer way to be alive, and it offers less pain, greater highs, and fewer lows. To exaggerate a bit, which I love to do, it could be said that an individual practicing high level wellness is stronger and better looking, has higher morale, better circulation, superior bowel movements, and more antibodies to resist illness. Such a person is warmer in winter, cooler in summer, and sleeps better all year around.

Other Wellness-Related Concepts

In addition to these 10 principles, I'd like to share some concepts that can be useful to you as you develop and put into practice your own wellness philosophy. Perhaps a few of these will help you seek out and incorporate similar ideas about wellness living that complement your own lifestyle.

One important concept pertinent to wellness is that of "strokes." Dr. Eric Berne, the founder of Transactional

---

5.　Naturally, a bit of discrimination is in order in applying this principle. If you are unconscious and bleeding heavily, you would not expect or desire the relationship to be equal. Let me assure you that, in such circumstances, there is not a thing wrong with being a patient!

Analysis, believed that we all need to be touched, recognized, and engaged in activity which we think is of consequence. These needs are part of our biological and psychological "hungers"; these hungers are satisfied with strokes. Any act that says to another, "I know you're there," is a stroke.

We know that reinforcement—whether it be positive or negative—is an important basis of behavior. Applying this concept in the wellness frame of reference, you could suspect that if you abuse your body by smoking or pursuing other high-risk behaviors, you are acting from *stroke deprivation*. This means, according to the TA folks, that your more basic needs are not being met. The idea is that if you respect your body, exercise, eat consciously, meditate or otherwise relax, and feel good about your life and purposes, you will not need stroke substitutes. On the other hand, if you are bored, depressed, manic, or generally unhappy with your existence, you will substitute destructive personal behaviors for the strokes that would otherwise come from realizing human needs. A wellness approach focuses on meeting human needs in positive ways and includes finding ways to earn recognition, create stimulating personal environments, give and receive care and affection from others, and evolve and grow toward a greater consciousness. Only when your needs are met are you in a position to deal with destructive tendencies and habits.

Another concept that will complement your understanding of high level wellness is that your mind, body, and spirit are integrated and inseparable. In pursuing wellness, the total *you* must be involved, including your self-concept, your work, your primary and other relationships, your environment, and so forth. An entire movement based upon this idea has taken shape, as you saw for yourself on our visit to the holistic health centers. At the center of this holistic medicine is the perception that you are a "whole" person requiring internal balance and harmony and external balance with your various environments. In addition to—or in place of—giving the usual tests (Travis says that with the exception for a few checks; blood pressure, TB screening, breast exams, and Pap smears for women over 25, glaucoma testing if glaucoma runs in the family, and sigmoidoscopy after age 50, the annual physical is not much help in staying healthy), a wellness-oriented physician might want to know something about what could be called your "serum fun level."

Also conducive to wellness is the idea that illness is a message from within. I believe, as do many physicians and students of a wellness philosophy, that illness goes deeper than the germ theory in that it has purpose and meaning in relation to our inner states. "Host-resistance," immunity systems, the psyche, temperament, and character are all interconnected as factors in illness and disease, and it is important that healers be sensitive to and interested in helping you unmask the meaning of your illness. Often, this meaning is not subject to discovery for varied reasons, but then the search itself can transform illness into an enriching experience.

I have mentioned that wellness is more enjoyable than the medical alternative; one way you can understand why I think this is so is to look at the "modalities" or approaches to working with clients used in the holistic health centers and contrast these efforts with the treatment techniques of the medical system. The wellness folks have developed a variety of new techniques and they have also designed variations on some very old and sound approaches, particularly in working with problems connected with physical fitness and stress management. The fitness emphasis incorporates yoga, stretching exercises, jogging, and assorted "new games" emphasizing participation and fun over competition and winning; stress management includes massage, psychosynthesis, meditation, and biofeedback as popular outlets or modalities for many pursuing wellness lifestyles. I'll describe these and other modalities when we explore the five wellness dimensions.

One characteristic distinguishing high level wellness from the too-often-discounted "prevention" theme so long in evidence is that the preventive posture is defensive and largely reactive. That is, it is designed to protect you against illness or disease; wellness, on the other hand, achieves the same end by advocating health enrichment, or health promotion, and life enhancement. The one is static; the other dynamic. One holds the line, the other moves forward.

One concept of special interest to a lot of people actively

pursuing a healthier lifestyle is revealed in the growing evidence that right-brain development offers potentially rewarding paths to a higher consciousness. The left brain, which controls the right side of the body, is associated with our rational capacities; the right brain, controlling the left side of the body, is said to be key to the intuitive, integrative, emotional, and nonlinear facets of our being. This concept, of course, has many implications regarding the development of the underutilized right brain for greater levels of well-being.

The idea of wellness as an *integrated* lifestyle is hard to overemphasize. Each of the five dimensions of high level wellness; self-responsibility, nutritional awareness, physical fitness, stress management, and environmental sensitivity, is fundamental to a complete lifestyle schemed in well-being. You need to have something going for you in each of these areas, for if you specialize in one or more to the neglect of even a single dimension, you will forfeit the effects of an integrated approach, which are synergistic (i.e. creating a whole greater than the sum of its parts).

As another of the principles suggests, knowing your body is critical to a wellness lifestyle. It is hard to fully appreciate and care for a stranger, and yet too many Americans know more about the workings of their auto engines or the lifestyles of movie stars (and congressmen) than they do about the biology of their own bodies. This casualness can lead to overindulgence and undernutrition, disregard of tension signals, high-risk behaviors (e.g., cigarette smoking), and an overdependence on doctors to cure illness and disease symptoms. The more you know about the purposes and functioning of your own heart and arteries, lungs and breathing apparatus, muscles and bones, kidneys and bladder, digestive system and liver, the less likely you are to permit your own degeneration by a careless lifestyle.

There is another wellness-related concept I ought to mention that hits close to home. I guess I'm as much a victim of the "youth is wellness, age is worseness" stereotype as the next person. I have gone to great lengths to avoid recognizing that I'm over 30, and I have often admitted no more than that I am between 35 and death. But I am beginning to recognize that acceptance of this aspect of life makes growing older more enriching than trying to stay young in years, and that the best youth is found in vigor, not chronological immobility. And, dear reader, that's another aspect of wellness; learning that you don't need the "fountain of youth" when your life is a sea of well-being. Poncé de Léon wasted much time looking for magic potions which never have existed, when all the vitality he ever needed was readily available from within. A quintessential concept of wellness, therefore, is that the vigor obtained through a health-promoting integrated lifestyle is more conducive to and indicative of youth and a fitness for living than is one's birthdate. Like Senator Proxmire, converts to wellness often can say, "I feel better at 57 than I did at 47.[6]

Speaking Up for Wellness

Now that you know the principles and concepts of wellness, you're ready to see close up what they can do for you. I asked a few of my wellness-oriented friends to tell me what their lives are like now—how they feel and how things are different than they used to be.

Michael Griffin, who has benefited from an organized program of self-responsibility (EST), talked of wellness as a state that "transcends pleasure and pain. I value experience more now in the sense that aliveness can be achieved with both pleasure and pain." Michael described the sensations of wellness as "peacefulness, warmth, and centeredness, which are possible even in the context of negative and painful feelings, such as sadness, loneliness, and the like. In a wellness framework, I find it easier to love myself and to have that as a less abstract, more 'real' experience. An example is in losing weight through a natural nonefforting energy or by experiencing a sense of joy by virtue of eating sensibly. Finally, I should mention that I have made a shift away from being involved in senseless, compellingly destructive behaviors like drinking alcohol and pursuing women I don't really care about. In other words, I have

---

6. William Proxmire, *You Can Do It: Senator Proxmire's Exercise, Diet, and Relaxation Plan* (New York: Simon and Schuster, 1973), p. 28. Isn't it curious that people show such great concern for grey hairs and wrinkles—which do not shorten their lives in the least—and so little concern for health habits which will induce premature aging and untimely death.

shifted away from seeking out 'pleasurable' activities which in a deeper sense are actually painful or do not contribute to my self-esteem."

Jeff Gero, a friend and former New York City real estate salesman living in California, said that wellness for him is not just the absence of illness but participation every day in doing things to feel better. Jeff told me, "I know how to recognize when I'm running down and when to give myself special attention. I feel much more in control of my health and life today than I did in the past when I lacked an overall wellness philosophy and knowledge of health-promotive techniques. I no longer act out nervousness through destructive behaviors—it just is not necessary anymore. I use my energy more productively because I'm more in touch with what I have and how to use it. I'm seldom idle—there are innumerable exciting things to do with 'spare' time, such as yoga, exercises, and other stress-reduction patterns. I eat less and feel better. The idea of returning to what you call a 'worseness' lifestyle is unthinkable. I believe it is important to do something positive for oneself each day; something special just to affirm your respect for and appreciation of who you are."

Jeff added that many of his friends are beginning to adopt a wellness lifestyle, which he described as a "conscious choice to take care of yourself." When I asked him to tell me what the change has meant for him in an everyday sense, he replied: "As my consciousness changed and evolved, I became so much more aware of health habits, my primary relationships grew deeper and more valued, and I learned to use my *mind* to stay healthy. My thoughts help me stay healthy; when I feel low I visualize myself running and having fun. In no time at all, this begins to affect my body and gives me strength and new energies. My mind goes and my body follows."

One of my advisers and a close friend, Don Gerrard, who incidentally is completing a book on the history of medicine (he has already written and/or published 22 as head of Bookworks in Berkeley, California), told me he feels "fantastic" about his wellness-oriented lifestyle. Don said his life "keeps coming together more and more all the time." An important ingredient of Don's wellness lifestyle is being a part of an always-growing "support community." Don, like Michael and Jeff, is an articulate individual; to give you the fullest possible sense of how another person experiences himself inside and out while pursuing a high level wellness lifestyle, I'll just quote for you what Don told me:

By being of support to other people, which is the vital force element in my life at this time, I find that people are tremendously supportive of me in return.

I am aware of a nonsectarian spiritual channel running through my life, and am also aware that living my life for a higher purpose than just meeting my immediate needs gives me constant satisfactions. That higher purpose is in giving to others *in my way*, which for me involves health education and the inspiration needed for self-motivation.

In 1970 I worked 12 hours a day. I could not sleep well at nights, I was not able to relate to people on a close level, in fact, I was using people as an extension of myself. My only friends were business associates. My friends were those who could further my business.

After a while I began to develop severe anxiety responses; heart palpitations, sudden losses of energy, irrational fears, and trembling. After six months of this, I took an inventory of my life at the urging of an acquaintance, and began to experiment with some different patterns.

I started by practicing deep relaxation and learned to allow myself to just experience my anxiety symptoms. When they came on, I would just be in that space—I would just go ahead and be afraid or tremble or whatever it was. Soon thereafter, the symptoms ended and have not been back.

I more and more since then have turned my work toward health and am continually learning to make a living from those very activities I need to live a wellness lifestyle. It is apparent to me that there are plenty of other people who are in similar situations to what I described as my former pattern, who would benefit from starting similar wellness approaches. When I started, I quit smoking, got into stress reduction through exercise, stopped drinking coffee, and began taking responsibility for what was right and wrong with my body and feeling states. In the years since these beginnings, I have evolved into many other approaches and patterns, including an hour of daily hard exercise and an hour of meditation. More important, I have a growing interest in personally contributing to the health of other people, which I find adds to my own health and wellness lifestyle. I find the more I give out the more I get back.

If I were going to die this afternoon there is nothing I would change. I would live as I am now. While the earlier stress symptoms have disappeared as chronic health difficulties, personal problems are still there, but I see them in a new light. They are just a part of my pattern. They are no more or no less interesting to me than the problems of my closest friends. In summary, creating a growing health community is the key to my wellness lifestyle of living, thinking, and being.

Another way some persons relate to wellness is exemplified in the remarks of my friend José Armas, a community organizer based in New Mexico. José talked of social wellness, consistent with his concern for the Chicano communities in the southwestern part of the country:

> Wellness in health is like the elements of social wellness: it is dependent on taking affirmative action (as opposed to having a reaction orientation). Wellness means having a broad perspective of the different dynamics which *cause* conditions rather than dealing only with symptoms. You always operate at a disadvantage when you wait for things to happen first before taking responsibility. Dealing with symptoms will always be costly and unending, and will inevitably lead to minimum results, at best. Dealing with causes is more intricate, but it is also more conducive to social wellness. The responsibility for social wellness rests with both the individual and the community—the responsibility can never be passed to other people.

Because you are unique, I can not promise that a wellness lifestyle will bring you greater force and depth in relationships, higher social consciousness, increased energy levels, more "aliveness" or any of the other specific benefits described by some of my healthy friends. But I would confidently forecast reduced stress, increased fitness, better feelings of physical health through changed food patterns, more awareness of environmental subtleties, and a greater sense of self through acceptance and constant practice of personal responsibility. With all these dimensions going for you, it is hard to imagine that there would *not* be positive repercussions on your energy levels, sense of joy and zest for life, purposes in being, and friendship networks, among other gains.

I know it is not easy to make sudden, dramatic changes in your life. Practices of long duration, habits formed in early years, cultural and many other barriers to new lifestyle patterns all mitigate against a rapid transformation from worseness to wellness. You should expect to spend time in what health planners call the assessment and preliminary program design stages. That's a fancy phrase for fooling around, experimenting, and learning by trial and error.

At first, the going will be slow and the returns not apparent. There will be no competition to spur you on, no crowds to applaud your better diet, your relaxation pauses, your growing wellness library, or your early efforts at jogging or other fitness initiatives. In fact, there are some who may find your self-reliance more than a little threatening—such as an unsupportive spouse, employer, or physician. But as a rule, I am confident that most of your friends and acquaintances will respect your commitment to your own well-being and will share with you some of the satisfaction that goes with a wellness lifestyle. Mini-rewards along the way will come when people credit you for being such a positive influence (without trying) on their lifestyle, and a model of support in their own efforts to improve their well-being.

When getting started, however, you may need a little help from your friends. A method that has proven successful by the Alcoholics Anonymous people, and adapted by weight-reducers, smoke-abaters, and other symptom-treaters, can help you make progress on a wellness routine. The method is simple, but dramatically important: namely, find a sympathetic, supportive, and available friend or "buddy."

A buddy who himself or herself is energized by wellness possibilities and who is at a similar place in the pursuit of a well-being lifestyle is a helpful ally. He or she is not any more of a prerequisite than a holistic health center—you *can* pursue wellness by yourself. But it is easier and more fun with a buddy. Especially if the "buddy" selected happens to be your lover, mate, and/or best friend.

Measuring
Your Wellness

A lot of effort has gone into attempts to measure the health of Americans. Unfortunately, most of what goes in and out of the computers concerns mortality (death) and morbidity (illness) levels, and the extent of activity limitations caused by disabilities. As you can see, these data do not a picture of health status make! It's just a lot harder to develop a system that enables us to understand how healthy people are than it is to add up all the usual indices of nonhealth.

Part of the problem, I suspect, is that we usually think of health as a state of not being sick. And how can you measure something until you define it in positive terms? Fortunately we have such "plus" definitions of health. Let's pause for a minute to glory in a few.

Ten years ago, a Navy scientist wrote of "promotive medicine" as an alternative to curing disease that would focus instead on promoting "positive adaptive responses." He viewed health as a developmental process and talked about good health as "joy in living":

> Being healthy is having confidence in the future. The healthy man's future does not happen passively to him; it is an active extension of his life. For him the future is created by his choices and decisions. Instead of the future coming to him, he takes himself to it and his living becomes a joint creation. Health is a participation in that creation, a participation in one's own being, a commitment to one's living in the world. To be healthy is to celebrate one's life.[1]

1. Bob Hoke, "Promotive Medicine and the Phenomenon of Health," *Arch Environmental Health* 16 (February 1968):270–71.

More recently, Dr. Henrik Blum, a preeminent authority on health planning and author of the leading text in the field, has reviewed a myriad of "health-plus" definitions, and concluded that most include a goal of "maximizing potential."[2] This is also phrased as self-fulfillment, self-expression, satisfaction, or desire to live; the key idea in Blum's view of health is that well-being is an optimal relationship between the physical, emotional, and social functioning of the individual. Blum's description of good health in a larger context is of interest at this point:

> Good health is only one among many descriptors of a person's ability to function in the midst of a great variety of biological and social goals and desires. It is subject to myriad variables. Most obviously, capacities normally change with age and with exposure to social and physical environments. What is a normal expectation of physical performance for a young laborer might be life-threatening to a middle-aged scholar. Good health is basically the capacity for those tasks for which a man has been socialized and trained. It is different for every walk of life and varies for each individual with the shifting assignment of family or professional duties, of recreational and social activities.[3]

J. I. Rodale said it another way. Describing perfect health as euphoria, Rodale waxed poetic in describing well-being as a time "when your soul is singing within you, when you feel as if you would like to fly with the wind, when you do not know that there are any organs in your body."[4] To Rodale, the "high spirits of health" were a buoyant state, not merely a "tolerable to middling" condition.

To Ivan Illich, positive health is a process of adaptation shaped to a socially created reality. It emcompasses an "ability to adapt to changing environments, to growing up and to aging, to healing when damaged, to suffering, and to the peaceful ex-

---

2. *Health Planning* (New York: Human Sciences Press, 1974), p. 97.

3. Ibid., p. 101.

4. "J. I. Rodale Said It," *Prevention* (May 1976), p. 77. (Quoted from *Prevention*, October 1954.)

pectation of death."[5] Health is a task; success in the endeavor is a result of self-awareness, self-discipline, and one's inner resources. Illich concludes his extraordinary book *Medical Nemesis* with the following commentary on health and its meaning:

> Healthy people are those who live in healthy homes on a healthy diet in an environment equally fit for birth, growth, work, healing, and dying; they are sustained by a culture that enhances the conscious acceptance of limits to population, of aging, of incomplete recovery, and ever-imminent death. Healthy people need minimal bureaucratic interference to mate, give birth, share the human condition, and die.
>
> Man's consciously lived fragility, individuality, and relatedness make the experience of pain, of sickness, and of death an integral part of his life. The ability to cope with this trio autonomously is fundamental to his health.

My own ideas of wellness and health are quite similar to those expressed by Hoke, Blum, Rodale, and Illich (that's why I quoted them!). But, my orientation is somewhat different, so I'll describe as briefly as I can what I intend when I use the terms *high level wellness* and *health*.

Quite simply, high level wellness is a lifestyle—focused approach which you design for the purpose of pursuing the highest level of health within your capability. A wellness lifestyle is dynamic or ever-changing as you evolve throughout life. It is an integrated lifestyle in that you incorporate some approach or aspect of each wellness dimension (self-responsibility, nutritional awareness, stress management, physical fitness, and environmental sensitivity). Such a lifestyle will minimize your chances of becoming ill and vastly increase your prospects for well-being.

Health is also a dynamic state, and is an outcome of the wellness lifestyle. Health has three components or levels of freedom, as I see it: the physical, the emotional, and the mental. The physical I think of as freedom from pain and limiting ill-

5. *Medical Nemesis: The Expropriation of Health* (New York: Pantheon Books, 1976), p. 273. See review in the Wellness Resource Guide.

ness—a state of well-being. The emotional component of health is freedom from disabling stress and excess passion—a state of serenity, calm, and, as often as not, of zest for living. The mental aspect of health is freedom from selfishness and aimlessness—a state of compassion and purpose.

This does not exhaust all the possibilities of wellness and health. I know that, and you do, too. But the brief discussion does let you know what I mean when I toss these terms around throughout this book.

At this point it's your turn. I would like to pause to give you time to consider the extent to which you are already into wellness—or worseness.

The Wellness/Worseness Continuum

Perhaps you are already practicing a high level wellness lifestyle. The following inventory is designed to help you assess on your own how far down the path to well-being you already are. Naturally, this inventory is only suggestive—not definitive. It applies mostly to Americans in urban areas—not everybody, and you may not agree with all my judgments regarding the definition of wellness behaviors. That's OK; my intent is simply to highlight some of the regular-type aspects of wellness in the phrasing of questions. Footnotes are provided wherever I thought an extended explanation might clarify points of view.

By asking yourself these questions, you'll be exploring (perhaps for the first time) your wellness values, habits, and knowledge, and discovering your weaknesses. As you fill out the questionnaire, take note of those things about yourself that you would like to change and give special attention to the discussion of those areas later in the book. You may want to come back to these questions at some later date to see if your answers have changed. If, in a year or two, they haven't changed—well, there's a message there, too.

Although there is no rigid scoring system for this questionnaire, I can give you some guidelines. If your score is over 50, your prospects for realizing dramatic gains from adopting a wellness lifestyle are excellent. If you score under 50, the same is true, of course, but you have a hard road ahead. Good luck to both groups. If your score is over 70, then you must already be conscious of health-enhancing practices which you apparently make a part of your life. Work on those areas you're low in or at least do some checking to decide whether the risks of illness and premature disability justify—for you—the continuance of certain patterns. If your score is over 80, you are doing well.

Self-Responsibility*

	Yes	No

1. Have you, in the past 12 months, read at least one book on each of the five wellness dimensions?[6] (Note: The dimensions are self-responsibility, nutritional awareness, stress management, physical fitness, and environmental sensitivity.)

2. Would you question a physician who prescribes a drug or medicine as to whether it is really necessary? If not persuaded that it is essential, would you ask for nonmedical alternatives, seek another doctor, or simply disregard his advice and not buy the drug?

3. Do you wear seat belts when you drive, and do you require the same of children who ride with you?[7]

---

* Score one point for each affirmative response in this category. In questions having more than one part, give yourself a point only if you answer both parts in a wellness way.

6. For examples, see the high level wellness honor roll list of publications given in the Wellness Resource Guide.

7. Children are specified rather than all persons because wellness respects free choice so long as people are free (i.e., mature in this case) to make decisions and those decisions do not interfere with the health rights of others (as, for example, does smoking in restaurants).

		Yes	No
4.	Do you respect and obey the 55 MPH speed limit, at least most of the time? (Nobody's perfect.)	___	___
5.	If you could buy health insurance that provided less for sickness care but allowed payment for wellness initiatives (e.g., a course in meditation or several sessions on biofeedback, or a massage every 3 months), would you buy it, other things being equal?[8]	___	___
6.	Is your life working? Are you satisfied and often fulfilled by your work, mate(s), leisure activities, and general sense of purpose?	___	___
7.	Are there people in your life with whom you can discuss your personal problems, concerns, and disappointments?	___	___
8.	Do you look forward to leisure time, weekends, outings with children, as well as occasions to be alone?	___	___
9.	Are there values which you place before promotion, prestige, profits, and success? And, do you reflect on these other motivators in your day-to-day existence?	___	___
10.	Do you feel well-acquainted with your body? Do you know what your extremities look like? Are you generally aware of the way in which your body processes food, what physiological events take place when you are stressed, and what happens during strenuous exercise?	___	___
11.	Can you laugh at yourself?[9]	___	___

8. Biofeedback, massage, and a variety of other modalities are discussed in part two as useful and enjoyable ways to control stress and otherwise obtain insights and skills for staying well.

9. Joan Gomez, author of *How Not to Die Young*, states that this ability represents the highest achievement of civilized man and is a complete safeguard against inner arrogance.

12. Do you reject or at least try to minimize use Yes No of laxatives, tranquilizers, pain killers, reducing pills, and aspirin? Are you cautious in your intake of refined white sugar and bleached flour, artificial flavors, color additives, and preservatives? — —

13. Have you, in the past year, completed any wellness evaluation forms, tests, or other measures of health such as this questionnaire? (Examples include Health Hazard Appraisal, wellness inventories, nutritional and eating habits survey, tension measurements, Life Change Index, or value surveys.) — —

14. Can people really choose to live well? Or are personal choices (e.g., to smoke, drink, etc.) dictated by environmental factors, peer pressures, ingrained habit, or the "rewards" of negative behaviors? (Check yes if you believe choices can be made.) — —

15. Do you use dental floss at least once daily, brush your teeth (properly) after every meal (if possible), visit a prevention-oriented dentist not less than annually, and minimize your exposure to dental (and all other) x rays? — —

16. Can you turn people down, say no, or otherwise disappoint others in giving priority to your own needs without feeling guilty? — —

17. Do you find death preferable to maintenance on a machine with heroic procedures and potent drugs when the prognosis for recovery is acknowledged by all involved as nil? — —

18. Have you ever attempted a journal, diary, or   Yes   No
other record of your feelings, internal states, inner qualities, or other introspective aspects, even for a few days?   ____   ____

19. Do you know the optimal rate level for one or more of your own vital signs (e.g., pulse, temperature, respiration, and blood pressure)?[10]   ____   ____

20. Do you believe your own attitude and the resistance of your personal organism based upon your attitude and will are as important in healing as the drugs, medical procedures, and equipment which doctors can marshall?   ____   ____

21. Do you feel that your life follows a "winner's script," that it is filled with positive strokes and guided by an adult ego state?[11]   ____   ____

22. Do you agree that little that is worthwhile comes without effort, self-discipline, time, perseverance, and the foregoing of other options?   ____   ____

23. Do you believe that you can dramatically arrest the usual pattern of slowdown and degeneration due to aging?   ____   ____

24. Do you think that you have a realistic view of your strengths and weaknesses? Are you confident of the validity of your own self-assessment?   ____   ____

---

10. Normal ranges are: pulse = 60–80 beats per minute; respiration = 12–18 breaths per minute without conscious awareness; and blood pressure = 100/60–150/90.

11. The terms are used as employed in the field of transactional analysis, a "rational method for problem-solving."

High-Risk Behaviors*

	Yes	No
1. Do you now smoke cigarettes, cigars, or pipes?[12]	___	___
2. Is it frequently difficult for you to fall asleep at night?	___	___
3. When you have a headache, do you take aspirin?	___	___
4. Do you take any medications on a regular basis?	___	___
5. Do you drink alcohol?	___	___
6. Are you assessed double fares on streetcars, buses, cabs, and airlines because of excess weight?[13]	___	___
7. Would you drive when angry or depressed, do you keep loaded firearms in your home, or do you generally think of yourself as an aggressive person capable of physically assaulting someone other than in self-defense?	___	___
8. Do you drink coffee or tea (nonherbal)? (Check yes if either of the above applies.)[14]	___	___

---

* Score 1 point for each negative response in this category.

12. Occasional marijuana, while redundant to one into a wellness lifestyle and still risky in certain benighted locales, is OK for purposes of this questionnaire. If you smoke pot, but nothing else, check no.

13. Obesity (weighing 10 percent or more over your desirable weight) is a most visible symptom of unhealth. Your heart has to work harder to pump blood through the extra adipose tissue, so the blood pressure increases. This pressure adds to the risks of artery breakage (stroke), kidney failure, and respiratory infection, to note just a few of the hazards of obesity.

14. Coffee, tea, cola, and chocolate are addictive drugs having no food value. All contain caffeine which stimulates the nervous system and causes stomach acid secretions leading to heartburn and bleeding ulcers. Herbal teas, fruit juices, and carob are among the nourishing and tasty alternatives.

9. Do you bite your fingernails, toenails, or other extremities?

        Yes   No

10. Do you feel uncomfortable in touching and being touched?

11. Have you experienced what seems to be a cluster of significant life changes in the past year? (Examples might include death of or rejection by a spouse or mate/friend, outstanding personal achievement, retirement, injury or illness, loss of a new job, change in financial status, and/or move to a new community.)

12. Do you find anything humorous in the portrayal or parody of "social" or any other form of drunkeness?

13. Do you put up with something less than warmth and compassion from medical people without complaining or taking action later?

14. Do you frequently listen to loud rock music?[15]

Environmental Sensitivity*

1. Are you concerned about future population/resource problems to the extent of thinking or doing anything related to these

---

* Score 1 point for each affirmative response in this category.

15. Are you ready for this? Evidence is accumulating which suggests that a lot of such music correlates with irritation, headaches, depression, insomnia, marital problems, and even impotence. Not only the loud noises, but the fact that such music has little plan or design and is loaded with random shock sounds are all factors in these adverse effects. So "nourish" yourself with Mozart, Beethoven, Schubert, and others, the "rhythms and tones that drive out the pollution and flush away the accumulating toxins of life." (Mark Bricklin, "Things Here and There," *Prevention*, July 1976, pp. 87–89.)

	Yes	No
issues, e.g., practicing birth control, or limiting your contribution to two or less?[16]	___	___

2. If you have a meeting one mile away and about 15 minutes to get there, are you likely to walk or bike rather than motor?[17]   ___ ___

3. Are you aware of, sympathetic to, and/or in any way involved in efforts (e.g., consumer boycotts) to reduce or eliminate the use of pesticides, chemicals, additives, and other contaminants in our food supply?   ___ ___

4. Do you avoid the purchase or use of aerosol sprays?   ___ ___

5. Are you aware that air pollution (including smoking) increases your need for vitamin E, or that high stress levels place added demands on the body for vitamin C?[18]   ___ ___

6. Do you use public transit whenever possible and reasonably convenient?   ___ ___

7. Do you consider yourself informed on community and national events? Do you vote regularly? Are you, in short, aware of and interested in what's going on in the world outside of your normal sphere of direct influence?   ___ ___

---

16. Births exceed deaths on the globe by 200,000 per day, or 70 million per year. The growth curve is exponential; resources and land are finite.

17. Assumes other things are equal. I wouldn't expect you to walk if thunderstorms were swirling and gusting about. But jogging to the liquor store does not count.

18. John Feltman, "A Nutritional Shield Against the Arrows of Stress," *Prevention*, September 1976, pp. 88–93.

8. Do you permit smoking in your home or car?[19]

    Yes   No

9. Do you try to develop and maintain a deep tan?[20]

10. Would you say that some of your friends and associates are at least as concerned about and involved in a wellness lifestyle as you are?[21]

11. Do you make special efforts when you travel to avoid fatigue, maintain sensible diet patterns, and otherwise continue healthy behaviors conducive to well-being

Appropriate Use of the Medical System*

1. Do you think an annual physical checkup is a valid measure of your health?

2. Do you believe that more doctors, health insurance, new drugs, and more hospital equipment and facilities will lead to better health for people?

3. Each American man, woman, and child is currently spending about $600 annually for medical care. Do you think this is a good buy?

---

* Score 1 point for each negative response to questions 1 through 6 and 1 point for each positive response for questions 7 through 10.

19. Tobacco smoke consists of long-chained hydrocarbons—tiny particles which easily become entwined in fabrics, upholstery, draperies, rugs, clothing, and human lungs.

20. High levels of exposure to the sun are closely associated with skin cancer.

21. It is a lot easier to live well if you are not surrounded by others hell-bent on destroying themselves.

4. When you have the misfortune to require   Yes   No
   the facilities of a hospital, do you assume
   that the institution you choose or your doctor assigns you is organized in your best
   interests?[22]   _____   _____

5. Would you agree to undergo surgery if your
   doctor recommended it?[23]   _____   _____

6. The "perfect nursing-home patient" is said
   to be one who is sedated, confined to a bed,
   and qualified for maximum government
   reimbursement. Would you permit a relative or friend to be institutionalized without
   personally investigating the orientation of
   management?[24]   _____   _____

7. Do you believe that the client-physician
   relationship should be a learning experience
   wherein the client is helped to understand
   the nature of the problem and its origin,
   what is recommended, why, what he might
   expect, and how might the difficulty be
   avoided in the future?   _____   _____

8. Does the principle set out by Roger
   Williams make sense to you as an axiom
   which should govern medical encounters?   _____   _____

22. The American Hospital Association has, since 1973, urged the nation's 7,
000 hospitals to enact and provide to all clients a "Patient's Bill of Rights." Only
one-fourth of U.S. hospitals have done so. Also, a random survey in 1975 of 261
hospitals throughout the country showed that 64 percent were deficient in
meeting federal standards of cleanliness, fire and explosion protection, adequate staff and equipment, or in standards of record keeping.

23. In an experiment to determine the necessity of surgery, Blue Shield of
Pennsylvania will pay for a second medical opinion to test the validity of the
first. The program will encompass nearly one million Blue Shield subscribers.
Does Blue Shield suspect something we don't?

24. James D. Whitaker, "Drug Abuse among Elderly Called Alarming by
Doctors," *Washington Post*, 13 June 1975.

The principle is that:

> One would assume that top priority in the treatment of disease should always be given to those medications which are most similar to nature's own biological weapons, and that one should be cautious about introducing alien chemicals into any patient's system . . . . The basic fault of all these weapons is that they have no known connection with the disease process itself. They tend to mask the difficulty, not eliminate it. They contaminate the internal environment, create dependence on the part of the patient, and often complicate the physician's job by erasing valuable clues as to the real source of trouble."[25]

9. Would you favor a national health insurance plan designed to foster self-responsibility and demedicalize care, in part by focusing on the single needs of the many (e.g., primary care) and not on the high-technology-treatment services for the few?[26] (Please read footnote before answering.)   Yes   No

10. Have you heard about or in any way been involved with the local health-planning agency in your community established under law

25. Roger Williams, *Nutrition Against Disease* (New York: Bantam, 1971), p. 8.

26. All proposals now before the Congress center around cost implications and issues of control and access to medical services. All take for granted the wisdom of existing approaches to "health." Each would result in a continuation of a "health" system which is hospital-centered and technologically weighted toward disease-treatment and care-giving. The opportunities inherent in the present health-care system "crisis" to reassess basic questions and directions could be lost. Little or no attention has been given to promoting the kind of ethic represented by wellness concepts. All NHI proposals, as Leon Kass, M.D., has noted ("Regarding the End of Medicine and the Pursuit of Health," *The Public Interest*, Summer 1975, p. 41), continue the "no fault principle." "They therefore choose to ignore, to treat as irrelevant, the importance of personal responsibility for the state of one's health. As a result, they pass up an opportunity to build both positive and negative inducements into the insurance payment plan, by measures such as refusing or reducing benefits for chronic respiratory disease care to persons who continue to smoke."

(P.L. 89-749 and P.L. 93-641) to improve   Yes   No
the medical system and the health status of
the people?   ____   ____

Nutritional Awareness*

1. Do you avoid or severely limit your intake of
   enriched white flour products and "sweets"
   made with refined (white) sugars?   ____   ____

2. Are you concerned about and do you make
   reasonable efforts to reduce the amount of
   coloring agents, preservatives, and other
   chemicals in your food supply?   ____   ____

3. Is your breakfast larger than your lunch, and
   is your lunch in turn larger than your dinner
   (and any snacks thereafter)?   ____   ____

4. Do you take food supplements (vitamins)
   regularly?   ____   ____

5. Are you careful to maintain a high-roughage
   diet?   ____   ____

6. If you became convinced that junk foods
   (e.g., soda pop, sugar-coated cakes, etc.)
   sold in school dispensing machines were in
   fact nonnutritive and quite possibly harmful
   to your children's health, would you organize a parents' group to pressure for the removal of such synthetics in favor of fruit
   juices, fruit drinks, or other nutritious alternatives?[27]   ____   ____

---

*   Score 1 point for each affirmative response in this category.

27. There are several recent documented cases where this has been accom-
plished. See, for example, *Prevention*, April 1976, pp. 126–31; June 1976, pp.
70–73; and August 1976, pp. 61–65.

7. When you go on auto or other trips with   Yes   No children, do you pack unsalted nuts, seeds, fruits (fresh or dried), honey rolls, and other tasty alternatives to the way station junk bins?   ___ ___

8. Do you avoid eating out in restaurants?[28]   ___ ___

9. Would you serve your infant (or anybody's infant) homemade baby food only, avoiding the commercial products?[29]   ___ ___

10. Do you often make your own flour (e.g., from whole wheat berries), or yogurt, or fruit drinks? Or do you often add unprocessed bran to your foods? (Check yes if any of the above apply.)   ___ ___

11. Do you read the labels on all packaged foods?   ___ ___

12. Do you conscientiously attempt to reduce your sugar intake?[30]   ___ ___

---

28. Most restaurants in this country, like most hospitals, are dangerous places; it's hard to come out better off than when you went in. In addition to the economic issue of extraordinary cost for value received, the food in most restaurants is uninspired and hazardous to your health. Most menu items are overloaded with fats, sugar, salt, enriched white flour, preservatives, additives, and are frozen, to boot. The risks are increased by the presence of cigarettes and other pernicious weeds. Given what's in front and all around them, it is small wonder that patrons are led to drink, which further increases the risks.

29. Consumers Union recommends homemade foods, and so do I. The homemade products are half the price, do not contain preservatives and other possibly harmful additives, have less carbohydrates, salt, sugar, and are obviously fresher and thus more nutritious. *Prevention* (April 1976, p. 151) reports the following excerpt from a Public Broadcast System "Consumer Survival Kit": "A commercial jar of bananas . . . contains sugar, modified tapioca starch, salt, citric acid, and water and costs 2.6 cents an ounce. A fresh ripe banana—100 percent fruit—costs 1.1 cents an ounce."

30. Sugar has no redeemable qualities as a nutrient. It is a pure carbohydrate, calorie-ridden, druglike refined substance that is absorbed rapidly, to the body's peril. It places a traumatic demand on the pancreas, which puts out insulin to the extent that the endocrine balance is upset. Americans consume an average of 120 pounds of sugar per person annually. Now you and I and lots of our friends are surely not going at it like that, so imagine the quantities of the stuff some people must be putting away. The thought's enough to cause a toothache.

		Yes	No
13.	Do you have any idea of your optimum daily caloric, protein, fat, vitamin, and/or mineral intake?	___	___
14.	Within the last year have you taken a nutritional survey and discussed the results with a qualified professional in this area? (Unlikely that he/she would be an M.D.)	___	___
15.	Do you abstain from red meat or try to minimize your consumption of it?	___	___
16.	Are you aware of the ecological impact of the American beef-eating habit?[31]	___	___
17.	Do you enjoy chewing your food instead of snapping at it and gulping it down?	___	___
18.	Are you aware of protein "complementarity" wherein nonmeat animal protein sources (e.g., dairy products) or different plant protein sources having mutually complementary amino acid patterns can be mixed in the same meal *to increase* the protein value of the meal?[32]	___	___

Physical Fitness*

		Yes	No
1.	Are you comfortable with and proud of your body?	___	___

---

* Score 1 point for each affirmative response in this category.

31. Frances Moore Lappé (*Diet for a Small Planet*) has shown that an average steer reduces 16 pounds of grain and soy to one pound of meat on the table; that 90 percent of all this nation's corn, oats, and barley are consumed by livestock; and that animal waste amounts to 2 billion tons per year. One estimate is that livestock contribute 10 times more water pollution than people generate and three times more than is produced by industry. Paavo Airola (*Are You Confused?*) and others maintain that Americans consume far more protein than is necessary or healthy. Excess protein causes toxic residues of metabolic waste products, biochemical imbalances, diminished strength, and intestinal putrefaction.

32. Frances Moore Lappé in the book noted above terms this phenomenon a case in which the whole is greater than the sum of the parts.

2. Do you exercise vigorously at least 30   Yes   No
   minutes nearly every day (i.e., five out of
   seven days)?   ____ ____

3. Do you include some flexibility and stretching exercises in your daily routine?   ____ ____

4. Are you motivated to play sports primarily
   for the pleasure, sociability, and/or exercise
   they provide? (Check no if you believe your
   major reward comes from the joy of winning,
   or perhaps the excitement of risking defeat.) ____ ____

5. Do you belong to a YM/WCA, health spa, or
   other fitness-oriented organization?   ____ ____

6. Does your company, employer, or work
   place provide or encourage exercise programs for employees? (If not applicable,
   check yes if you believe that exercise times
   should be a built-in part of the workweek.) ____ ____

7. For the most part, have your experiences
   with athletics from the time you were a
   young boy or girl been positive?   ____ ____

8. Do you have any idea of the processes by
   which exercise and attendant increased fitness benefit the body?[33]   ____ ____

9. Do you regularly cycle, play handball, basketball, or soccer, or do you engage in swimming, rowing, running long distances, or
   other sustained vigorous activity?[34]   ____ ____

---

33. Blood pressure is lowered, resting heart rate decreases, muscles (including the heart) become stronger, the number of active small blood vessels carrying blood to the cells of muscular tissues are greatly increased, and the blood
itself is improved (carries more oxygen and blood platelets are less sticky).

34. These sports all provide the "training effect"—that is, the intensity
needed for strengthening the heart muscles and circulatory systems.

Stress Management*   Yes   No

1. Do you meditate or otherwise try to center, balance, or quiet your mind on a regular basis?   ___   ___

2. Have you experienced a massage (for relaxation) within the past six months?   ___   ___

3. Are you acquainted with Rolfing, bioenergetics, the Feldenkrais methods of structural integration, clearing, or any similar "hands-on" modalities focused on balance, centering, and increased awareness?   ___   ___

4. Have you undergone or are you familiar with any of the various forms of biofeedback?   ___   ___

5. Did you know that insomnia, general fatigue, stiffness of muscles, back pain, headaches, ulcers, colitis, gastritis, heart disease, cancer, and strokes are all highly correlated with stress?   ___   ___

6. Do you respect your own accomplishments?[35]   ___   ___

7. Are you free, most of the time, from tension, frustration, insecurity, aimlessness, and dissatisfaction with your work and vocation?   ___   ___

8. Have you taken at least two weeks of vacation in the past year?   ___   ___

9. Are you aware of foot-tapping, leg-shaking, and assorted rhythmic movements with fingers and/or pencils, and similar habits? Do

---

*   Score 1 point for each affirmative response in this category.

35.   Hans Selye, M.D., author of *Stress Without Distress* (New York: Signet, 1974), p. 75, claims that dissatisfaction with life due to disrespect for one's own accomplishments is one of the major sources of distress.

	Yes	No
you recognize these behaviors as nervous mannerisms indicative of stress? Are you alert to the meaning of such gestures in yourself? (Check yes if this response applies to at least two of the above conditions.)	___	___
10. Do you sleep soundly, seldom feel tired, enjoy a good appetite, and deal satisfactorily with pressure?[36]	___	___
11. Do you make a conscious effort to arrange your mealtimes so that an easy, relaxed atmosphere is part of the eating experience?	___	___

Other Measures of Well-Being

Unlike the test you just took, a number of available wellness evaluations focus on just one of the many dimensions of wellness. Several of these self-tests are designed to help you understand the extent and causes of stress in your life, and to help you learn how to reduce or eliminate such stresses.

Voice Stress Analysis

This evaluation is marketed by Introspective Technology Services (ITS) of San Francisco, and costs $25. The Voice Stress Analysis takes only about 15 minutes to complete. You circle yes or no to 50 questions, and then read both the question and your yes or no answer into an automatic recording system. The recording is fed into a computer voice analyzer, a biofeedback device which measures changes in vocal cord vibrations when you experience stress. The voice analyzer measures minute changes in voice pattern (micro-muscle tremors) based upon

---

36. John H. Knowles, M.D., who is president of the Rockefeller Foundation and a former professor of medicine at Harvard and general director of the Massachusetts General Hospital in Boston, wrote in a Time bicentennial essay ("The Struggle to Stay Healthy," 9 August 1976, p. 62) that about "80 percent of the doctor's work consists of treating colds, minor injuries, gastrointestinal upsets, backaches, arthritis, and anxiety. One out of four people is 'emotionally tense,' and worried about insomnia, fatigue, too much or too little appetite, and his ability to cope with modern life."

voice frequency vibrations, which in turn enable the ITS staff to pinpoint your stress patterns and attitudes. ITS then recommends a series of exercises which you can take to deal with those emotions and attitudes, some of which are hidden sources of conflict, that are producing stress within you.

A sampling of the questions on the Voice Stress Analysis may be of interest to you:

I neglect to complete things that I start . . . . Yes   No
I reject others' points of view . . . . Yes   No
I lack a sense of humor . . . . Yes   No
I have unrealistic expectations . . . . Yes   No
I often invalidate myself . . . . Yes   No
I make promises that I know I can't keep . . . . Yes   No
I am unsupportive of others' goals . . . . Yes   No
I take compliments poorly . . . . Yes   No
I am faultfinding . . . . Yes   No
I fail to acknowledge others for their
     contributions . . . . Yes   No
I have ideas that I don't dare disclose . . . . Yes   No
I fail to state my goals clearly . . . . Yes   No
I am often inflexible . . . . Yes   No
I don't express my anger towards others . . . . Yes   No
I make excuses . . . . Yes   No
I am unmotivated . . . . Yes   No
I am undisciplined . . . . Yes   No

The following excerpts from the ITS Voice Stress Analysis brochure provide insight into the philosophy behind the evaluation while providing useful information on the dynamics of stress management. In addition, the ITS people nicely reinforce the ethic of self-responsibility so vital to a wellness lifestyle:

Stress reduction starts when you accurately identify the issues that are stressful. It accelerates when you apply this understanding as a guide to action. Once you recognize your points of stress, you develop a more realistic self-image. Just the act of identifying these points tends to diminish confusion and reduce stress, since you now know where to focus your attention to produce results. And what to do to produce results becomes clearer, since you now know what you are trying to change.

What you do with this knowledge is, of course, up to you. Only you can produce change in your life. The purpose of this service is to provide you with data from your own body, free from human error, opinion, evaluation, or interpretation, concerning what you do in your life to bring stress upon yourself.

I completed the Voice Stress Analysis, read the questions and my answers into the telephone recorder, and waited for the analysis. A few days later it arrived. Here are a few excerpts from the stress analysis report on yours truly:

1. You have stress on being *undisciplined*. You see yourself as more erratic than you'd like to be in your personal discipline. You often waste large amounts of time and then become trapped in the crunch of a deadline. Many times you consider your willpower sadly lacking and your schedule a disaster. You could benefit by reading *How to Get Control of Your Time and Your Life* by Alan Lakein.

Or your stress in this area may come from adhering to a rigid discipline you have imposed upon yourself against your natural inclination for more flexibility. Begin immediately by reviewing your attitudes and thoughts about discipline, followed by a strict (but practical) allocation of your time.

List 20 reasons you shouldn't do anything about this.

2. You have stress on the issue of *humor*. By your own standards, you are often not as light and humorous as you could be. Your inability to laugh about some things (especially yourself?) indicates you spend too much time reviewing the past or worrying about tomorrow. What would happen if you let go of your woes and had a good laugh at your own seriousness?

Or you may suspect you are using humor as a device for "taking the heat off" and diverting attention from the situation at hand. What other ways could you find to confront uncomfortable situations? Start noticing the times you get people to laugh.

People with no sense of humor are no fun because:

3. You have stress on the issue of *inflexibility*. You have a tendency to be more rigid than you'd like to be, a good deal of the time. Regimentation and inflexibility can be a problem to you in light of all the surprises and changes which occur in your life. Look at the anxiety and impatience you encounter and see if lack of flexibility isn't the source of much of your distress. Suppose nothing ever again happened as planned . . . would it make a difference?

Find one thing to change your mind about every day.

This analysis did not, at first, strike me as fitting my personality and certainly not my self-concept, though item 1 does apply. But perhaps these are in fact hidden sources of conflict "exposed" by the minute changes in my voice pattern.

The folks at ITS have also developed special stress assessments for the following subjects: communication, love, sex, money, power, personal integrity, job/work, study, body, and efficiency. (Cost: $50 each). In addition, ITS has created a 10-day Stress-Reduction Program in workbook-form based on the results of the Voice Stress Analysis, and is planning to market workshops, consultations, and research using the technology of computer stress analysis.

The ITS work demonstrates yet another approach to understanding how well you are before you get sick.[37]

Life Change Index

Another popular measure used in assessing stress levels is the Life Change Index developed by Dr. Thomas H. Holmes, a pioneer in identifying stress-related illnesses.[38] Dr. Holmes has

37. For more information about the Voice Stress Analysis and the other stress products of ITS, write or call (415 921-3875) the company at 2172 Green St., San Francisco, CA 94123.

38. Dr. Holmes is on the faculty at the University of Washington School of Medicine in Seattle, Washington. The test reproduced above was published in the *Chicago Tribune* on 27 April 1976, as part of a series on how the "good life" is killing Americans. The article was entitled "Stress—The 'Wild Beast' Enemy Facing Modern Man."

rated 43 life changes; his index has been used to accurately predict a person's risk of becoming ill. The life events and item values are listed below, along with an explanatory note.

Will stress in your life make you sick?
Score yourself on the Life Change Test.
If any of these life events have happened to you in the last 12 months, please check Happened column and enter Value in Score column.

Item no.	Item value	Happened (√)	Your score	Life event
1	100	————	————	Death of spouse
2	73	————	————	Divorce
3	65	————	————	Marital separation
4	63	————	————	Jail term
5	63	————	————	Death of close family member
6	53	————	————	Personal injury or illness
7	50	————	————	Marriage
8	47	————	————	Fired at work
9	45	————	————	Marital reconciliation
10	45	————	————	Retirement
11	44	————	————	Change in health of family member
12	40	————	————	Pregnancy
13	39	————	————	Sex difficulties
14	39	————	————	Gain of new family member
15	39	————	————	Business readjustment
16	38	————	————	Change in financial state
17	37	————	————	Death of close friend
18	36	————	————	Change to different line of work
19	35	————	————	Change in number of arguments with spouse
20	31	————	————	Mortgage over $10,000
21	30	————	————	Foreclosure of mortgage or loan
22	29	————	————	Change in responsibilities at work
23	29	————	————	Son or daughter leaving home
24	29	————	————	Trouble with in-laws
25	28	————	————	Outstanding personal achievement
26	26	————	————	Wife begin or stop work
27	26	————	————	Begin or end school
28	25	————	————	Change in living conditions
29	24	————	————	Revision of personal habits
30	23	————	————	Trouble with boss
31	20	————	————	Change in work hours or conditions
32	20	————	————	Change in residence
33	20	————	————	Change in schools
34	19	————	————	Change in recreation
35	19	————	————	Change in church activities

Item no.	Item value	Happened (✓)	Your score	Life event
36	18	————	————	Change in social activities
37	17	————	————	Mortgage or loan less than $10,000
38	16	————	————	Change in sleeping habits
39	15	————	————	Change in number of family get-togethers
40	15	————	————	Change in eating habits
41	13	————	————	Vacation
42	12	————	————	Christmas
43	11	————	————	Minor violations of the law

Total score for 12 months___

Note: The more change you have, the more likely you are to get sick. Of those people with over 300 Life Change Units for the past year, almost 80 percent get sick in the near future; with 150 to 299 Life Change Units, about 50 percent get sick in the near future; and with less than 150 Life Change Units, only about 30 percent get sick in the near future.

Note that even life events that could be desirable changes, such as a new job or vacation, produce stress.

Health Hazard Appraisal (HHA)

This is the best-known and one of the more sophisticated instruments currently used by wellness practitioners.[39] It is designed to make you aware of the causal link between lifestyle and potential loss of health. Using well-accepted mortality data, the computerized HHA is used to provide information on where you stand in selected risk categories; that is, how likely you are to die of lifestyle-related diseases or accidents.

The HHA takes about 20 minutes to complete; the questions are designed to provide clues to the health risks to your survival and well-being in the next 10 years of your life. By compiling your present risks and showing you the implications of these behaviors, the HHA is helpful in encouraging you to adopt lifestyle reforms, before illness strikes. Questions in the HHA probe the following areas: medical history, smoking, illness symptoms, extent of auto travel, medicines taken, out-of-the-ordinary risks (flying a private plane, sky diving, etc.), alcoholic consumption patterns, anxiety symptoms, and other areas.

39. Developed by Drs. Lewis Robbins and Jack Hall of Methodist Hospital of Indiana. See J. La Dou, J. N. Sherwood, and L. Hughes, "Health Hazard Appraisal in Patient Counseling," *Western Journal of Medicine*, 122 (February 1975):177–180.

To give you a sense of how it works, let's say you are a 35-year-old white female 20 percent overweight, working at a sedentary job, rarely exercising, eating junk food, and smoking nine cigars a day. You would receive a print-out which would rather dramatically present you with the bad-news implications of your lifestyle. In your case, the HHA would probably indicate high risks in the following disease categories: arteriosclerotic heart disease, hypertensive heart disease, and diabetes. The instrument would also list you at three different ages: the first would be your chronologic age (your actual age, 35 in this example); the second your appraisal age (based on your lifestyle, about 45, meaning you stand the same risk of dying as a person of this age); and the third your compliance age (the appraisal age you could attain, about 37, if you followed all the lifestyle reform recommendations given in the analysis). If you are already into wellness and you take the HHA, you will find that your appraisal and compliance ages are quite close, and well below your chronologic age.

Nutrition, Health, and Activity Profile

A number of nutritional surveys have been devised to assist people interested in knowing more about this dimension of well-being. In my opinion, the best of the lot is that used at the Wholistic Health and Nutrition Institute (WHN). It is called the Nutrition, Health, and Activity Profile.

The profile is a four-page computerized questionnaire designed to teach nutritional basics while emphasizing the importance of other wellness dimensions. After you complete this survey (it takes about 20 minutes), you will get a conversationally written analysis of your dietary intake. This profile provides you with a short course on the value of protein, carbohydrates, fats, fiber, vitamins, minerals, calories, and so forth, and assesses your nutrient consumption relative to accepted standards. Suggestions are offered in areas needing attention with an emphasis not so much on existing problems as upon ways to improve longevity, overall fitness, and resistance to disease. Interspersed throughout the analysis are recommendations for readings appropriate to your situation. Features that I especially like about the Nutrition Health and Activity Profile are the emphasis upon other wellness dimensions that complement a growing nutritional awareness, the suggested readings, the conversational style of the analysis, and the citations of research evidence when advice is given on controversial subjects (e.g., the link between coffee consumption and ulcer formation).[40]

YMCA's Fitness Evaluations

One of the oldest wellness operations in America, the YMCA, offers a service that certainly deserves mention in any listing of tests that measure well-being and motivate health-conscious behavior. I refer to the fitness evaluations done at YMCAs throughout the country at minimal charge, and usually free to members. You might be interested in how the evaluation works.

Basically, the Y's fitness evaluation is designed to acquaint you with the value of pulse-conscious exercise. It begins with the taking of your pulse, and an explanation of what given pulse ranges suggest about your level of fitness. Your pulse, incidentally, is nothing more than a reading of how often your heart beats against a column of blood in your circulatory vessels. But this reading provides you with information vital to your health. It is an index of changing body temperature, energy and oxygen consumption, muscle and emotional functioning, and overall condition. It is, perhaps, the most single valid indicator of your well-being.

The method used at YMCAs is quite simple; I'll review it briefly, using my pulse data as an example. You can use this approach on your own if you want to be sure you are deriving the optimal cardiovascular returns from your workouts, without pushing yourself beyond reasonable limits.

In the calculation, the first step is to simply insert the figure 220—this is an accepted norm or *standard maximum heart rate*. Then subtract from this rate years of age (38). The result is a

---

40. For more information and/or if you wish to complete a Nutrition Health and Activity Profile ($19), write to N.E.W.S., % James M. Cloud, Building C, 150 Shoreline Highway, Mill Valley, CA 94941.

maximum attainable heart rate (182). This is the highest pulse rate I could achieve without losing consciousness. (I doubt if I have ever been close.) To get the *resting heart rate*, I would next subtract from this maximum attainable heart rate my *resting pulse rate* (44), which, by the way, is best taken upon waking from a normal period of sleep. This provides a subtotal (138) from which is derived the optimal "work load" or *level of intensity*, the pulse range an average person needs to obtain a "training effect" on the heart and related systems. The accepted range is from 60 to 80 percent of the subtotal, so the final step in the calculation is to compute both 60 and 80 percent of the sub-total (83 and 112), and add to these percentages the resting pulse rate, which in my case is 44. Thus, the pulse range I need to achieve a training effect is 127 to 156.

To summarize (using my figures), here is how you can perform this part of the YMCA evaluation for yourself:

Standard maximum heart rate	220
Minus your age	−38
Equals your maximum attainable heart rate	182
Minus your resting heart rate	−44
Equals a subtotal (needed to calculate intensity levels)	138

To calculate your optimum level of intensity (optimum work-load range) of 60 to 80 percent, simply take these percentages of your subtotal and add to each your resting pulse. Thus:

Subtotal	138
60 and 80 percent of subtotal	83 and 112
Plus resting heart rate	+44 +44
Equals the optimal range of pulse intensity levels	127 to 156

As you probably know, the easiest way to check on your workout intensity is to time your pulse for six seconds and multiply that by 10 to get beats per minute. Do it a few times and you will get quite skilled at it.

★   ★   ★

These are a few examples of varied measures that actually tell you something about your health, rather than just another battery of tests showing how sick you are. These measures help you *avoid* illness, and they reflect the special concerns of positive health-oriented practitioners and others having particular interests in stress management, nutritional awareness, self-responsibility, and other wellness dimensions.

But such measures are valuable for reasons other than what they indicate about your health status: they also show that the habits and patterns governing your behavior are more important than all the hospitals and doctors and pills between here and China. And the measures underscore the point that *health is so much more than not being sick!* Health in this context can be thought of and followed as a dynamic state of being in which you are actively involved in the quest of a balanced lifestyle. When your life is working, when you are able to cope, and when you feel in touch with your best potentials, you are enjoying a richer level of health than when you are simply not sick, but not all that well, either! *Health is more than the absence of illness*, when you can enjoy the varied efforts which you choose to extend in pursuit of a healthy lifestyle.[41]

---

41. *Health* is an Anglo-Saxon term that shares its root meaning with *hale, hearty, holy, heal,* and *whole.*

The Five Dimensions of High Level Wellness

Wellness is a way of life which you design to enjoy the highest level of health and well-being possible during the years you have in this life. The wellness philosophy sketched in the previous pages, the activities taking place at the resource wellness centers and through the holistic health programs, and the principles and concepts of high level wellness are all potential elements of *your* wellness philosophy. Take what you need and choose what you think will work for you—I know you will add a lot to what I have started.

Up to now, we've been delving into the nature and philosophy of high level wellness, merely mentioning the key dimensions of wellness along the way. It is now time to explore these areas so you can begin working them into your own wellness lifestyle. While I discuss each of these dimensions separately, you must integrate all of them if you expect to create and profit by a wellness lifestyle. That's why I am presenting all five in part 2, though I realize that it is easier to bring together these critical dimensions of well-being in a book than it is in your life. (Becoming an exercise superstar, for example, is self-defeating if you eat like a bear and overlook or do little to moderate the tensions and stresses you experience every day.) With this caveat in mind, let's take a closer look at self-responsibility, nutritional awareness, stress management, physical fitness, and environmental sensitivity—the five dimensions of high level wellness.

Self-Responsibility

All dimensions of high level wellness are equally important, but self-responsibility seems more equal than all the rest. It is the philosopher's stone, the mariner's compass, and the ring of power to a high level wellness lifestyle. Without an active sense of accountability for your own well-being, you won't have the necessary motivation to lead a health-enhancing lifestyle. That is, you are not likely to put the energy into nutrition, stress management, fitness, and environmental shaping that is required for optimal health. So, in the sense that you will not grow in other areas if you neglect this dimension, self-responsibility represents your keystone to a life of high level wellness.

In my opinion (and that of many others), the single greatest cause of unhealth in this nation is that most Americans neglect, and surrender to others, responsibility for their own health. I won't bore you with the statistics on the nation's morbidity and mortality patterns, nor will I belabor the indices showing how the U.S. ranks below 10 to 20 other developed countries in assorted measures of "health" (absence of illness). The lack of widespread acceptance and practice of an ethic of self-responsibility for our own health and well-being is evident not only in these "bottom-line" indices related to neglect, but in the reliance of our citizenry on a medical system to provide, maintain, and restore "health." Ivan Illich offered the following opinion in concluding his classic analysis of the role of medicine in discouraging personal autonomy:

> The level of public health corresponds to the degree to which the means and responsibility for coping with illness are distributed among the total population. This ability to

cope can be enhanced but never replaced by medical intervention or by the hygienic characteristics of the environment. That society which can reduce professional intervention to the minimum will provide the best conditions for health. The greater the potential for autonomous adaptation to self, to others, and to the environment, the less management of adaptation will be needed or tolerated.

A world of optimal and widespread health is obviously a world of minimal and only occasional medical intervention.[1]

You need a strong sense of personal accountability for your health to avoid high-risk behaviors, what the Transactional Analysis folks call "stroke deprivation" habits (e.g., over-eating). The evidence is overwhelming that these behaviors are predisposing factors in the chronic diseases of heart failure, cancer, stroke, diabetes, and other debilitating disorders killing and maiming vast numbers of Americans. You might pause just a moment to recognize the extent of just two such high-risk habits.

- Smoking—The per capita annual consumption of cigarettes in 1974 was 4,270; in recent years, teenagers and women have increased their smoking levels.[2] The President's Science Advisory Committee in 1973 placed 16 percent of all mortality on this habit alone; well-established evidence links smoking to cancer of the lung, larynx, lip, oral cavity, esophagus, bladder, and other urinary organs; chronic bronchitis and emphysema; and arteriosclerotic heart disease.

- Alcohol consumption—Nearly half the U.S. population drinks; nine million are alcohol abusers. Alcohol is a factor in half the motor vehicle fatalities, half of all homicides, and a third of all suicides. The annual cost in lost productivity, damages, etc. is put at $15 billion.[3] Cirrhosis of the liver is

---

1. *Medical Nemesis: The Expropriation Of Health* (New York: Pantheon, 1976), p. 274.

2. U.S. Department of Health, Education, and Welfare, *Forward Plan For Health: FY 1975–81.* DHEW Publication No. 76-50024 (Washington, D.C.: DHEW, 1975), p. 100.

3. Ibid., p. 101.

one principal result of alcohol abuse; others include malnutrition, lowered resistance to infectious diseases, gastrointestinal irritations, muscle diseases and tremors, and
brain and/or nervous system damage.

I'm optimistic that a person can overcome these and other
high-risk habits and move ahead to wellness behaviors if he or
she chooses to do so. The place to begin is here—by learning to
act upon the conviction that *your* health is primarily within *your*
own hands. That's what self-responsibility is about.

Don't you think that a lot of people stay with "worseness"
behaviors just because they are not aware of alternatives that are
equally gratifying? The fact is that a wellness lifestyle fueled by a
strong sense of personal responsibility *can be more satisfying*
than any combination of the high-risk behaviors.

But if this is so, why hasn't self-responsibility caught on in a
big way? As you might have noticed if you are already following
a self-reliant path, you have to go out of your way, sometimes, to
pursue wellness. For example, to buy "health" foods we have to
go to small, expensive, usually out-of-the-way stores rather than
the neighborhood supermarket (where, by inference and
oftentimes fact, "unhealthy" foods are sold—at more attractive
prices); to breathe unpolluted air in planes and buses we have to
demand "nonsmokers' rights." In other words, in various ways
society reinforces worseness standards and behaviors, making
the wellness proponent go to special lengths to assert responsibility for his/her well-being.

Another reason we avoid consciously accepting, and actively pursuing, responsibility for health-enriching lifestyles is
that it can be burdensome to challenge assumptions which inhibit our health. Without credentials or experience in medicine
or the health sciences, we often feel intimidated by physicians
and other providers of care who, for whatever reason, discourage a sense of independence and personal accountability.
Advertisements assure us drugs are "doctor-tested"; who are we
to say they might not be good for us? If one Ph.D. biochemist
expert, who may be a consultant to the food industry, appears at
a school board meeting on removal of the junk food vending ma-

chines and states there is no proof that Twinkies are a health hazard, what parent will feel able to contest this assumption? Our knowledge about what is good for us is paved over with accepted practices and health "truths" which most of us unthinkingly value and act upon, and seldom challenge. There has probably been far more unhealth caused by our acceptance of false assumptions than by the unavailability or poor quality of medical care.

Yet, the biggest factor accounting for insufficient self-responsibility in our society is probably the lack of effective health education to date. It is not enough for doctors, health educators, and others to recognize the role of individual behavior in illness, disability, and premature death, or to repeat the obvious fact that medicine can do little to promote well-being. It is just as essential that health education be targeted specifically on discovering and promulgating ways to motivate us to accept responsibility for our own health, and not remain centered on negative messages that often cause us to "tune out" and avoid acceptance of our own accountability. Health education as a broad field of interest has been underfunded (receiving about ½ of 1 percent of the federal health budget), poorly researched, highly fragmented, and, too frequently, unimaginatively presented. Fortunately, the federal government is now giving much more attention to health education, and its high potential for fostering self-responsibility is thoroughly outlined in a major new report.[4]

Society may not change while you are reading this book, but you can decide to investigate the alternatives to dependency, overcome the social obstacles to a wellness lifestyle, and challenge the assumptions that reinforce ill-health. With a well-developed sense of self-responsibility, you can be free to live your life without crippling dependencies and life-threatening addictions to doctors, drugs, and disease-causing habits and neglects. While nobody can persuade you to accept such a goal if you are not ready for it, or convince you that reaching it is effort-

---

4. *Preventive Medicine USA*, a compilation of task force reports sponsored by the John E. Fogarty International Center for Advanced Study in the Health Sciences, NIH, and the American College of Preventive Medicine (New York: Prodist, 1976), p. 851.

less (for it is not, otherwise everybody would be living accordingly), you'll find the benefits of asserting your sovereignty and autonomy can be more than sufficient to reward the effort.

Self-Responsibility Principles

1. You are in charge of your own life.   Others have influence, can make things easier or more difficult, but in the end you must make your own choices and accept responsibility for what good or ill and health or disease occur in your life. When you emotionally and intellectually come to terms with this reality, then you are free of the need for scapegoats, villains, victims, or excuses. The linkage between your well-being and your lifestyle is much more obvious when all the ostensible variables are removed. When you view yourself as the cause of your health, your prospects for wellness are vastly increased.[5]

2. You are different from everybody else.   What keeps you from becoming ill is more or less what does the same for others, but your path to high level wellness within each wellness dimension must be unique, as you are unique. And you are extraordinary and special in every way; your nervous system, brain, body-build, personality, life history, likes and dislikes; everything about you is different. So are the alternatives that are available to you, including resources and role models. Thus, expect that your approach to nutritional awareness, stress management, physical fitness, and environmental sensitivity will also be different from anyone else's, though certain basic principles do apply in all dimensions for all human beings.

3. You are motivated by a desire for happiness.   Each of us pursues health and high level wellness not for their own sake, but in the context of our values and purposes. And, for most of us, these include seeking happiness, however differently we

---

5. Naturally, there are exceptions. Some people do lose their health through ill-fate, misfortune, "bad" genes, "acts-of-God," and so forth. There are no profits, satisfactions, or other gains to be had from "blaming-the-victim." But, since you can not guard against these unseen and unforeseeable catastrophes, don't worry about them. And don't let them ruin my principle!

perceive this hard-to-define state. We can learn to pursue high level wellness because it makes us feel good about our lives. We need less guilt and gloom; "our days are numbered even in the best of times," wrote historian Kenneth Clark. The present and future can be your own "best of times."

4. You need a sense of purpose.   To pursue high level wellness and to avoid the pitfalls of destructive lifestyles, it is essential to develop a means of self-expression that fits your unique talents and skills. An aim in life can help you obtain the kind of rewards needed for fulfillment and balance, and is crucial to your feeling "centered" and reasonably content with your life. Ben Franklin's adage about there being "nothing wrong with retirement—as long as it does not interfere with one's work," is often cited in this context. Hans Selye, author of *Stress Without Distress* (see the Wellness Resource Guide) believes that a goal or purpose in life is fundamental to positive health and well-being; most wellness advocates cited throughout this book place this principle at the top of their lists of components in a balanced lifestyle.

5. You are OK—and on your way to being even better.   The way you feel about yourself has a powerful effect on how you treat yourself. Smoking, heavy drinking, overeating, and other forms of self-abuse are highly correlated with low self-esteem. Thus, the way to change these habits is to learn what a prince or princess you are, fully worthy of love, respect, and acceptance. I know this can be difficult, especially when there are so many people who would have you believe otherwise. The consciousness-raising programs I'm going to describe and most others that I know about have as their basic mission the goal of encouraging self-acceptance. It is hard to be well when you are sick of yourself.

6. At times, you might prefer illness to health.   This may seem strange at first, but a lot of serious researchers and physicians believe that many people unconsciously choose to be ill. We do this because it seems to offer an escape from an unpleasant reality, because it brings forth desired attentions and special considerations from others, or because it helps to mask or excuse an inadequacy, or otherwise enables the "patient" to escape taking responsibility. In William Glasser's phrase from *Positive Addiction* (New York: Harper and Row, 1976, p. 5), people sometimes choose illness because it "hurts less this way."

7. Stop, examine, and choose.   Do you ever find yourself making decisions, taking actions, and experiencing feelings on the basis of outdated tapes? Remember, you draw from life what you seek; *you* get to select the payoffs. Do you want sympathy, attention, or both? Or, do you prefer payoffs such as joy, happiness, and the other elements of high level wellness? Unlike wallowing in worseness, choosing wellness requires a clear intention or consciousness that this is your preference, and a recognition of your responsibility to go for it. And, a part of choosing well is acceptance of others and yourself. There are times when this is difficult, or when confronting some pattern about yourself is painful and troubling. But the more you do accept yourself, the easier it will be to work with and enjoy others. So, open all the windows you can find, look out at other ideas, and make sure the beliefs you carry around are really yours. If they are yours, be sure they are the kind you want to bring along on your life trip.

8. Go for positive happiness, wellness style.   What is happiness but a state of well-being, a momentary sense of what Maslow termed "self-actualization"? You know very well what it is like to feel genuinely happy! It's such a positive kind of self-realization, even if it lasts only a moment. For most of us, this kind of happiness comes and goes; sometimes, the glow lasts a little longer than usual. Such feelings are highly valued in our culture, where so much human action is in pursuit of objectives we think will give us happiness (e.g., more money, greater power, fame, love). But there is another kind of happiness, a negative form, that some people derive (probably without realizing it) from high-risk behaviors. Though such "worseness" behaviors as smoking, drinking, and junk-food tripping have a demonstrated long-term negative impact on health, they often bring short-term emotional reactions that substitute for a positive form of happiness. But I believe that a personal, conscious decision to pursue wellness has the potential for bringing greater *positive* happiness than any of the transient, short-run, negative approaches. Wellness-oriented people practicing active self-responsibility seem to prefer positive to negative decisions in their pursuit of the highest kind of happiness. After all, why spend most of your time avoiding failure and ill health when you can be cultivating success and well-being? Looking at the quality of your own periods of happiness is another add-on to a wellness lifestyle.

9. Great decisions under distress seldom are.   Don't make decisions when under great duress or other high emotional charge, whether the feelings are positive or negative. And don't mix judgments and feelings; postpone decisions until your emotions subside. In the meantime, think about your lifestyle, and ask yourself some questions:

> • Is my behavior providing as much happiness as I could obtain from a wellness way of life? Do I feel good about the way I treat my body?
> • Have I consciously set up the patterns I follow, or did things just develop as they are?
> • Have my habits been influenced by others in ways I might not choose for myself—and if so, am I willing to do something about it?
> • Do my friends contribute to and reinforce a health enhancement way of living, or model and encourage a worseness lifestyle?
> • Are my exercise, diet, relaxation, and personal environment uniquely designed to fit me at this time in my life?
> • Do I think of myself as the sovereign authority who primarily determines how, what, where, why, and when things will happen for me?

Thinking about such questions will help you relax, will provide a diversion at a time when it is best not to make decisions, and will promote an important habit of wellness inventory-taking.

Further Perspectives
on Self-Responsibility

Right now you might be asking, why should I take on so much responsibility for myself? What are friends for? Are we not interdependent people, brothers and sisters needing each other for caring and everything else, including survival? Isn't self-responsibility as defined herein reminiscent of man-as-an-island thinking, which seems rather jejune in the late 1970s? Like almost anything else, self-responsibility can be overdone. I have tried to emphasize the importance of being connected with others, open to expressing your needs, able to respond with affection and caring to friends, and deeply aware of the value of being interdependent and part of a human network. All this is possible with and complementary to an active sense of self-responsibility for your own life. Only you, no one else, will directly experience the health consequences of the way you live, thus no one else should share your ballot when you decide in so many ways how your lifestyle franchise will be cast. Since those you love most dearly (e.g. children, mate, parents) will be indirectly affected by your choice, you have added incentive to expect the best from yourself.

People who practice high level wellness take responsibility for their own health in many ways, not all of which seem health-related in the usual sense of that word. Specifically, they always try to choose that one course of action which will provide the most happiness; others just muddling through life are more likely to spend their days deciding which decisions will bring the least displeasure. For example, a wellness-oriented jogger decides if he or she will derive more satisfaction from running on a given day or selecting some other exercise routine; someone else might think he or she *ought* to do one thing or another, and then feel guilty about the choice foregone. Positive selections are easier if you accept the idea of self-reliance and recognize that you make the decisions based upon your own best interests, not outside pressures or expectations from others that are not consistent with your own wellness philosophy.

You're in what could be called a trap of nonresponsibility if you believe you cannot change your diet, your destructive habits and patterns, your inability to engage in vigorous exercise for pleasure and fitness, your stress levels, or the environment in which you live. You created that trap by your own limiting definitions of your possibilities and potentials. Why not decide you want to change those worseness standards? Reown your power, take charge of your fate, and design a lifestyle that works for you. Incorporate something in each wellness dimension that underscores your own autonomy, and enjoy the rewards of being in charge of *you*. When you recognize the capability you have to be *the* responsible party in your life, you automatically then-and-there obtain control of your future lifestyle.

Part of self-responsibility is knowing how to use the medical system effectively, as well as learning to create a lifestyle that enables you to stay healthy and out of the medical system to the extent possible. I thought Tom Ferguson, editor of *Medical Self-Care*, expressed a lot of good sense on the subject of self-responsibility when he wrote his introductory comments for the first issue of the magazine:

> I never planned to edit a magazine. I'm a fourth-year medical student planning to become a family practitioner. But during my first year on the hospital wards, I was continually amazed by how little responsibility most patients took for their own health.
>
> About half the patients I saw that year had a preventable illness. Every time I saw a smoker with lung cancer or emphysema, a heavy drinker with liver disease, a fat, sedentary businessman with a heart attack, or a woman who'd only come to the doctor when her breast cancer was long past any chance of cure, I realized that medical care is not something to be left to doctors and other health workers.
>
> This magazine is dedicated to those patients, and to those of our readers who will profit by their example and avoid becoming patients at all.[6]

---

6. Ferguson, Tom. "Editor's Page," *Medical Self-Care* (Summer 1976), p. 2. For more information about this magazine, write to Box 31549, San Francisco CA 94131.

In addition to using the medical system effectively, when you really need to use it at all, asserting self-responsibility for your own well-being should include two other courses of action. One is to independently read a few books which reinforce and provide guidance on the ethic of self-responsibility: you can begin, if you wish, with a review of a few of the books I recommend on self-responsibility in the Wellness Resource Guide in the back of this book. The other course of action is to consider participating in one of the increasing number of "consciousness-raising" or human potential-enhancing programs offered throughout the country.

Programs Fostering Self-Responsibility

Common Ground, a quarterly directory of growth, healing, and other programs containing profiles of consciousness-raising classes and service offerings in the San Francisco Bay Area provided 178 separate listings in the Autumn 1976 issue,[7] and the list contained just a fraction of the varied programs offered to the public in this region! Now I realize that this may be atypical of the situation in most parts of the country, but wherever you live, some resource activities and programs which underscore and reinforce the ethic of self-responsibility are probably available.

Without endorsing specific programs or even implying that any of the following would do you any good at all, let me just highlight a few approaches that are not confined to the San Francisco Bay Area or even California. Informative, sardonic, and largely fun accounts of individual encounters with programs similar to those I'm about to note are provided in books by Adam Smith and Jerry Rubin.[8] In addition, a few popular books on dif-

7. Available from New Dimensions/Common Ground, 461 Douglass Street, San Francisco CA 94114. One dollar (at the time of my writing) gets you on the mailing list.

8. *Powers Of Mind* (New York: Random House, 1975) and *Growing Up At 37* (New York: M. Evans and Co., Inc., 1976).

ferent aspects of EST and Transactional Analysis deserve read-ing.[9]

For our purposes, it is not necessary or useful to get into the debate as to whether these various programs represent what Theodore Roszak terms "the biggest introspective binge any so-ciety in history has undergone", or what Peter Marin deplores as "the new narcissism" that supports the "deification of the isolated self."[10] For some, these programs have worked in the sense of enhancing their abilities to cope with, accept responsi-bility for, and take charge of what happens in their lives. For others, most perhaps, although I do not know the success and "failure" rates, the promised returns do not pan out. As in everything else, you have to make judgments based upon your experiences and knowledge, and how well you are in touch with your own needs.

EST, or Erhard Seminars Training—Founded by Werner Erhard, EST has nearly 160 staff members and over 5,000 volunteers in cities throughout the U.S. It is difficult to describe what it is you "get" (a key word in the training), but the objec-tives are no less than to transform your life and help you to learn the rewards of being the sole author of your well-being. Each EST trainee has an opportunity to experience the positive feel-ings that come from becoming responsible for his own subjective emotions, ideas, and approaches. ("EST is experienced better than it is explained," say its followers.) EST teaches that reality does not often conform to our assumptions and to the artificial meanings imposed over the years by outside sources (e.g., doc-tors and parents). The program offers a composite of many tech-niques and modalities from the consciousness movement, and

---

9.   See Adelaide Bry, *EST* (New York: Avon, 1976) and William Greene, *EST: Four Days To Make Your Life Work* (New York: Pocket Books, 1976). Also, see the following on varied applications of Transactional Analysis: Eric Berne, *Games People Play* (New York: Grove, 1964), Thomas Gordon, *Parent Effectiveness Training* (New York: Peter Wyden, 1970), Thomas Harris, *I'm OK–You're OK* (New York: Harper and Row, 1969), Jut Meininger, *Success through Transactional Analysis* (New York: Signet, 1974).

10.   Quoted in "Getting Your Head Together," *Newsweek* (6 September 1976), p. 57.

centers on breaking down philosophical assumptions and beliefs we have about reality and our place in the world. EST sessions are difficult for many people: the training imposes restrictions, induces exhaustion, fosters mental strain, and mounts attacks on the ego to prepare trainees philosophically for the principles EST teaches in the area of self-responsibility. Some consider it a fast brain food chain. As of 1977, the cost of the program was $300. For more information about EST check the classified telephone directory in the largest city near you, or write to EST headquarters at 1750 Union Street, San Francisco CA 94108.

Psychosynthesis—Developed by Roberto Assagioli, this approach focuses on subpersonalities and the "true self." Subpersonalities are various roles we have been conditioned to assume (parent, patient, producer); the true self is our genuine "center of awareness." Psychosynthesis says that when one or more subpersonalities become dominant, our true self is thrown off balance and we therefore function less well in relation to our capacities. Like EST trainers, psychosynthesis practitioners utilize a wide variety of techniques and forms of therapy, including music, stress management, guided daydreams, self-analysis, and many others. The true self is considered to be interdependent, autonomous, and prepared for personal governance in adapting to the demands of modern living. If you would like to learn more about psychosynthesis, write to the Psychosynthesis Research Foundation, Room 314, 527 Lexington Avenue, New York NY 10017.

Polarity Balancing—Devised over 40 years ago by Randolph Stone, a doctor of osteopathy/chiropractic/naturopathy, this modality centers on the study of how energy works in the human body. It deals with balancing these life energies; the idea is that disease and illness occur when energy currents and fields are interrupted. Polarity therapy is directed at mind/body exercises which help the client relax and regain (or maintain) normal body energies. Adherents of this approach offer an extensive explanatory theory, varied manipulations, and numerous techniques for fostering awareness. Emphasis is upon both diet and yoga as ways of cleansing and invigorating the body and its energy processes. For more on polarity, write to Polarity Institute at 401 North Glassell Street, Orange CA 92666.

Bioenergetics—Started by Alexander Lowen (a student of Wilhelm Reich, who birthed a similar method that bears his name), bioenergetics also combines many methods from psychoanalytic practice to "unlock energy flows." The idea underlying bioenergetics is that the human body is a system of energy which must flow without impedance or blockage if the individual is to enjoy a healthy existence. Bioenergetics asserts that when we do not realize our potentials, accept full responsibility for our lives, and function in a manner conducive to effective coping, it is because we have locked certain tensions and emotions in our bodies; that is, we have energy blocks. The release of these contained energies is the objective of bioenergetics. The techniques employed include vigorous body movements, sound and breathing patterns, mild stress postures, and assorted exercises which emphasize "expressive mobility." If you would like to learn more about bioenergetics, write to Alexander Lowen, M.D., Director, Institute of Bioenergetic Analysis, 144 East 36th Street, New York NY 10016.

ARICA—Founded by Oscar Ichazo, ARICA also is related to the idea of ego formation and social conditioning as the bases of human "blocks" preventing us from fully experiencing the universe, and ourselves and others. As multidisciplinary as EST, psychosynthesis, and bioenergetics, ARICA also incorporates techniques from Eastern cultures. ARICA's programs are 40-day intensives, with periodic workshops designed to facilitate clients to achieve and maintain the "divine life" or "satori" (Buddhist term)—a lifelong sense of inner harmony and peace. Exercises include dance, music, chanting, and meditating while surrounded by visual displays or wall symbols called "yantras." If you would like to learn more about ARICA, write to the headquarters office at 24 West 57th Street, New York NY 10019.

Silva Mind Control—Developed by José Silva, this approach to self-awareness and personal growth emphasizes mental relaxation as a way to overcome health-destroying stroke deprivation behaviors and personal programs aggravated by "negative thoughts." The techniques employed in a series of four 12-hour classes include meditation, self-hypnosis and auto-suggestion, and guided fantasy. Clients "visualize" solutions to their difficulties and learn to cultivate skills of "sensory perception" in order to know the essence of things. If you would like to learn more about Silva Mind Control, write to the national center at P.O. Box 1149, 1110 Cedar Avenue, Laredo TX 78040.

Transactional Analysis—Primarily set forth by Eric Berne, TA is a theory of human interaction designed to assist people to analyze their current behavior in relationship to learning which took place during child and parent-dominated periods of life. In TA terms, everyone has three sets of "ego states": parent, adult, and child, each with its own ways of thinking, feeling, and acting. Although each set is capable of growth and change, in many of us grown-ups the parent and child are not much different from what they were when we were small. Our parent states may lead us to express critical, judgmental remarks towards others (as our own parents perhaps did towards us); our child states may motivate us to feel or behave as we did when we were very young, sometimes inappropriately; and our adult states may be misinformed, and lead us into self-defeating decisions. According to TA, the more we learn to adapt our child and parent states to the present, with a well-informed adult usually in control, the sooner we may learn to live in harmony with ourselves and with each other. Terms such as life "scripts," "strokes," and "games" (manipulative strategies) have been popularized by TA. TA is expressly organized to foster self-awareness, genuineness, and an active sense of self-responsibility. The focus is on the present and on ways to obtain knowledge of why we react as we do and ways to change based upon understanding of the dynamics of our "transactions" with others. Paul McCormick, editor of Transactional Analysis Press, kindly helped me with this brief summary. If you would like to learn more about TA, write to the International Transactional Association, 1772 Vallejo Street, San Francisco CA 94108.

My own view of programs like the above is strongly favorable. I personally have many friends who claim that EST,

ARICA, or Transactional Analysis have helped them take control of their lifestyle patterns and affirmed their right to happiness. One program or another has also provided individuals known to me with the tools and concepts they felt they needed in order to be more effective at what they chose to do with their lives. Two of my friends, Michael Griffin and Gay Larned, have recently become EST graduates, and both are among the most self-aware, confident, and fully human individuals I have the good fortune to know. They credit the EST program with facilitating a lot of the growth and knowledge that has contributed to the process or state that they seem to enjoy so much today. I have a friend in Aspen, Colorado who serves as an elected county commissioner in that lovely part of the country who speaks of EST in glowing terms; in part because of the impact of the training upon his career. Michael Kinsley told me his first reaction at the end of the training was pretty neutral, sort of a "Well, that was interesting in an academic kind of way." That is, Michael had "observed rather than experienced the process." Gradually, however, the effect of the training was to "erode many barriers and irresponsible patterns in my life which had been barriers deadening my experience of living." Michael said he experienced a transformation of his ability to speak before groups because of an increased level of self-confidence and capacity for work. Knowing what he does today, Michael said he would borrow money if necessary in order to take the training. For Commissioner Michael Kinsley, EST apparently meant a lot.

Testimonials of this nature are just as readily available from individuals positively affected by other programs. For example, a young health-planner friend named Jeanne Allen told me that her work with the ARICA program brought her "closer to the realization of my own simplicity and beauty. I have become more sensitive to the needs of my body, and more willing, on a continuing basis, to respond to those things which my body seems to need; regular exercise, healthful foods, massage, love. Experiencing the integration of my body, mind, and spirit through ARICA work is making my attitude toward self-change more positive. I work better, I live life better."

Personally, I have not taken any of these programs except TA, and that was a long time ago. I am not attracted by the regimented training program by which the EST folks help students to "get it," and I'm a bit turned off by the mumbo jumbo (my bias) of ARICA and Silva Mind Control. I do not care for the "cult of the personality" aspects surrounding the leaders of each of these three programs, and most of the others. So, I have not enrolled. But I am in favor of all self-responsibility programs in the sense that I am glad they exist, and I know they do a number of folks a lot of good. If you are interested, I hope you will investigate the program of your choice.

There are, of course, many other programs which I could have included in my illustrative listing. I struggled with a few regarding whether to include or omit them, and decided to require a yes answer to two questions: do I know enough about the program to sketch the content and purposes, and does the program seem reasonable? Answering the last question took days of my time, and I still have not completely resolved the ethical issues involved. If I think programs involving rebirth and attendant physical immortality, harnessing tidal energies, orgone boxes, prosperity-consciousness raising, psychomotor therapies, marathon growth sessions, primal organic processes, and other seemingly "far-out" endeavors are either hokum, freaky, untested, or all of the above, should I exclude them? Or should I make the considerable effort to experience everything or more nearly everything that is out there, wherever it is? I decided against the latter; among other reasons because such an undertaking might have taken at least 10 years to complete! In addition, I might have had to write a few exposes, and that was not the kind of mood I wanted to adopt. Furthermore, I might have made some serious errors of judgment based upon my own limited consciousness.

I suppose one could develop a consumer guide for assessing the new modalities. Such a guide would contain information on how to compare them or at least feel some confidence that a given program, technique, or approach is worthy of your investment in time, money, and/or lost opportunities to try other things. Here are some of the questions I would like to see answered in such a guide and some points I would like to see made. (You might find them helpful as you investigate on your own.)

• Are the promises understandable and realistic? Be suspicious of mystification and/or extravagant claims. The most respected wellness resource people understate potential benefits, communicate clearly, and carefully avoid raising hopes that may prove unattainable.

• Is the emphasis on the technique, program, or other outside factors, or upon you? If it's not on you, it sounds like a gimmick. The best approaches are those wherein you are a full partner since *the* key to success in wellness is your motivation.

• Who are the people behind the program? What is their track record? Are their fees reasonable? What did they do before inventing the current method? The consciousness of the leaders is as important as any technique.

• Who has benefited by this approach? Have you talked with unbiased individuals aware of the modality, under pressure-free circumstances? What can experienced participants say about both the positive and negative aspects of the program? An above-board wellness practitioner will welcome and respect your interest in talking to his or her clients.

• The more objective and dispassionate participants are, the more credence you can place in their assessments, and the more confidence you, in turn, can invest in the approach.

• If you do enlist in a program designed to foster self-responsibility, be especially attentive to whether it is actually doing you any good (or any harm). Do you feel better? Are you more effective at what you do in your life work? Have others made any observations to this effect?

• Watch out for the guru who offers his approach as the single answer to high level wellness. There is no single modality that can offer total well-being, as you well know. We must all design individual programs that are comfortable for each of us, and we need to incorporate some activity in each of the five wellness dimensions. Guard against the "swallow it whole" syndrome—take what applies to your situation from any program, and leave the rest for later. Or for someone else!

So, dear reader, if I have not described your favorite program, it is probably because I do not know much about it. It is too early in the wellness era to be writing off new initiatives, particularly since (unlike surgery) few of them are likely to cause (holistic) iatrogenesis. Those who enjoy unmentioned modalities and attribute to them benefits such as being "born again" physically or spiritually, or both, are entitled to their rewards. I'm happy for them, I wish them well, and I may someday join them, particularly if I could be guaranteed the kind of humane, caring, and loving reentry being developed by Dr. LeBoyer and his growing ranks of supporters.[11] But for the present, I will keep my peace and retain skepticism toward the unknown, and recommend that you consider a similar cautious openness until you feel comfortable with the facts. Good luck, and remember, the search itself can be a lot of fun.

It seems only fitting to conclude this section on the dimension of self-responsibility with a quote from one of my own favorite gurus or wellness spokespersons, Harry Browne of *How I Found Freedom in an Unfree World* fame.

> You are the sovereign ruler who has chosen which city to live in, which job to take, which people to associate with, which rules to live by. Others may have made requests—even demands—but it was you who made the ultimate choices regarding your action.
>
> But what is most important, it is also you who will make the choices in the future. Whatever you did in the past, you did for the best reasons you knew at the time. But today, you have more alternatives to choose from. And tomorrow, you'll have even more. There's no reason why you have to repeat your choices of the past—unless they proved to be best for you.[12]

---

11. For more information on the LeBoyer method of childbirth, write to the Holistic Childbirth Institute, 1627 10th Avenue, San Francisco CA 94122.

12. New York: Avon, 1973, p. 166.

Nutritional
Awareness

You probably know that the major diet-related health hazard in our country is the combination of overconsumption and undernutrition, and a long list of ills is associated with this deadly duo. A U.S. Senate Select Committee, in fact, recently concluded years of testimony, studies, and investigations on the state of our national eating habits. Its conclusions sum up the nutritional situation as well as any book or other report on the subject:

> We have reached the point where nutrition, or the lack or the excess or the quality of it, may be the nation's number-one public health problem. The threat is not beri-beri, pellagra, or scurvy. Rather we face the more subtle, but also more deadly, reality of millions of Americans loading their stomachs with food which is likely to make them obese, to give them high blood pressure, to induce heart disease, diabetes, and cancer—in short, to kill them over the long term.[1]

The Senate Report identified 5 of the 10 leading causes of death as being diet-related. These 5 are diseases of the heart, cerebrovascular diseases, diabetes mellitus, arteriosclerosis, and cirrhosis of the liver.[2] A chart from the same source depicts the

---

1. U.S. Senate (Select Committee on Nutrition and Human Needs), *Nutrition and Health: An Evaluation of Nutritional Surveillance in the United States* Washington, D.C.: Government Printing Office, 1975), p. 5.

2. Ibid.

imbalances between an optimal balanced diet and the current U.S. rate of fat, protein, and carbohydrate consumption.

No other dimension of wellness has received as much atten-

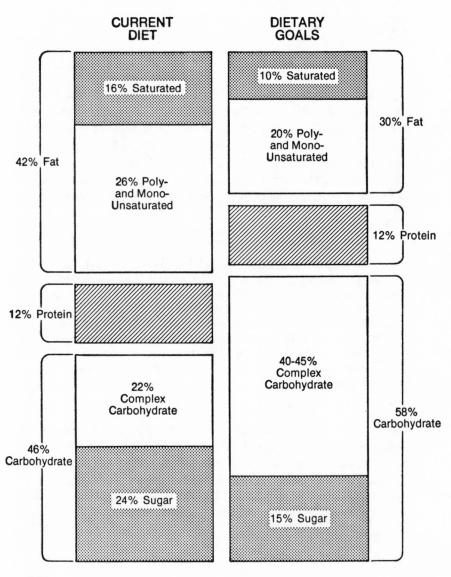

tion as nutrition. Books on the subject could fill the largest libraries; the best-seller lists usually include at least one title on diet, a wonder food, or a nutritionally oriented way to better health. Yet, wise food selection and sensible diet patterns are more the exception than the popular way. Why? Well, eating properly is usually more trouble, often costs more, almost always requires a bit more than average nutritional awareness, and commonly takes more time. In addition, the "best" foods are too frequently either unavailable or inconvenient to obtain. Like everyone else, you undoubtedly find temptations to please the senses and overlook the cells constantly before you. And like me, you are probably considered a "health nut" if you avoid food additives, refined white sugar and flour, and the unhealthy foods which our friends seem to enjoy so much. What price must you pay to eat in accordance with a wellness lifestyle? Is the special effort really worthwhile?

I hope to convince you that it is.

Nutritional Awareness Principles

1. Go out of your way for natural, "live" foods. Natural foods are usually harder to obtain than "convenience" or "fast" foods, but it is well worth your trouble to make the extra effort. A number of especially beneficial foods do more than their fair share to help your body work well. Some which are highly recommended include:

(a) *soybeans*. Soybean sprouts, which can be grown in your kitchen, have an enzyme called *invertase*, which can help convert an otherwise impoverished diet into carbohydrates directly assimilable into usable energy.

(b) *fresh fruits and raw vegetables*. Whole fruits and vegetables are better than the juices, which lose something in the heating processes for canning and bottling. They are best of all when taken from your own pesticide-free garden.

(c) *yogurt*. Easy to make and delicious to eat plain or sweetened with honey and/or fresh fruits, yogurt facilitates digestion and increases resistance to infections.

(d) *garlic*. An antiseptic that decreases the amount of harmful bacteria in the stomach and reduces blood pressure for those having hypertension, garlic is also delicious (and leaves little mouth odor if mixed with or followed by fresh parsley).

(e) *honey*. The "nectar of the gods," honey preserves vitamins and contains valuable minerals (copper, iron, calcium, sodium, titanium, and potassium). It also contains all 10 essential amino acids, and is a mild laxative, a gentle sedative, and a natural alternative to sugar as a sweetening agent.

(f) *apple cider vinegar*. Dr. Jarvis's favorite tonic, apple cider vinegar is both a healing agent and an antiseptic, though I do admit it tastes terrible.

(g) *nutritional yeast*. Containing all the B vitamins in natural form, some varieties of brewer's yeast are also over 50 percent protein.

(h) *wheat germ*. Usually removed from packaged goods in order to preserve shelf life of the product, wheat germ has an abundance of vitamin E, B vitamins, and important trace minerals.

(i) *watermelon*. Familiar to nearly everybody, watermelon is an excellent diuretic for eliminating toxins.

(j) *sunflower seeds*. Loaded with vitamins, minerals, and trace elements, sunflower seeds are rich in fiber and are an excellent source for polyunsaturated oil high in linoleic acid. They are easy to digest, and taste wonderful alone or in salads.

(k) *bran*. Last, but anything but least, bran has increasingly been recognized as the single most valuable ingredient in promoting a healthy digestive tract.[3]

2. *Vary your diet.* Choose different types of foods throughout the week (milk and dairy products, meats, fish, leafy vegetables, seeds, root vegetables, and fruits), but do examine the arguments pro and con on the controversial subject of food combinations. Study nutrition; it is a fascinating subject and awareness is vital to your health. Every time you learn something new, you will be pleased and reinforced in the process of becoming your own most trusted expert on what is and what is not "good" for you.

---

3. For a full discussion of the benefits of living foods, including most on the list given here, see Ivan Papov, *Stay Young: A Doctor's Healthful Program for Youthful Health and Vigor* (New York: Grosset and Dunlap, 1975).

3. Avoid dangerous foods and food additives.   The prevalence of known and suspected carcinogenic elements entering our food supply as artificial colors, additives, preservatives, stabilizers, and other processed chemicals, is well established. (An NBC television documentary in the summer of 1976 entitled "What Is This Thing Called Food?" provided a summary of the extent of this pollution, noting that 5,500 different chemicals go into the U.S. food chain.) Nitrates, a leading factor in cancer of the colon, are found in most bacon, sausage, luncheon meats, and frankfurters; and petroleum derivates such as BHA, BHT, and artificial flavors and colors are standard ingredients in so many of our foods. In addition to the hazards of altering meats, fruits, and vegetables through chemical restructuring, the dangers of chemical interactions are a matter of increasing concern. Neither our government nor the manufacturers have established the safety of these contaminants, so why take chances? Don't buy these counterfeit products; they cannot do you any good, and they are good bets to cause a lot of grief.

4. Boycott refined, processed foods.   Examples are packaged cereals, candies, commercial ice creams, colas, etc. They consist mostly of empty calories devoid of nutritional value, including vitamins, amino acids, and minerals. You have relatively little control over climatic conditions, growing and harvesting methods, packaging and distributing practices, and processing conditions that affect the nutrient values in our foods, but you do not have to buy that which you know is deficient in vitamins or other needed food elements. And you know that refined, processed foods are relatively empty products compared with untampered-with, "unmanufactured" fruits, vegetables, certain meats, fowl, dairy products, seeds and grains, and so forth. In fact, thanks to various kinds of processings as much as 80 percent of the food value in the 3,500 calories the average American eats each day is lost. So please, don't let the processors fool you with Orwellian word-games like "enriched," applied to milled grain products because thiamine, riboflavin, niacin, and iron have been put back into the product. These foods are as "enriched" as you are when you receive a tax refund for $100 after you paid many thousands during the year. You cannot keep your tax

117

money, but you do not have to accept breads and other foods, the essential nutrients of which have mostly been taxed away by the processors.

5. Learn to dislike the refined carbohydrates.   Think of it this way: sugar provides calories—period. It is absorbed directly into the bloodstream, requiring an immediate insulin treatment from the pancreas, which upsets the endocrine balance within the body. Refined sugar is highly concentrated; it lacks other food factors or proteins needed for the metabolic process to function properly. The body therefore must draw on its own reserves to metabolize the sugar, which causes a loss of vitamin B_1, B_2, B_6, niacin, magnesium, cobalt, and other properties. A buildup of lactic and pyruvic acid can occur if the sugar is not completely metabolized, and this leads to tissue degeneration.

The empty calories are worse than no food at all, for they take the place of other calories which could provide nutritional fuels for hungry cells. And, refined sugar has no fiber, which means it does nothing for digestion and a lot for tooth and gum disease. While the average citizen may consume 120 pounds of the stuff annually, you do not have to! The refining story on white flours is similar. The valuable germ and the outer bran coat of wheat are discarded in the milling process, with the consequent loss of vital nutrients and the "gain" of empty starches. Both these refining processes are significant susceptibility factors in the formation of degenerative diseases. In this context, you can recognize that soda pop, pastries, synthetic ice creams, potato chips, white-flour spaghetti, white bread, etc., probably do not taste as good as you thought they did, especially when such tempting and nutritious alternatives are available (honey/molasses, fresh fruits, whole-grain breads, seeds, and all the rest).

6. Keep it simple and take your time.   It is not necessary to give up supermarkets, grow everything yourself, and otherwise act like an ascetic to eat well, nor do you have to transform your food habits overnight. On the contrary, it is best if you can make the basic changes over time as you gradually feel more strongly about the importance of sound diet for better health. Realistic goals help your evolution toward wellness remain a pleasant activity rather than a grind.

7. Eliminate coffee, tea, alcohol, and other addictive drugs.
For many, this seems easier to prescribe than to practice, which of course it is. But, over time, the effort to reduce and eventually eliminate harmful addictions in your life is well worth the discomforts involved. Not much needs to be said about the destructive aspects of alcoholic drinks (including wine) or other hard drugs of one kind or another, but many people are surprised to learn of the hazards of coffee and tea (and cola and chocolate drinks). All contain caffeine, which stimulates the sympathetic nervous system, induces acid secretion in the stomach, leads to heartburn, bleeding ulcers, and related disorders, and generally causes nervousness if consumed in sufficient quantities. How strange that we drink the stuff at all. It really does not taste good (why else do so many put cream and/or sugar in coffee and tea but to make the caffeine palatable?). And it can keep you from sleeping, make you nervous, rob your body of thiamine, and scald your throat. There's probably only one good explanation why so many of us are in the habit of drinking coffee, despite the incredible cost rises: it is a drug to which we can and have become habituated! A high correlation has been found between coffee consumption and illness in general, and the same correlation holds as well for tea; both utilize stored body sugars from the liver at an excessive rate, alternately raising and then lowering blood sugar levels. It's better to learn to enjoy juices, herbal teas, and other substitutes which nourish rather than draw from your body.

8. Concentrate on quality in proteins. When protein foods contain all eight essential amino acids, they are referred to as first class proteins. Such proteins come in both animal and vegetable products; however, foods containing the essential acids in relative amounts most preferred by the body (i.e. complete proteins) are meats, dairy products, and seafood. If you use both animal and vegetable sources of protein, vary your sources for best effect. Keep in mind that if you want to eat more economically and more ecologically, you don't have to eat foods with complete protein in them, you can, instead, mix whole grains, legumes, and other inexpensive foods in combinations to obtain what Frances Moore Lappé calls protein complementarity (see the review of her book in the Wellness Resource Guide). Your need for protein varies with many factors, including your overall state of health, stress level, diet, and your liver's capacity for synthesizing the proteins, among other variables. Who really knows whether you need 20, 56, 80 or some other minimal number of grams of protein each day? Does the Food and Drug Administration really have the answer with the recommended daily allowances (RDAs)? Many think not. There is a constant debate on this quantity issue; as in nearly everything else, you are the one who must assess how much protein you need given your unique lifestyle and energy demands.

9. Enjoy fresh fruit and uncooked vegetables every day, if you can.   The fresher your food, the more enzymes and nutrients are in it. Naturally, the more organic and less cooked your fruits and vegetables, the better.

10. Try to get high-fiber roughage every day.   The low-fiber diet of high starches, fats, oils, sugars, refined flours, and other extensively purified carbohydrates converts into fecal matter which remains in the lining of your colon for three or four days. This use of the colon as a stagnant holding tank can lead to nausea, heartburn, excessive gas, bloating and distention, abdominal pain, rectal irritation, and constipation. Worse, it eventually can produce one or more of the degenerative diseases, particularly coronary heart disease, cancer of the colon or rectum, appendicitis, hemorrhoids, diverticulosis, varicose veins, phlebitis, and obesity.[4] So if you needed another reason to shun the porno "foods" (commercial ice creams, white flours stripped of dietary fiber, sugar-strewn breakfast cereals, hamburgers, hot dogs, refined pastries and desserts, etc.), you have it. The best ways to ensure that you get the 24 or so roughage

---

4. For a thorough review of the evidence supporting this statement, see David Reuben, *The Save Your Life Diet* (New York: Ballantine, 1975), pp. 155–172. This book is reviewed in the Wellness Resource Guide.

grams recommended daily are to take a teaspoon or two of bran each day, use whole grain products, enjoy fresh fruits and raw vegetables, and avoid junk food.

11. Don't overlook Grandmom's homilies—they still make good sense.   Sometimes age-old wisdoms seem old-fashioned and irrelevant to the very different culture of the space-conquering, supertechnological, sophisticated society of today. It may seem that way to some, but don't you believe it. Grandmom was right, and the basics still hold. You need, for example, to chew your food slowly and thoroughly (this gives fiber time to absorb liquid), to eat only when you are hungry, to drink lots of water, and to learn to use nature's herbs for natural vitamins and as alternatives to chemical medicines and synthetic pills. It helps to eliminate booze, get a good night's sleep, exercise regularly, and avoid worrying too much. You and I knew all these things, and so did Grandmom. But sometimes I forget, and I thought you might welcome a reminder, also.

12. Take just a moment for reflection with your food.   This needn't be religious or God-oriented reflection; it can simply be a thoughtful mood in which you link the act of eating to your sense of life's meaning and purpose. You might try eating alone by choice occasionally. When you do, find a place that feels good and comforts you, take one course at a time, and be unhurried while you enjoy the process of dining with yourself. Much of what we think of as hunger is a desire for attention, sensual pleasure, relief from anxiety, and gratification. Explore the tie between your food feelings and inner harmony. Pay special attention to how each morsel tastes, and how it feels when you swallow. You may find that this approach helps you avoid eating foods that do little for your health, gaining weight from overeating, or leaving the table tense and unsatisfied.[5] After a while, eating will become a more integrated part of your life, and less a means of entertainment.

---

5.   See Don Gerrard, *One Bowl: A Simple Concept for Controlling Body Weight* (New York: Bookworks/Random House, 1974).

13. Find a mate or friend with whom to share nutritional adventures and discoveries. Make time for the joy of cooking, and the satisfactions of good eating. If you already have a mate or friend as interested in nutritional awareness as you are, wonderful. If you live with a porno-food junkie, convert him or leave him (you can love him too, but get him out of the house). Eating well is seldom accidental; you have to work at it, learn new things, experiment, avoid certain foods, and cultivate others. It is hard enough without having to deal with and be distracted by a low level worseness diner.

14. Keep the joy of eating a pleasure, and never an obsession. You do not have to count calories, monitor scales, measure portions, or undergo the folderol of weight-watching grinds to be healthy and fit. Just eat sensibly, as noted above, and get plenty of exercise, rest, and enjoyment in your life. Be suspicious of quick-weight-loss schemes (results are always temporary), and avoid any diet plan that destroys your enjoyment of food. Do little things that help to make good food as pleasurable as the less nutritious alternative. For example, if you are serving fresh apple-strawberry juice instead of cabernet sauvignon, use your most delicate, exquisite wine glasses as containers for the juice. Psychologically, it makes the transition easier, and can make the juice seem all the more flavorful and worth savoring. There is probably someone in the crowd who can give a "rating" to the juice, commenting in the manner of the savant on its body, character, clarity, aroma, and so forth. (And he or she will be so much easier to take than most wine experts.)

15. Start every day with a full and nutritious breakfast. While you are at it, enjoy a satisfying lunch and dinner, also. Skipping meals (except when fasting or systematically undereating) often leads to food distractions throughout the day. Don't leave the table stuffed, but don't go away hungry, either. As for breakfast, be aware that little or no breakfast can cause dangerously low blood sugar levels, interfering with concentration and stimulating you to a junk-food splurge as hunger pangs increase.

Personalize Your Approach to Nutrition

Attention to the dimension of nutritional awareness is a form of insurance against disease and debilitation. It will lower your risk of becoming ill at any age, and seems especially important when you reach the middle years and beyond. When you nourish the environment of your body's cells, you better your chances to feel, think, and be well.

But how do you evaluate and synthesize the mind-boggling tonnage of books and articles which offer such thoroughly documented, *conflicting* advice? When the manufacturers turn out a roomful of Ph. D.'s to protest that sugar-coated Zonkers are good for your children,[6] how is a houseperson to defend his or her own wisdom which advises otherwise? And what can be done to prevent total frustration when a world authority writes a book to dispel all confusion and leaves you more baffled than ever?

As always, you must develop the confidence to decide for yourself after hearing the varied claims, asking questions, and doing what you must to learn enough to make your choice. The challenge of developing a nutritional ideology suited to your unique needs and life conditions can be a fun pursuit. It may take a while, but think of this aspect of wellness as a continuing educational process. It should be interesting and satisfying to develop individual diet pathways as your understanding increases year after year. You will be amazed to discover, someday, that you are an "expert" yourself, and then you will be even less threatened or upset by the conflicting opinions of other experts.

My own approach to nutrition, which, of course, would not work for you since you are different from me, nonetheless may be of some interest. Since I have emphasized that there is so much more to the process of nourishing oneself than just eating, I'll start with some basics. To begin, I dine when I am hungry, I almost always enjoy what I eat, and I try to avoid eating while

---

6. See, for example, Max Huberman, "Freddy Still Running (A Confession from Dr. Frederick Stare)," *Let's Live* (November 1976), pp. 22–23. Max Huberman is the president of the National Nutritional Foods Association.

exercising, rushing for a plane, or grappling with a difficult problem. I scrupulously try to avoid refined and processed foods with preservatives or artificial colors, I no longer even like sugar-rich "treats," and I have little use for alcoholic drinks. But I do love certain rich foods (made with honey, not sugar), and I do consume a substantial number of calories, which would be excessive were I not such an exercise nut and therefore able to assimilate and otherwise speed the goods through my system.

For breakfast, I have fresh fruits, two cups of herbal tea, bran muffins, occasionally eggs and whole wheat toast, an eight-ounce container of homemade yogurt, and a large bowl of granola. (Naturally, the muffins, granola, yogurt and everything else I buy or make contain honey or molasses, not white or brown sugar.) After vigorous exercise during the noon hours, I am ready for lunch, usually another container of yogurt, two glasses of papaya juice, about four ounces of unsalted sunflower kernels or some other nuts, seeds, or grains. Sometimes I'll add a few slices of chicken or other white meat, though I am cautious about animal proteins. For dinner, I almost always have a large salad flavored with shrimp or crab, mushrooms, onions, tomatoes, bean sprouts, and avocadoes. I also have a glass or two of certified raw milk, and some vegetable side dishes, such as artichokes, corn-on-the-cob, yellow squash, or whatever else is in season or looks good when I pass the vegetable stand. A fresh fruit is usually my dessert, along with a cup of herbal tea. Oftentimes, I vary this salad routine with seafood; I enjoy eating just about anything that lurks in lakes and oceans. (There are exceptions, I'm sure, but none come to mind.) I retire a few hours later satisfied, but not full.

I take supplements, although I vary my intake at different times. Usually, I take 1,200 milligrams of vitamin C, 400 International Units of vitamin E (natural), and multipurpose grain concentrates daily; sometimes I take vitamin B complex and bone meal tablets. In addition to these supplements, I often add a teaspoon of bran to my granola.

I realize that I have a long way to go before my diet constitutes a fully balanced, moderate level of nutritious sustenance. But I am happy with the way I eat at this time, I get pleasure from every meal, and I am pleased that, however imperfect, my current diet is so dramatically healthier for me than the way I used to eat! So don't you worry if some expert gets nauseous when he hears of your diet; find what you like, enjoy it, and be open to change as you evolve and your understanding grows. I fluctuate between 175 and 180 pounds, which is okay for me and comfortable for my "skinny mesomorphic" 6 ft. 3 in. frame.

I do not expect any of you to follow my diet. It took me years of experimenting to find what I like, and I am sure I'll be enjoying a somewhat different diet regimen next year. For example, I would like to obtain much more of my food from soils treated only with natural fertilizers and will be making a special effort to get more raw, uncooked meals than I seem to obtain today. But the basics will not change; I will still avoid refined sugars and flours, processed or chemicalized anything, and continue to eat lots of fruits and vegetables. I hope you will consciously work into your own unique diet that regimen which best nourishes and pleases you.

In the Wellness Resource Guide at the end of this book, I list a few publications which I found helpful in my own quest for better nutritional understanding. Maybe some of them will be of interest to you. In reading about nutrition, in becoming more aware by attending lectures, listening to radio and TV programs that address the subject, and in talking with friends and counselors about this basic but potentially complex area, be particularly attentive to the following issues, with which I am still struggling, or perhaps evolving.

One such issue is whether to eat animal products. The predominant perspective in the recommended readings is to avoid meat, or at least to drastically limit the intake of red meat products with high fat content. The case against red meat rests on the ecological inefficiencies of livestock maintenance, the nutritional quality of meats as compared with vegetable protein sources, the costs of meat versus the alternatives available, the toxins in meats due to commercial livestock practices, and the digestive and assimilative complications associated with meat consumption. It might take a while before you work this one out;

at the present time I am a "fallen-away" carnivore. That is, I was raised and trained to consume vast quantities of meats of all kinds; some suspected I had a special calling in this area. But, alas, over the years I drifted away from the faith and now go back to animal flesh only when it is inconvenient to do otherwise. I'm not a hard-core vegetarian, I enjoy white meats about once a week. But, for the most part, I find my body feels better when I avoid meat, so I avoid it, usually. I favor the approach recommended in the "Prevention System,"[7] namely, a diet that includes certain meats sometimes, but not the smoked or processed variety. This means avoidance of delicatessen and fried meats, and inclusion of organ meats (particularly liver). Such a diet obviously is not vegetarian—among other reasons why I continue to eat some meat is that it is simply too difficult to get enough nutrients (e.g., iron) from a strict vegetarian diet. As you can tell, I'm really on the fence on this one, balanced in a manner to please neither cattlemen nor my "new age" flower child friends who equate meat-eating with cannibalism.

Another controversy surrounds the problem of weight control. What *is* the best weight-loss diet? I surely do not know, but I am interested to learn what standards and criteria are used by those who claim to have the answers. Best for whom, under what conditions, and what are the risks?

Most of the books on the subject present you with one diet and make claims for that diet that sound somewhat reminiscent of the way snake oil used to be marketed. Since I do not strongly favor any one diet, and because I suspect that you might respond to one kind of regimen quite differently from the way your neighbor would respond, I suggest you evaluate several. There is at least one book that can help you do this; in fact it's called *Rating the Diets* and was written by Theodore Berland and the editors of *Consumer's Guide* (Chicago: Rand-McNally, 1974). Another source you could use is a special issue of *Cosmopolitan* (Spring 1976) that described "Thirteen Fabulous Diets that Really Work." (But please, choose one at a time.) Per-

---

7. Robert Rodale, *The Prevention System for Better Health* (Emmaus, Pa.: Rodale Press, 1976), p. 33.

sonally, I am suspicious of *any* diet plan that is focused on *temporary* food restrictions and which neglects the larger aspects of a person's life. The best diet plan, in my view, is one that is custom-designed for the whole you by the most authoritative expert on the subject—you. Such a plan, worked out over time and adjusted throughout your life, would take account of such principles as those suggested in this discussion and as your needs and preferences evolve. The design of such a diet would be influenced by your activity levels, past eating patterns, metabolic rate, psychological and economic strengths, barriers to good eating, and other factors unique to *your* life that do (or should) affect your food habits. A magazine article on diet plans can fit as a tiny piece of a big puzzle, but you should start with an understanding of the bigger picture.

What about the water controversies; mineral, spring, distilled, hard, soft, and so forth? Is one kind best for everybody all the time? Are there enough benefits to justify the effort and expense of securing other than whatever tap water is available locally?

Personally, I obtain not enough satisfaction from the claim that our tap water sets the world's standard. (Maybe that's why Europeans drink so much wine and beer.) While tap water quality varies throughout the U.S., enough concerns have been expressed to give me a lot of pause. In some places, bacteria and contaminants leak into reservoirs from domestic septic tanks, fertilizer and insecticide runoffs are a seasonal hazard, and water departments routinely add fluorine and chlorine (to bleach solid matter and combat odors). Sometimes all this gets a bit much: one southern California resident who switched to bottled water said the local water tastes as though "it's irrigated three artichoke farms, just after manure-spreading, before it reaches us."[8] But, on the other side, bottled water is a mixed blessing. For one thing, it's expensive (from $.50 to $8.00 per gallon, the latter for a first-rate imported variety). For another, it's also usually treated quite a bit (distilled, filtered, processed by deionization or electrodialysis, and/or supplemented with cal-

8. "How to Avoid Getting Soaked When You Buy Bottled Water," *Moneysworth* (28 March 1977), p. 12.

cium, sodium, magnesium, or carbonates), and sometimes has a "funny" taste. In any case, tap water versus some variety of the costlier (but almost always better) bottled alternative is another one of those "unsimple" choices we face in life. At this date, I'm still drinking tap water, and wondering. So, how can I make a suggestion as to what you should do, when I sit here on the middle of the fence? I'll drink (?) to that.

Supplements are perhaps the most trying of all concerns because there seems so much to learn. What should you know about each of the vitamins, the amino acids, and the minerals? How important are they? What are their functions and sources? Do we all need supplements and, if so, which ones in what amounts? Does it matter whether vitamins and minerals are derived from natural or synthetic sources? How does a person make sense of this overwhelming subject? I have a lot to learn (that is why I am describing my ideas regarding supplements on this page rather than as a nutritional awareness principle), but I'm willing to share my impressions. Essentially, I believe that few of us manage to obtain a balanced and adequate diet on a regular basis, and therefore we need supplements. I favor natural vitamins and minerals rather than synthetic ones, not because I have seen convincing scientific evidence that the cheaper synthetics are less effective or sometimes hazardous (as some claim regarding the separation of the B vitamins), but rather because of my belief system. I just think that foods from vegetables, fruits, and grains; the earth—are preferable to those derived in laboratories. I trust the wisdom of nature; I'm suspicious about whether man's tampering can really improve on the original products. And as to the importance of knowing what you are doing in taking vitamins: I would give a rating of nine on an ascending scale of one to 10 to the value of knowing at least the basics. You'll find interesting information on all the aspects of supplements noted above in the books on nutritional awareness listed in the Resource Guide at the end of this book. You will probably do a lot of experimenting before settling down on an approach to this issue.

We hear so much about fasting. What is its value and what are preferred approaches? When do you need supervision by a nutritional expert skilled in the fasting art and science, and what is the optimal length of time for a fast? Here is another area where only you can decide what makes sense for you.

While I do not fast, I certainly am impressed with the claims for fasting made by those who do. It is said that fasting fosters the healing process, facilitates mental efficiency, and enables spiritual awareness. According to Airola and others, fasting rejuvenates and revitalizes and helps to cure and prevent disease. During a fast, dead and dying cells are eliminated and the building of new cells is accelerated. Toxic waste products that interfere with the nourishment of the cells are expelled and optimal metabolic rate and cell oxygenation are restored.[9] That's a capsule account of a complex and fascinating subject; it does deserve your investigation. I know a lot of people who fast regularly for the purposes noted above. Andrea Miller, for example, periodically does one- and 10-day juice fasts. While Andrea's experiences have convinced her that the benefits claimed for fasting are valid, she did acknowledge that the process is sometimes uncomfortable, to put it mildly. Andrea talked of "stages" experienced during one-day fasts; the first being a time of high nervous energy, the next relaxation, and the third a tired period. "I go to bed around 8:00 P.M. on one-day fasts; by falling asleep I don't think about how hungry I am." During longer fasts (10 days), Andrea feels tired for three or four days, and the temptations to give in to mental urges to eat are almost overwhelming. But after this period, the fast becomes a pleasant time of "good moods without noticeable energy losses." If I ever do fast, it will be under the close supervision of someone who knows the process quite well. Before I would experience these changes, I would want to be sure I was ready for a fast, and be assured by a trusted guide that the changes experienced were OK and that no harm was being done. If I chose the right guide and a short, nondrastic beginner's fast (three to five days), I might even enjoy the experience.

There is an increasing amount of attention being given to

9. Paavo Airola, *Are You Corfused?* (Phoenix, Arix.: Health Plus Publishers, 1972), p. 112.

the merits of "supernutrition" or "megavitamin" strategies wherein cells and tissues are bombarded with huge doses of nutrients to treat or help avoid disease. Do you believe that 3,000 milligrams of vitamin C will saturate your bloodstream and all the tissues of your body to the extent that toxins and poisons will be neutralized, pathogenic bacteria will be killed, the healing process will be speeded, tissues will be better oxygenated, and other benefits will accrue? This is one claim of the hundreds made for variations on the theme of vitamin and food enrichment strategies. Like the other issues it seems to warrant some investigation and consideration as you develop your own approaches.

Dr. Richard Kozlenko, a cofounder of WHN and a consultant in nutritional awareness, told me that superhigh or "megavitamin" strategies are only justified in cases of definitive enzyme deficiency or errors in metabolism. Expressive vitamin/mineral intake over time will, according to Dr. Kozlenko, "upset the natural system of nutritional adaptation, cause tolerances for the nutrients to develop, provide diminished benefit, and eventually upset a person's unique biochemical balance." On the other hand, Dr. Kozlenko does strongly support a "high vitamin potency" strategy involving an intake of vitamins and minerals 10 to 20 times greater than that expressed in RDA values. And, as a minimum, Dr. Kozlenko urges clients to adopt an "urbanization offsetting" allowance to compensate for the vitamin deficiencies, mineral imbalances, and poisoned-enzyme-systems metabolism that could otherwise result from pollutants in the modern food chain and the lowered air quality.

In your nutritional awareness studies, do not overlook the value and the use of herbs, and all the intricacies of herbal selection, cultivation, cooking, and applications for healing purposes (homeopathy).

Learn as much as you can to judge the concern about pasteurized (cooked) milk, which is said to be devoid of enzymes and most vitamins and to contain minerals, fatty acids, and proteins that are less digestible and more difficult for the body to assimilate than those in uncooked milk. If this is so, and my research suggests that it is, it might be worthwhile to go to the extra expense and trouble to find certified raw milk, noninstant powdered milk, and other alternatives to the products of big dairies. Or, as the Wellness Resource Center suggests, take the position that milk products are not even necessary for adults.

And what do you suppose are the best rules to apply regarding food combinations? Is it OK to mix raw fruits and vegetables, starches and carbohydrates, and to eat different kinds of proteins at one sitting? My friend Marscell Rodin, who wrote *The Organic Gourmet: A Guide To Preparing Organic Gourmet Natural Foods* (Mill Valley, Calif.: COFU, [160 Miller Avenue] 1976) told me there are two occasions when combinations are critical: (1) when eating raw foods, because the beneficial but potent enzymes have not been destroyed or depleted as in cooked food; and (2) when you suffer from a digestive problem (e.g., ulcers). Marscell added: "The proof is always in the result upon you— how does a combination make you feel, how well does it get along with you?" He believes it is all right to mix fruits and certain salad-type vegetables (lettuce, cucumbers, celery) and to mix most proteins if doing so does not cause digestive discomfort. Marscell favors a "mono" diet (one food at a time), and thinks it is a good idea to start every meal with a fresh fruit drink half an hour before ingesting solids. There are many opinions on these and similar "combination controversies." The question of most consequence seems to be, "What feels good for you?"

Is it necessary to know the vitamin, amino acid, and mineral contents of all the major foods available in this country (there are five different kinds of meat and poultry, 40 to 50 popular vegetables, 24 varieties of peas, beans, and lentils, 20 different fruits, and nine grains)? Probably not, but it is better to know more than less; the greater your understanding, the better your chances of eating wisely.

I think a policy statement given to clients at the Wellness Resource Center covers the basics:

> Below is a general guide suggested by Wellness Resource Center as of January, 1977. We reserve the right to change our position as we evolve ourselves.
>
> Proteins: Most Americans get too much protein, though often those proteins are poorly balanced in amino acid content.

Fats: Again, most Americans get too much. Minimize animal fats, use cold-pressed oils, and supplement with soybean lecithin (1 tablespoon of granules per day).

Fiber: It is very hard to get enough without taking bran as a supplement. Use 2 tablespoons of bran per day, mixed with dry cereals or oatmeal, stirred in juices, baked in bread or by any other clever means of disguising its sawdustlike consistency. Other good sources of fiber are sesame seeds, sunflower seeds, almonds, and peanuts with skins in that order. Carrots and celery have surprisingly little fiber value.

Carbohydrates: Natural carbohydrates (sugars and starches)—grains, fruits, vegetables, root vegetables, and legumes—should be eaten in abundance. Refined carbohydrates like sugar, white flour (often called unbleached wheat flour to fool you into thinking it's whole wheat flour) and alcohol ought to comprise less than 10% of your diet. Use honey as a sweetener sparingly.

Vitamins and Minerals: You ought to meet the RDAs with food sources (since many nutrients are yet to be discovered and isolated and are therefore less likely to be present in supplements). We recommend these supplements as a guide. We have not as yet endorsed any particular brands, as much misrepresentation exists in the field. Our suggestions for daily supplements include: (the higher up on the list, the more certainty we have about its efficiency)

Vitamin C — 500 to 1,000 mg.
Vitamin E — 400 I.U. for women
600 I.U. for men and post-menopausal women (mixed tocopherols are preferable to alpha tocopherols)
B Vitamins — Brewer's yeast is the best balanced B vitamin source. Various brands of the little critters taste milder than others. Fragilis is one of the milder ones. Work up to two to three tablespoons per day, one teaspoon at a time. Too much too soon can produce indigestion. Liver and wheat germ are other sources, but livers often have poisons

	in them and *fresh* wheat germ is nearly nonexistent. Stress, coffee, and alcohol use up extra B vitamins.
Vitamin A	— The only vitamin that can be toxic in large doses. Individual needs vary greatly. A good diet will probably provide enough.
Vitamin D	— Produced by sunlight on skin that has not had its natural oils recently washed off. Caution: Tanning can produce early wrinkles and elephant skin.
Minerals	— A good multimineral supplement (kelp base) is best.

Notice the nondogmatic, nonextremist counsel given. I appreciate this low-key approach to a subject wherein science is so often invoked to support completely disparate positions.

All this information, as you can imagine, will take a while to examine and evaluate. But I think you will enjoy the process. The important step is to become informed, to accept change as you evolve, to develop a continuing interest in your own changes, and to live and dine in a manner which brings both nourishment and enjoyment.

Stress Management

You might have heard the crack attributed to Norman Vincent Peale to the effect that people are so stressed today that they don't sleep in church anymore. I don't know if that is an accurate quote, but it conveys the same concern about stress that experts are voicing when they describe it as a hazard of modern living. Just what is this stress problem, and what are the consequences of too much stress? More important, what can be done about it and how does stress management fit into the context of high level wellness?

Hans Selye defines stress as "the nonspecific response of the body to any demand upon it."[1] By "nonspecific response," Selye means that the body goes through a number of intense biochemical reactions and readjustments without regard to the nature of the stress-causing event. Stress triggers what are called "adaptive functions" directed at establishing normal physiological states. One effect of stress over a long period of time can be *distress*, which is associated with some rather difficult problems, including tension, insecurity, and frustration. Selye claims that these conditions lead to migraine headaches, peptic ulcers, heart attacks, hypertension, mental illness, and suicide.[2] That is the negative side of stress: the positive aspect is that stress can be enjoyed, and is considered an essential element of life. It's just a matter of learning to manage *it*, rather than letting it control *you*.

In addition to creating those problems already mentioned

---

1. *Stress without Distress* (New York: Lippincott, 1974), p. 111.

2. Ibid. pp. 14, 18.

by Selye, long-term stress has been singled out by Herbert Benson and others as a factor in strokes, bowel irritations, diabetes mellitus, and assorted skin disorders.[3] Emotional stress causes the body to go out of balance, the immunity system to break down, and cells to malfunction and deteriorate more rapidly than normal. If you combine poor management of stress factors with reckless nutrition, disregard for exercise, dependence on the medical system, and an adverse environment, you get a lifestyle guaranteed to produce disease and premature death.

It is rare when an expert in one field acknowledges the importance of another field, and rarer still when an expert notes that another area is even *more* important than his own. This, however, is what Dr. Paavo Airola has to offer in the conclusion of one of his ten books on nutrition:

> I believe that relaxation and peace of mind are very important health-promoting factors, perhaps the most important. These are what modern man needs most of all in order to live a long and happy life in good health.
>
> It has been scientifically established that emotional stresses and disturbances can cause practically every disease in the medical dictionary, including arthritis, ulcers, constipation, asthma, strokes, diabetes, high or low blood pressure, angina, glandular disturbances, etc. Extensive research into medical literature made by J. I. Rodale indicates that "happy people rarely get cancer." Unhappiness, deprivation of love, loneliness, emotional stresses and tensions can interfere with your normal body functions and may lead to serious illness.
>
> There are many factors that contribute to optimum health. Nutrition is *one* very important factor. But relaxation, peace of mind, positive outlook on life, contented spirit, absence of envy and jealousy, cheerful disposition, love of mankind, and faith . . . are all-powerful, health-promoting factors without which optimum health can not be achieved.[4]

3. *The Relaxation Response* (New York: Avon, 1975), p. 29.

4. *Are You Confused?* (Phoenix, Ariz.: Health Plus Publishers, 1971), pp. 208–209.

In addition to reducing your prospects for experiencing one or more of the conditions of utter worseness noted above, an understanding of and a capability for effectively managing stress has other important benefits.

When you recognize that stress is inevitable, desirable, but potentially harmful, you are automatically better prepared to cope with events and circumstances that otherwise could cause distress, or tension and anxiety. One part of stress management is having some skill or technique that you can use to recover mental and bodily relaxation in times of duress. This stress-management skill will also help you to be more alert, creative, and productive. Becoming acquainted with your own stress moods and having a sense of the amount of stress you can manage under varying circumstances will enable you to use body rhythms and feeling states to perform to your best potential without risking energy breakdown. In addition, if you can learn to relax your muscles you will enjoy better circulation and an overall inner strength.

There are three technical aspects of stress management that you might find of interest. These are: (1) the significance of different cycles of electrical activity in the brain; (2) the concept of the "fight or flight response"; and (3) the idea of a "general adaptation syndrome."

Four basic terms are used to describe cycles of brain activity; beta, theta, delta, and alpha. Brain activity can be measured in varied speeds and intensities. When you are fully conscious, your brain waves register between 13 and 32 hertz, or cycles, per second; when you're asleep, your range is four to eight cycles per second. Deep sleep is ½ to four cycles per second. The awake phase is called *beta*, sleep or nonconsciousness is termed *theta*, and deep sleep is *delta*. Most of your waking time is in the beta condition, the upper range of which corresponds with nervous tension, stress, and distress. But there is another state of consciousness which many associate with more natural, creative brain activity; the alpha condition at eight to 13 cycles per second. If you learn how to induce an alpha state, you can blank out distressors, regain normal blood pressure and cholesterol levels, lower nervous tension and anxiety, and gain a mental peace conducive to creativity. John McCamy and James Presley recommend that you get at least 30 minutes a day in this alpha state of consciousness.[5]

The term *fight or flight response* has been used by Selye and others to describe an inborn characteristic which has been part of the human condition for millions of years—a characteristic which well served your ancestors who needed an internal "shot" before fighting, running or, alas, being eaten. Essentially, situations which you interpret as highly stressful evoke an involuntary surge of adrenalin or other hormones through activation of your sympathetic (involuntary) nervous system. This automatic or involuntary response raises your blood pressure, breathing rate, heart rate, and metabolism, increases your muscle blood flow, and brings about related physiologic changes.[6] Under certain conditions (e.g., athletic competition), the fight or flight response enables appropriate behavioral adjustments. Unfortunately, frequent activation of this response without suitable behavior outlets can lead to a variety of illnesses. Learning to manage the fight or flight response should be one of your objectives.

Selye developed the concept and coined the term *general adaptation syndrome* to describe stages of biological stress resistance. The first stage he called *alarm reaction*. This is followed by *resistance*, and then *exhaustion*. In the first stage, your body undergoes certain biochemical reactions as a part of a nonspecific response, and your overall resistance is lowered. In the next stage, resistance increases due to the body's alarm reaction. In the third stage, which occurs if the stress continues over a period of time, your body's adaptation energy will become exhausted, and then you will be in big trouble (i.e., dead).[7] Adaptation energy is finite; stress over time will deplete your body of the resources it needs to defend itself and you.

---

5. John C. McCamy and James Presley, *Human Life Styling: Keeping Whole in the 20th Century* (New York: Harper & Row, 1975), pp. 120–139.

6. Ibid.

7. Seyle, *Stress Without Distress*, p. 27.

Stress-Management Principles

1. Take stock of your own power.   You already have the resources within yourself to control your stress, you just need practice at exercising that power and at taking control. Distress, when you think about it, is not really outside of you—it is in your subjective response to a situation. This being the case, you can learn to recognize and almost completely manage your feeling-level by working on the notion that you have the power to control your own stress response. Rather than permit your body to undergo harmful biochemical reactions, you can develop the ability to interpret stress events in a positive way. Your response can then contribute to instead of detract from your well-being. There is a statement attributed to Marcus Aurelius which seems to affirm this stress-management principle quite well: "If you are distressed by anything external, the pain is not due to the thing itself but to your estimate of it. This you have the power to revoke at any time."

2. Make up your own guidelines.   There is an amazing variety of stress-management principles, techniques, approaches, "mental sets," and rules by whatever name, that are offered as guides in this area. Consider as many as you wish, but don't be afraid to make up your own, also. I enjoyed reading the 12 "mental sets" outlined by McCamy and Presley, but I think you could get more from developing your own, after considering theirs, mine, and a number of others along the way. Those offered in *Human Life Styling* include recognizing the beneficial aspects of stress, the importance of doing one thing at a time, trying to do your best and not worrying beyond that point, expressing feelings honestly, and being positive; even to the extent of seeking growth lessons in "bad" experiences. Other principles given are treating all people with respect, taking steps to improve important relationships, accepting the reality of the world as it is (including the inevitability of death), being in touch with your needs, remembering that there are always options, choosing to be well, and living in what McCamy and Presley term the "golden now."[8] These ideas seem helpful and

---

8. *Human Life Styling*, p. 124.

consistent with a wellness orientation to life. Another "mental set" worth noting is the list of "rules for right living" by Satchel Paige, a famous baseball player who had his own ideas for stress management:

1. Avoid fried foods which "angry up" the blood.
2. If your stomach disputes you, lie down and pacify it with cooling thoughts.
3. Keep the juice flowing by jangling around gently as you move.
4. Go very lightly on the vices such as carrying on in society—the social ramble ain't restful.
5. Avoid running at all times.
6. Don't look back. Somethin' might be gaining on you.

3. Take it easy. How many times do you actually benefit by worrying about a problem? Is it necessary to worry to resolve a difficult situation? I believe worrying is neither profitable nor constructive. Instead, it is a distress condition which can cause you to slip out of sync or balance. The alternative is to do what you can about a situation, and go on to other things. Affirm to yourself that you will do your best to manage the difficulty, that this is all you can do, and that things will work out well. Positive affirmations (e.g., "Today I will complete a first draft of my report") can do more to help you deal with difficulty than negative hand-wringing, and they bring on none of the destructive stress effects of worry.

4. Try ways to quiet yourself. The benefits of being able to create a calm and serene peacefulness through meditation or some other relaxation method of your choosing, when you need or choose to do so, are considerable. There are many ways to quiet yourself. Under the stress management category in the Wellness Resource Guide I have included books which provide a thorough listing and assessment of most of the more popular varieties of techniques for quieting. Some of these are Transcendental Meditation (TM), the Relaxation Response; Autogenic Training, Progressive Relaxation, hypnosis with suggested deep relaxation, sentic cycles, and various forms of yoga and Zen Buddhism. Meditation lowers the body's oxygen consumption, blood lactate level, carbon dioxide elimination, heart and respiration rates, fatty acids in the blood, and acts beneficially on other processes connected with the sympathetic nervous system. It also increases the likelihood and duration of alpha brain-wave cycles, and reduces muscle tension throughout the body. All this, of course, is just the reverse of the effects of the unattended (i.e., not acted upon) fight or flight response, so the importance of a quieting technique as a way to manage stress is apparent. By having a quieting skill, you are able to reduce the effects of excessive sympathetic nervous system activity so frequently called into play by modern living. Unlike the fight or flight response of automatic adrenal flow evoked by stressful conditions without conscious effort, a quieting technique enables relaxation whenever you decide that a quiet period is needed. So shop around a bit. Try the least expensive approaches first, and experiment with different forms of quieting until you find one you enjoy enough to practice regularly. It just might be a method you've devised yourself.

5. *Enjoy what you do to manage stress.* If repeating a strange-sounding mantra 20 minutes every morning and 20 minutes every evening (i.e., TM) is not your thing, don't toss out the dimension with the bathwater. Try something else—there are as many approaches available as you have time to put into the search. Some of my favorites, which are only partially satisfactory and not a complete program of stress management, are massage, hot tubs and saunas, exercise, chanting, biofeedback, and music. Someday I'm going to try hypnosis. Some of my friends go for "visual imagery"—thinking of a place where you feel good, relaxed, and at peace. It might be a mountainside, a beach, a friend's bedroom—whatever place you have actually experienced relaxation and calm. Gradually, instruct each part of your body to let go, become soft, and rest. Then relax with whatever images come up for you. Stay with this for three to five minutes, and take another minute or two to come out of the relaxation pattern. Try it; if you are not big on the more involved and disciplined forms of meditation, visual imagery or a variation on it may be for you.

6. Design an environment for quieting. It is possible to meditate, relax, or quiet yourself in just about any setting regardless of external conditions, if you have the discipline and commitment to practice under adversity. An office, home, bus, plane—it makes no difference if you work it out in advance and practice a little bit. It is necessary to plan and otherwise structure events and places if you want quiet periods to occur and to be useful. I find I can enjoy a quiet environment if I make a regular time for the experience, find a place away from distractions, repeat a special work in my mind and dwell upon it, practice breath awareness, assume a completely relaxed posture, and allow a passive frame of mind. All this takes but a few minutes a day. Use whatever works for you and remember to set the stage—before you go out on it.

7. Set your sights on inner peace. There is one theme heard in several studies of long-lived people, and that is the importance of serenity, a sense of purpose or place—in short, the feeling of being valued and respected by society.[9] Try to find modes of self-expression which you find satisfying, that you are or can become good at, and on which you can work hard and long. Such resources make possible inner peace, which more than anything else can protect you from the steady assaults of stressful living. Kurt Vonnegut, Jr., once wrote that "we need all the uncritical love we can get," and I must tell you I have a related theory. Based upon incredibly complicated, extraordinarily scientific, and wonderfully intuitive reasoning, I have personally determined that you need not less than 6.5 hugs and/or warm strokes daily. More than this number will do you no harm; in fact, I recommend you get, and give, as many as you can while getting on with the affairs of the day.

8. Plan your response to stress. Remember the list of 43 separate stress-causing events and their stress ratings, provided by Dr. Holmes in the Life Change Index? Many of these events

9. See Grace Halsell, *Los Viejos: Secrets of Long Life from the Sacred Valley* (Emmaus, Pa.: Rodale Press, 1976), and Alexander Leaf, "Every Day Is a Gift when You are Over 100," *National Geographic* (January 1973), pp. 93–118.

have occurred in your life, will again, and will provoke a certain level of stress, depending upon your reaction. You do not have to wait for such events and their attendant stress loads to bear down on you before doing something to minimize their impact on you. You can, if you choose, anticipate a "crisis" (e.g. a promotion, a success, a disappointment, a "peak moment" such as a speech you will be giving) and determine that you will manage it with greater equanimity or calm. Also, you can slow down for a while; do not, if possible, do what you really don't want to do. Postpone moving, changing jobs, mates, and routines to the extent possible, until you are ready to deal with the stress of these decisions. Minimize hazardous activities, eat well, get plenty of rest, exercise for fun at an enjoyable pace, treat yourself to a massage, and work especially hard at avoiding high-risk behaviors (which bring only brief, symptomatic relief and can exacerbate the true issue). Ask your friends for extra strokes; in every way possible, be good to yourself. And, of course, be ready to initiate the stress-reduction method of your choice.

9. Work on being open and (politely) assertive. Suppressed feelings, anxieties about appropriate behaviors and disclosures to others, self-doubts and low esteem are among the major stressors which lead to illness and disease. Work on developing a wider repertoire of assertive and personal disclosure skills; your friends and associates deserve to understand how you feel and it is self-fulfilling and conducive to your well-being to let them know. When you can act in your own best interests, stand up for your rights without fear and anxiety, express your emotions, and still respect the needs and rightful claims of others, you free yourself from a great deal of traumatic distress which cannot do you or anyone else any good whatsoever.

10. Consider "getting lost" occasionally—in a calming activity. You may get more relief at times from states of tension and anxiety by working at a craft, playing a vigorous sport, creating a work of art, or other such diversionary endeavors than by employing one of the forms of meditation or quieting techniques. Recognize this beneficial outlet, and go for your racquet, or whatever, when you sense the need for a respite from accumulating stress.

11. Consider changing parts of your life that bring chronic stress. There are objective conditions in some of our lives that deserve evaluation and possible reconstruction. You may become the most skilled meditator in the looney bin if you do nothing over the years about a tension-producing job or a profession you abhor, a husband/wife/mate who will always drive you up a proverbial wall (and vice-versa, which is just as distress-provoking), or some other disabling stress producer. Take responsibility for doing what can be done to lower stress levels in a more generic way, rather than just adapting to and/or modifying the specific effects of stress.

Approaches to Stress that Work

I have a technique which seems to work for me, and I do it every morning on rising, most evenings before retiring, and at any time during the day when I feel tense or uncomfortably "hyped." I have no idea whether it would work for anyone else, but I will mention it in case you might be interested. I simply sit comfortably in a chair, close my eyes, and (slowly) inhale and exhale as deeply and fully as I can. I try to feel myself relaxing, starting with my toes and feet and proceeding to my ears and head. (If you have never experienced fully relaxed ears, well, you're missing something. Like limp ears.) All this takes but two or three minutes, which I am willing to surrender for the calming effect it provides. On the other hand, the TM I learned years ago requires 20 minutes every morning and night (before meals), and I found too many distractions disrupted that routine. While I do not expect to take up TM again (I also have difficulty relating to a mantra, levitations, and other trappings), I do respect the results which others report from employing this and other relaxation methods. In the future, I expect to devote more time to quieting than I do today, and to put greater effort into constructing an environment suited for and conducive to my own approach to stress management.

Some of my best friends have other approaches which work very well for them. Dorothy Kelly, a yoga instructor and leader of stress-reduction workshops in nearby Larkspur, told me she finds a walk in the woods to be a certain method of "clearing" tension. Kelly (as she is called by all who know her well) described how she takes her flute into the woods whenever a spiritual sanctuary is needed, and plays to a bird! "The birds are always singing to us—it's not too often we play for them. I enjoy switching roles." Kelly also said that massage, yoga, and meditation have "saved my life" and that she tries to do a little of each, plus jogging, every day.

A lawyer acquaintance and holistic practitioner, Jerry Green, told me that stress comes to him from a sense of disorder experienced as a loss of "grounding" or orientation. This is usually manifested in his body as pain, stiffness, or a general sense of being "out of alignment." Jerry's remedy or approach? "I listen to music, sit in the sun, clean up my yard or garden, pay bills or organize my desk, and perform some movement patterns and yoga on the floor of my house. This seldom fails to bring me back in touch with myself. It helps me remember who I am." This approach seems particularly appropriate and noteworthy in Jerry's case because as a child he had a diagnosis of cerebral palsy. The message he received from the medical system was that there was no "cure," thus no emphasis was given to getting Jerry to take responsibility for doing what he could with the problem. For many years, he "carried" his left arm and walked with a limp. Today, after a few years as a student of movement patterns, yoga, structural integration, and other body therapies popular in the holistic health arena, Jerry has no noticeable disability. He is very active physically, both for pleasure and as a practitioner of body arts, massage, and other alignment practices.

You may find all the skills and techniques you need in practicing one of the well-known approaches to stress management and adhering to a few of the principles noted in this chapter. Or you might discover, as Kelly, Jerry Green, and I have, that a personalized variation on a theme is the most appropriate and effective approach for you. Either way, having stress-management consciousness and skills will take you a long way down the road on your life journey towards high level wellness.

Physical Fitness

It is hard to exaggerate the importance of physical fitness—but let me try. A client called upon his wellness-oriented physician and exclaimed: "Doctor, you must help me. My self-concept has deteriorated, I'm overweight, my energy level is low, and I can't sleep nights. Worst of all, my wife says I'm unbearable, and doesn't want me around the house anymore. What's wrong?" Without hesitating, the insightful physician said: "I know what your problem is: you are physically unfit. Here's what I want you to do. Run 10 miles daily for the next 15 days." Immediately, the client responded: "Doctor, that makes sense. I'll do it." And 15 days later, he called the physician and reported that he did as recommended, and the results were wonderful. That is, his self-concept was terrific, he had lost weight, had high energy levels, and slept soundly at night. "Fine, fine," said the physician, "but tell me, how are you getting along with your wife?" "How the hell should I know?" he replied. "She's 150 miles away."

Now this story is not true, but the benefits of regular exercise are so substantial as to require no exaggeration. Alas, the same is true of the problems of neglect. Did you know that, according to the President's Council on Physical Fitness and Sports, 45 percent of the American people never exercise?[1] I do not want to overwhelm you with the case for regular exercise, but inactivity *is* a serious health hazard that has been convincingly linked to hypertension, chronic fatigue, physiological inef-

1. For a summary on how Americans are exercising and what forms of exercise are most popular, see "Why 60 Million Americans Are on a 'Fitness Kick,' " *U.S. News and World Report* (14 January 1974) pp. 26–28.

ficiency, premature aging, poor musculature, and inadequate flexibility. These conditions, in turn, are major causes of lower back pain, injury, tension, obesity, and coronary heart disease. No matter how attentive you may be to your nutrition, however much you control and channel stress, and regardless of how much you practice self-responsibility and environmental sensitivity, you cannot be healthy if you are not reasonably fit. Not superfit, not to the degree that you are setting records, or not even an exercise nut like me. Just adequately conditioned and feeling good and fully able to derive considerable satisfaction from the sensory joy of being in touch with your own muscle tone. Whereas a lack of fitness can have an adverse effect on your morale, adequate toning will insure biochemical and other positive changes that have the effect of elevating your mood and reinforcing a healthy self-concept. You just cannot be as pretty or as devilishly handsome out of shape as in shape.

You probably realize that there is plenty of evidence that inactivity increases your chances of developing arteriosclerosis and other manifestations of heart disease, and that it negatively affects both the efficiency of your heart and the circulation of your blood.[2]

As if all this were not bad enough, you might as well recognize that lack of exercise leads to premature bodily aging, or pathological old age. The results? Infirmity, feebleness, frailness, low energy levels, sallowness, and loss of gravity. According to Dr. Morehouse (coauthor of *Total Fitness*), this kind of aging "literally pulls you down; your height diminishes, your body stoops, you dodder."[3]

Enough—you get the point. You are most likely already into fitness activities in some form, or at least have no quarrel with the value of regular exercise. It is just a matter of finding the time and energy to pursue fitness programs, and finding a suitable place where you can enjoy the activity of your choice.

2. U.S. Department of Health, Education, and Welfare, *Forward Plan for Health: FY 1975–81*, DHEW Publication No. 76-50024 (Washington, D.C.: DHEW, 1975), p. 108.

3. L. E. Morehouse and Leonard Gross, *Total Fitness in 30 Minutes a Week* (New York: Pocket Books, 1976), p. 21.

You know that I will make no effort to tell you what programs to follow. And you know I'm not going to suggest any shortcuts to instant vigor or total fitness by high noon. What I hope will be useful, wherever you happen to be on the "superfit–physical wreck" continuum, is a closer look at what I think are the "inner and outer" joys of being reasonably fit, and a number of fitness principles that seem to work for me.

The Inner and Outer Joys of Exercise

While the downside problems of neglect are reason enough for you to adopt an individualized fitness regime, more enjoyable motivations are to be found on the positive side of things. I have found that folks who take an active interest in keeping fit, whether as joggers, tennis bugs, or whatever, usually display an abundance of wellness characteristics. These include an increased ability to manage stress, greater self-confidence, better eating habits, fewer risk-behaviors, and an overall ability to relate effectively to other people. Joggers, for example, are said to be strengthened and their lives made more satisfying by the activity. In *Positive Addiction*, William Glasser writes that for those strong enough to find them, "fulfillment, pleasure, recognition, a sense of personal value, a sense of worth, the enjoyment of loving and being loved are not optional, they are the facts of life."[4] Fitness, says Glasser, is one nearly sure way to develop these characteristics.

And, of course, there are the physiological benefits, including the lowering of the heart rate, blood pressure, percentage of body fat, stress level, and cholesterol and lipids (fats) in the blood. Exercise even increases air flow through nasal passages,[5] no uncertain blessing for hay-fever sufferers. Fitness programs usually reduce joint stiffness, and the resulting stronger muscles provide better support for the skeletal structure, which in turn aids circulation. The energy output required to strengthen muscles causes the appestat mechanism to operate more effec-

---

4. New York: Harper and Row, 1976, p. 3.

5. James C. McCullagh, "Break Through Hay Fever Congestion with Vitamins and Exercise," *Prevention* (August 1976) pp. 148–156.

tively for appetite control. Exercise particularly benefits the heart, arteries, and lungs; the increased circulatory output and oxygen intake helps nourish the nerves and body tissues. Conditioned people usually have less acid in their stomachs, and exercise has even been shown to aid in the treatment of diabetes, glaucoma, depression, and other disorders.[6] As the Earl of Darby remarked: "Those who cannot find the time for exercise will have to find the time for illness."

Unfortunately, too many Americans do not exercise. To some extent, this may be due to unimaginative physical fitness education patterns in the past which emphasized varsity competition for the few to the neglect of intramural participation for the many. A commitment to intramurals could have demonstrated the fun and life-long advantages of varied exercise possibilities; the varsity sports orientation too often stressed competition, winning, and sports-as-war. The mass participation programs that did exist were commonly given to regimented calisthenic drills; a long way from the sports for fun, health, participation, and teamwork values being popularized by YMCAs and contemporary physical educators.

There are at least as many modalities or approaches to physical fitness as there are techniques and programs for self-responsibility, ways to eat wisely, and strategies for managing stress. Some of the most popular include jogging and running, biking, swimming, tennis, dancing, martial art forms, hiking and brisk walking, basketball, volleyball, and all kinds of other ball games involving graceful movements and strenuous exertions. All of these and hundreds of other physical activity forms are valuable and contribute something to the fitness of those who enjoy engaging in them. But some are better than others: any exercise that requires sustained effort and greater oxygen consumption affects the enzyme system by stimulating increased blood flow, muscular exertions, and lung respirations. This "aerobic" effect does more for your conditioning than lesser exertions. For example, if you exercise for 20 minutes at a pulse rate of about 140 beats per minute, you will probably derive more cardiovascular benefit than if you exercised four times as

6. Walter McQuade and Ann Aikman, *Stress* (New York: Bantam, 1975), p. 135.

long at only 100 beats per minute.

There is an actual case, on file with the President's Council on Fitness and Sports, that illustrates a most unusual and highly "nonrecommended" approach to fitness. A middle-aged executive, in dreadful condition and on a severely limited activity basis due to a succession of near-fatal heart attacks, decided to kill himself. To spare his family embarrassment and to safeguard their eligibility as beneficiaries of his insurance policies, he decided to do so in a nonsuspicious manner. So he donned a jogging outfit (borrowed, of course, he didn't own one) and started running at a fast pace. In a short period of time he collapsed, but did not die, or suffer an attack. So he tried again the next day, with the same results. He did so again, and on the fourth day, he did not collapse. He continued the practice, and by the second week he was feeling much better about his life and prospects, and decided to live, after all. As I said, this is not a recommended approach, but it makes the point that the human body is designed for action and movement. Unlike machines, it wears faster from disuse than use and, in fact, it operates better with more work than less work.

Goals you might want to consider in selecting a fitness approach might include increased muscle tone, better appearance, stamina, respiratory endurance, strength, vigor, and an increased capacity to resist stress. Weight loss is another very real possibility.[7] The trick is to develop fitness for the kind of life

---

7. The President's Council on Physical Fitness and Sports has produced a brochure on, "Exercise and Weight Control" which you can obtain for $.35 (c/o Superintendent of Documents, U.S. Gov't Printing Office, Wash, D.C. 20402). The brochure describes the value of exercise in maintaining proper weight. It contains a great amount of useful information on such matters as energy expenditures (expressed as gross energy cost in calories-per-hour by a 150-pound individual) for 34 different activities. The authors state that the key to effective weight control is keeping energy intake (food) and output (physical activity) in balance. Some of the points made I found especially interesting. For example, "remember that although it takes an hour's jogging to use up 900 calories, one does not have to do it all in one stretch; a half-hour, for example, uses up 450 calories. It is a fact that one must walk 35 miles to lose one pound of fat but the 35 miles need not be walked at one time. Walking an additional mile each day for 35 days also will take off that pound. This means one can lose 10 pounds in one year by walking an extra mile a day—providing, of course, that food intake and other physical activity remain the same. This really isn't an impractical amount of time or effort and to lose more or faster one needs only to increase the extent of activity."

you want to enjoy and for coping in the environment of your choice. Do you want just the minimum fitness necessary to avoid deterioration? Do you want enough of a fitness margin to help ward off fatigue? Or do you want to train for a strenuous activity (e.g., skiing, long-distance running, handball, etc.)? The amount of commitment you'll need to enjoy the pursuit of your chosen fitness level will vary accordingly.

One of the nation's best known fitness enthusiasts, U.S. Senator William Proxmire, puts the case for exercise very lyrically:

> If you exercise enough you will be leaner, stronger, more energetic. You'll love life, enjoy the smell of flowers, the taste of your food, the cold, and the bracing freshness of a morning breeze. You can literally exercise your way out of boredom, listlessness, anxiety . . . . And you'll look so much better. The heavy jowls, the sagging stomach, the yellowish or pallid complexion will diminish and then vanish with exercise. Exercise won't grow hair on your head, alas. And it won't give you the nose you want, won't make you taller, won't change your bone structure. But it will do just about everything else and everything else is plenty. It will put a warm, pink color in your cheeks. It will eliminate the bulges and sags and fat. It will put firmness in your muscles, put a brightness in your eye.[8]

There are more technical and dispassionate ways to state the benefits of exercise for physical fitness, but the Senator's description seems to the point. In summary, if you want to pursue a lifestyle of high level wellness, you really ought to think of fitness as both an integral and pleasurable part of your routine; valued not only for the good things it does for your body, but equally for the satisfactions it provides and the added zest it gives to nearly everything you do. The following principles should be of some help as you think about tailoring an approach to life-long fitness that suits your needs and expectations.

8. *You Can Do It!: Senator Proxmire's Exercise, Diet and Relaxation Plan* (New York: Simon and Schuster, 1973), p. 31.

Physical Fitness Principles

1. Make physical fitness a part of your life.   Reassess your values if you think you are too busy to exercise daily. Consider the disease- and illness-prevention aspects of being fit, the potential joys of personal progress and achievement inherent in varied physical outlets, and the sociability of sports participation. Consider these and other reasons why you have so much to gain and so little to give up by adopting an exercise regimen and making fitness a part of your life. Recall the expression that we all have two doctors—the left leg and the right leg. Keep thinking about these benefits-in-waiting until you are fully ready to commit yourself to some fitness-inducing endeavor. Then, do it, and when you get bored, switch to another exercise routine. With respect to muscle functioning, it's a case of use it or lose it!

2. Don't think of fitness as a crash program.   Finding a conditioning activity that is right for you and time to devote to it on a regular basis requires a commitment and some energy. Avoid trying to rush the development of endurance and attempting to hurry the realization of cardiorespiratory benefits. If you are in the process of relearning the enjoyment of rigorous activities, go slow and get back in touch with your inherent rhythms, gradually renew your strength, and carefully reestablish the sense of vigor you might have overlooked for years. Whatever you do, don't think of fitness as something you do on a Sunday afternoon—when it is warm and there is no exciting football game on TV. Becoming and staying fit can and should be gradual and enjoyable, especially during the first year of concentrated effort. Best of all, when you start out properly it always becomes easier, increasingly enjoyable, and more rewarding. Be wary of programs that offer quick (and effortless) fitness approaches. You know better than that. A 30-minute-a-week strategy promising total fitness is either a hoax or a come-on; the fine print always belies the blurb. And don't let anybody try to tell you that you need any fancy equipment, such as indoor cycling machines, rowing devices, or other mechanical contraptions. These sorts of things can be helpful but they are never essential, you can get all

151

the exercise you need walking or jogging, which requires very little paraphernalia except you.

3. Exercise is fun so don't cheat yourself by taking an activity too seriously. Competition can, in itself, be a stress producer. Chances are you get enough of that in other aspects of your life. There is a time and place for competition, of course, but don't let winning become an end in itself. Even if you "win" all or most of the time, you could be missing a bigger reward— the satisfaction that comes from genuine enjoyment of the exercise experience for its own sake. So forget about points, clocks, and schedules. Try not to be in a hurry about physical fitness and exercise routines, do not compete with yourself or others to meet some standards or guidelines, and do not worry about what is the average performance for your weight and sex. How can you enjoy something and get in touch with the earth and yourself if you are struggling to measure up to someone else's idea of *the* norm? The only norm you need be concerned about is *your* pulse rate, both at rest and when experiencing the training effect needed for conditioning. You ought to learn how to check your pulse (using either the carotid or radial artery), and make a habit of exercising at a pulse level that is from 62 to 80 percent of your maximum predicted heart rate. (For a reasonably fit person this training rate might be anywhere from 120 to 140 beats per minute, although age is another factor.) To learn how to calculate *your* training rate, see the section, Other Measures of Well-Being under Measuring Your Wellness. After a short while you will know when you have reached this level of effort, and pulse checking will be necessary less often. One other pointer—take time to "warm up" and "cool down"—three to five minutes is about right. But most of all, remember, you are unique. It should not matter what 50 out of 100 other people did. What counts is what you do, whether your chosen activity provides an exertion level useful for your endurance conditioning, and whether you are enjoying the activity enough to continue to pursue fitness as a lifelong adjunct to healthy being.

4. Learn to distract yourself—and enjoy exercise even more.
I have not monitored my pulse on a regular basis, but I have

discovered that my most effective workouts occur when I don't have time or opportunity to think about how much I'm huffing and puffing. For example, I get very tired after a few games of handball with an opponent at my skill level, yet I seldom think about how much effort I'm expending during the games. And it is these endurance activities of a sustained nature that best fortify my body against stress and contribute to efficient cardiovascular conditioning. So, find some activity that you really enjoy and get in the habit of forgetting about how much sustained vigor you are putting out. Then participate fully at the level you find most rewarding. By the way, though distraction can help mask your exertions, you really ought to expect to work at fitness to some extent. If it were effortless, total fun, and completely undemanding, everybody would be fit and trim and, as you might have noticed, that is not how it is. Thomas Jefferson was fond of quoting Euripedes on this point of energy investment: "For with slight efforts, how should one obtain great results? It is foolish even to desire it." So accept the idea that you must "put out" a bit to derive vital cardiovascular and other benefits from exercise. Just recognize that you are doing so because you value fitness, that such exertion is part of living life to the fullest, and that in exercising, as in making love, the more you give of yourself, the greater the capacity and interest you (eventually) regain. And, as this principle was intended to suggest, find an outlet wherein you don't have to constantly think about the energy you are sending out.

5. Get in touch with Mother Nature—and yourself.
Exercise is a great way to commune with the environment, with the gods, and with yourself. If you enjoy jogging, running (same as jogging, but faster), cycling, walking, and similar outdoor activities, create the best possible mood to go with the endeavor. Instead of (or in addition to) running around gyms or tracks or city streets, seek out a mountain, beach, park, farmland, golf course; the most attractive place available in your area; and combine a workout with a retreat for spiritual renewal. The benefits of doing so include fresh air, sunshine, vitamin D, and avoidance of shin splints or other leg or foot difficulties caused by pounding on concrete or other hard surfaces. And not to be

overlooked is another reward difficult to measure or describe—the opportunity to transcend ordinary experience. We are often limited more by our mental attitude than by our physical stamina and skill. With suitable surroundings, your approach to an activity can be calm and peaceful, without self-criticism, and can take you beyond limiting inhibitions and norms. The Zen-oriented might call this the "inner game" and speak of "going out-of-your-head" or out of normal consciousness.[9] I think of it simply as getting in touch with Mother Nature, and your own best friend. Yourself.

6. *A little activity goes a long way.*   A lot is better if you develop a yen for it, but if exercise is not your thing and minimal fitness or basic maintenance is all you want, do not despair. You can engage in professionally programmed exercise at any YMCA and most health clubs that will provide you with minimal musculoskeletal and circulo-respiratory endurance. Such a program will only require two or three 30-minute workouts a week. The health return you can obtain on such a minimum time and effort investment is considerable. As Morehouse and Gross point out in an early section of their *Total Fitness* book entitled "Fitness Is a Piece of Cake," "when your fitness is low, the least bit more of activity of any kind will change your strength, your muscular and cardiorespiratory endurance, help solidify your bones and resurrect your circulatory vessels." This approach is not what I prefer, but if you have tried all kinds of fitness approaches, games, and so forth, and just cannot "turn on" to exercise, this is your best bet. I don't recommend it, but it is one hell of a lot better than no exercise at all, the favored modality of most Americans today.

7. *Set modest expectations.*   It is better to promise little and surprise than to promise a lot and disappoint. Establish targets for yourself which you know you can reach. Too many have become discouraged by establishing heroic expectations, and then

9. For more on this concept, see George Leonard, *The Ultimate Athlete* (New York: Viking Press, 1974); and Michael Murphy, *Golf in the Kingdom* (New York: Delta, 1973).

finding themselves dreading the attendant difficulties and fear of failure. The too-common outcome in this case is loss of self-esteem and eventual loss of the will to pursue fitness. Remember, you are not training for the Olympics, though the rewards to you from physical fitness will prove far more valuable than a gold medal.

8. *Like a grape, you can get better with age.* There is no reason whatsoever to be nostalgic about an earlier time when you think you were fit. Whether you were or not, there are fitness levels within reach at 40 that could exceed your condition 10 years earlier. The same applies at ages 50, 60, and older.[10] For people who have not pursued a wellness lifestyle in their twenties and thirties, the prospects of "getting better" with age (through commitment to the wellness dimensions and principles) are excellent. If you doubt it, look at Senator Proxmire.

9. *Get involved in your activity.* Doing so will increase your appreciation for the activity and strengthen your commitment to it. Keep a casual record of your efforts, join a club or group that participates in your interest, buy the gear that goes with it, subscribe to the magazine about it, and in whatever ways possible structure your exercise time so as to make it an important part of your day.

10. *Learn how to breathe!* Sure you have been getting by, or you would not be here, but consider that there is far more than reflex inhaling and exhaling associated with a lifestyle of health enrichment. The yogis and many others (including champion athletes) have known the importance of deep breathing techniques, and you ought to pay attention to this process, also. (Nearly all the fitness books listed in the Resource Guide contain

---

10. Of course, the time must come eventually when your body simply wears out. I recall the story told by Dr. Alexander Leaf in the *National Geographic* article about long-lived people. Miguel Carpio, 123 years of age and the oldest citizen of Vilcabamba, continues his fondness for the opposite sex. According to his daughter, he "still likes to flirt with the girls, and was quite a ladies' man in his younger days." Says he: "I can't see them too well anymore, but by feeling, I can tell if they are women or not." Miguel has been heard to remark, "Oh, to be 108 again." ("Every Day Is a Gift When You Are Over 100," January, 1973: pp. 93–118.)

some commentary on the importance and techniques of thoughtful respiration before, during, and after physical fitness routines.)

11. Supplement your favorite fitness activity. Just as you reinforce, complement, and extend the range and quality of nutrients taken into your body as food, so should you supplement your exercise routine with well-rounded conditioning. Most sports, for example, do not provide stretching, flexibility, toning, shaping, and endurance for all the muscle groups (i.e., back, abdomen, and waist; lower extremities, hips, and buttocks; upper extremities and shoulders; and head and neck). For total fitness based upon overall body vitality encompassing musculoskeletal strength and cardiorespiratory endurance, try adding an activity such as about 10 minutes of rope jumping, isometric/isotonic routines, yoga postures, and other daily supplements to whatever it is you prefer as your daily workout. Do, however, minimize calisthenics. They are a bore, and sometimes cause the very problems you seek to avoid, particularly torn muscles and strained joints. Calisthenics are OK for trained athletes and for people with highly developed specialty regimens (who know what they are doing), but they can be hazardous for the rest of us. A gentle routine of flexibility and stretching exercises is preferred. I do a set of supplemental exercises each day that I learned from a business-oriented fitness newsletter entitled *Executive Health*.[11] The exercises are both isotonic (for endurance) and isometric (for strength). They are designed strictly as supplemental fitness outlets and do nothing for cardiovascular and respiratory fitness. But they can help people who sit a great deal to avoid pot-bellies and hernias. And some of them can be performed at a desk, while driving or riding in a car, or just waiting around. Isometrics consists of static exercises wherein you pit your own muscles against each other or some immovable object (do make sure it is indeed immovable). You do this for a maximum effort lasting only a few

11. See *Executive Health* brochure entitled "How to Avoid a Pot-Belly and Double-chin or Get Rid of Them for Good," vol. 6, no. 4. *Executive Health* is published monthly by Executive Publications, Pickfair Building, Rancho Santa Fe CA 92067. Subscriptions are $18 per year.

seconds. One procedure is to sit erect, breathe deeply, and draw in your stomach as hard and far as you can for six to 10 seconds. Next, lock your hands on your stomach, then force your stomach out against your locked hands (which are simultaneously holding your stomach in). Hold this for six to 10 seconds. Repeat this 10 to 20 times a day for six weeks and, according to the *Executive Health* folks, you will have a hard, flat stomach. But watch out if you have a heart condition or high blood pressure: this exercise will cause your blood pressure to soar briefly.

Isotonics is a system of movement exercises wherein you are building endurance on a time axis (as opposed to strength, which is derived from isometrics). The isotonic procedure I do is to sit on the floor, hands on hips, and extend my legs out straight at an angle to the floor of 30 to 45 degrees. I used to do this for six to 10 seconds, then I would rest and repeat it three times. I did this several times during the day, and almost always before retiring and after waking. Now I do this exercise less often (two or three times per day), but hold the position for about one minute. Naturally, you can vary these exercises to suit your preferences and your changing levels of fitness as you go along.

12. Express your fitness objectives in a contract.   Write an agreement with yourself to cover at least a three-month period, and check off compliance and progress as you go along. Also, note your feeling states, that is, what effect the workouts are having on your mental attitude, energy levels, and the overall balance between sore muscles and satisfactions. After three months, consider upgrading your targets, and continue to do so in stages until fitness is such a part of your life that the contract is unbreakable, and thus unnecessary to codify.

13. Be sensible.   If you are overweight, under treatment for a coronary disease, totally out of condition, or otherwise at a place where sudden exertion will surprise the hell out of your body, and create the risk of further damage and even doom, be cautious and prudent. Naturally, if in doubt, have your blood pressure measured and have both resting and treadmill electrocardiograms taken to check for any heartbeat irregularities (about $16 at a YMCA). Work into fitness slowly and find a qualified guide who can assist without keeping you dependent on him or her for an unreasonable period.[12] But guard against asking too little of yourself or you may succeed in subtracting rather than adding life to your years and years to your life.

Discovering Your Own
Strenuous Pleasures

Though I can't say the same for all the other dimensions, I have always been active in the area of physical fitness, so it is easier for me to continue to exercise and enjoy participation in varied sports than it is for many others. There must be some sports which I do not thoroughly delight in playing, some games that are of no interest, but I cannot think of any at the moment (maybe bowling). I spend at least two hours every day in one of three varied routines: handball, basketball, or long-distance running.[13] I supplement these efforts (which are strenuous pleasures, not toil) with occasional yoga and other stretching routines, weight-lifting, and other sports depending on opportunities (touch football, volleyball, tennis, etc.) and seasons (skiing, swimming, etc.). Physical fitness, in short, is an important part of my life, and I very much hope that, in your own way, you can make it a treasured part of your lifestyle, also.

Naturally, all this can be overdone. You would not want to emulate my friend, Walt Stack, for example. He wakes at 5:00 A.M. *every* morning, runs 10 miles, swims in the San Francisco Bay, and then rides his bike to work. Walt Stack, incidentally, is 69 years old.

---

12. A qualified guide does not mean a physician, unless the doctor has demonstrated a personal commitment to fitness and views exercise-counsel as an essential part of his/her practice. Otherwise, you may be discouraged from exercising or urged to be excessively cautious. The doctor might even say something dumb like "I never exercise; I get plenty of exertion serving as pallbearer for my friends who do."

13. Most of my running is done on Sunday mornings in San Francisco, with about 500 men, women and children in organized runs sponsored by the Dolphin-South End Rowing Club. If you are in town some Sunday morning and want a bit of exercise, consider joining us. The runs start at 10:00 A.M. at the clubhouse at Fisherman's Wharf at the foot of Hyde Street overlooking the Bay. Everybody "wins," and an enjoyable time can be had in the process of being good to your cardiovascular system.

Try to resist feeling that you should compare yourself with anyone else, especially fitness "crazies" like yours truly. I would never carry on as I do if I did not have a good time in the process and value the returns I get from my exercise activities. You can get just as much satisfaction doing less than half of what I do. I can even "prove" what I just suggested regarding the benefits of fitness. A few years ago, a physical activity program was designed and conducted involving 259 employees (age-range from 35 to 55) at NASA headquarters in Washington, D.C.[14] The investigators carefully looked at the results of the one-year program in terms of what impact the fitness programs had on work, health, and habits and behavior. They found a strong, positive, and consistent set of benefits in each of these three areas. The specific benefits included greater stamina, feelings of better health, weight loss, more positive work attitude, improved work performance, more adequate sleep and rest, less smoking behaviors, more selectivity in choice of diet, lowered food consumption, and decreased stress and tension. In addition, and certainly not of least value, was the "ripple effect" reported. That is, participants in the program positively influenced the health habits of family members, work colleagues, and friends. And, best of all, these benefits were derived from simple jogging and/or other fitness activities of only *three days per week at 30 minutes per exercise period*. So, as I said, you don't have to be a fitness fanatic like me to get a great deal of benefit from attending to this wellness dimension.

My friends all take different approaches to building fitness maintenance into their lifestyles. I'll mention a couple to show you how varied and interesting exercises can be, depending on your performance goals and lifestyle. Rick Carlson, a neighbor, a colleague, and a friend (who, incidentally, wrote *The End of Medicine*, which is reviewed in the Wellness Resource Guide) told me he has found the practice of Aikido to represent "a meta-

14. For a description of this study, see Donald C. Durbeck et al. *The NASA-USPHS Health Evaluation and Enhancement Program,* a monograph from the Division of Occupational Medicine (Washington, D.C.: National Aeronautics and Space Agency). Also of interest on this study is an article by Fred Heinzelmann and R. Bagley, "Response to Physical Activity Programs and Their Effects on Health Behavior," *Public Health Reports,* vol. 85, no. 10. (October 1970): pp. 905–911.

phor for life, generally. I am normally a 'doer,' and fairly aggressive. But in Aikido 'doing' doesn't work; 'being' does. Moreover, being aggressive doesn't help, either. Aikido teaches me that what I am doing has already happened and that my task is to flow into that place and not try to create it. It is for me, then, a very releasing, mellowing experience." Rick also jogs, stretches, and plays tennis and basketball, but his regular activity is Aikido. As his own words suggest, this form of physical expression also provides an element of spirituality for Rick, and an important means of stress management.

Quite another approach is that taken by an extraordinary woman (also a neighbor) named Dyveke Spino, a classical pianist, ski and tennis instructor, former fitness coach at Esalen, and now teacher at the Mill Valley Physical Therapy Center. Referring to her daily exercise on Mt. Tamalpais, Dyveke told me, "If I don't run that mountain I'm no good for anything." Dyveke has been the subject of several articles and now has her own radio show in San Francisco. A recent article provided a summary of Dyveke's approach to fitness, which she applies to herself as well as to her students:

> Write down everything about your daily schedule. See what works for you, and what doesn't. Then see what you desire for yourself, what it would be like if you had a body that could facilitate what you desire. Take a look at your environment—where are there green fields, running tracks, swimming pools? Locate them, explore them, begin to put them into your life. When you wake up, give yourself beautiful things. Read a poem, play some beautiful music, touch a leaf or an animal gently. You can do a sun worship exercise, hyperextending your body, stretching your spine, and you will get in touch with rigidity in your body. This is rigidity in your mind, cutting off your life force. Relax your mental sets. Let the healing aesthetic energy come in. Find a time of day that suits you, and a place you like, and go out and run on soft, unpaved surfaces. In forty minutes a day, every one of us can stay in a maximum condition of fitness.
> "We move in this entity called a body most of the time with so little awareness. Go within yourself, find the values you want to connect with, reflect on the edges of your own

body sense. Sometime each day close your eyes, let the light of a sun star come down into your head, into your body, filling your heart and lungs, filling your whole cellular system, and then go beyond your body after you have filled it with light, send out energy streamers to all the life forces around you.[15]

These approaches are, of course, not typical fitness regimes, but then you are not typical either. Go ahead and take what seems to work for you from here and there, experiment, add your own touches, create your own games, and exult in the glow that "feeling good" about your body brings to your mind. All the five wellness dimensions may be equally important, but this one can be more fun than the rest.

15.   Laughingbird, "Reown Feminine Power: Dyveke Spino," *New Age* (February, 1977) pp. 51–54.

Environmental
Sensitivity

An attitude to life which seeks fulfillment in the single-minded pursuit of wealth—in short, materialism—does not fit into this world, because it contains within itself no limiting principle, while the environment in which it is placed is strictly limited. Already, the environment is trying to tell us that certain stresses are becoming excessive. As one problem is being "solved," ten new problems arise as a result of the first "solution," As Professor Barry Commoner emphasizes, the new problems are not the consequences of incidental failure but of technological success.[1]

You know and I know there is trouble out there. Our environment seems under assault on all fronts. The Club of Rome has outlined possibilities of famines and industrial collapse, small conflicts far away often threaten the peace, scientists warn of J curves of exponential population growth, and disparities of wealth create social upheavals throughout the Western world. And to this you can add energy crises, inflation, unemployment, crime—there is plenty to worry about if you want to spend your time this way. Naturally, I don't recommend it. I'm an optimist,[2] and I believe that by pursuing the fullest life available to you in an environmentally sensitive manner, you can contribute at least as much to the universe as you can by worrying yourself

---

1. E. F. Schumacher, *Small Is Beautiful: Economics as if People Mattered.* (New York: Harper and Row, 1973), pp. 29–30.

2. I heard a fine definition of an optimist the other day. He or she is one who, watching a football game on TV and seeing his/her team's wide receiver break in the clear, move into open field position, and then drop the perfect pass, stays tuned—expecting that the receiver will probably catch it on the video instant replay.

ill about things going to perdition in a handbasket. What's more, you ought not to get too worked up about how the rest of the world is squandering the earth's resources if you are not doing your own small part to conserve and use wisely what there is. Self-responsibility extends beyond accepting what you can do for yourself to embrace a reasonable concern for the environment and other living things; this is another aspect of being an effective and well-adjusted adult. It just feels better to know that you are not contributing to the problems.

In discussing this dimension of wellness, I would like you to think of the environment as having three aspects—the physical, the social, and the personal. The first two components are rather familiar and self-evident: they refer to the extent to which all aspects of air, water, land mass, and other physical configurations combine with social conditions (economic, governmental, cultural, etc.) to act upon the individual and enhance or limit health and well-being. The personal component of environment refers to the extent to which your immediate surroundings either affirm or deny, or facilitate or inhibit, your efforts to pursue high level wellness. Another way to think of the personal component of this dimension is to talk of a "space" or spaces, which I define as all the stimuli or forces acting upon a person at any point in time. To the extent that you learn to design and shape the spaces under your control, you are planning your personal environment and making it easier to enjoy the pursuit and experience of high level wellness.

The air you breathe, the city or town in which you live, the quality of your home, and the attractions or shortcomings of your neighborhood are all examples of physical and social environments. The manner in which you organize your bedroom or work space, the kinds of friendship networks you create and sustain, and the nature of the feedback about yourself which you invite by your actions, are all examples of the personal environment, or spaces you consciously or unknowingly set up for yourself.

Most of us are relatively insensitive to our physical and social environments, and are even less attuned to the personal spaces around us which vastly affect our health and well-being.

163

If you commit yourself to a lifestyle of high level wellness, you will have to cultivate an awareness of the physical and social components of the environment. You will also deliberately design your personal environment.

There are severe limits to what most of us can do to change the physical and social aspects of our larger environments. The problems of population expansion, air pollution and other forms of pollution, atomic waste, urban blight, inflation, and all forms of social dissolution are beyond the province of the individual. But, while it is difficult to change, affect, shape, order, and design your relationship to these overarching physical and social environments, it is both easy and enjoyable to design the personal component of your environment.

The first step in doing so is to increase your sensitivity to all the stimuli that touch upon your senses at any point in time. These may be physical, mental, chemical, or anything else. You create a great deal of your physical, social, and personal environments by your choice of place, career, job, friends, and lifestyle. In turn, these environments, or spaces, affect all aspects of your life. There are many reasons why it pays to learn to shape a space. A positive environment will help you stay healthy and move toward high level wellness, whereas a negative environment will block your growth toward well-being and all manner of positive expression. The right kind of a space-fit "potentiates" you and helps you to choose the best for yourself. The wrong kind of fit can undermine your health and diminish the benefits you would otherwise derive from attending to all the other wellness dimensions.

When the personal component of your environment is not contributing to your well-being, you experience what an "eco-space design engineer" would call a "demand load."[3] A demand

---

3. I want to credit my good friend and advisor Leland R. Kaiser, Ph.D., an associate professor in the Department of Preventive Medicine, University of Colorado Medical Center, with encouraging me to think about and study eco-space design. A good deal of this material is based upon concepts first formulated in articles by Dr. Kaiser, which you may obtain by writing the good professor at the University of Colorado Medical Center, 4200 East 9th St., Denver CO 80220. The major articles by Dr. Kaiser which I recommend are: "Increasing Personal Effectiveness"; "Personal Qualities"; "Personal Dimensions: A Guide for Self Explorations"; "Planning for Survival"; and "Requirements of a Healthy Environment."

load is a burden, just as the name implies, and it can hold you down and drag you under. The weight of a poor fit between who you are and want to become versus how you are living and where you genuinely think you are going can upset you and create distress. So it is essential that you attend to this dimension in order to live a wellness lifestyle.

An ability to understand how you can shape the various aspects of your environment, a recognition of how you are in turn affected by those environments, and a skill in arranging those aspects of your spaces which you can control are all part of environmental sensitivity. The following principles are intended as guides to your own individualized approach. Use them to learn to shape spaces that will affirm you and help you become whom you want to be—spaces that will make it so much easier to pursue the principles and practices related to self-responsibility, nutritional awareness, stress management, and physical fitness.

Principles for Physical/Social Environmental Sensitivity

1. Do yourself and the world a favor—live lightly on the earth. You cannot save the world, or even change very much the physical and social environments. You *can* affect your own well-being by pollution-defensive and energy-conscious behavior. Consider not living in places where the carbon monoxide levels represent a clear and present danger to your health, not buying foods that raise the amount of DDT in your body fat, and otherwise doing what you can to avoid the hundreds of similar dangers to living creatures resulting from physical and social insensitivities.

Why not abandon the typical American energy binge, even if you can afford such increasingly expensive highs? Turn off lights and gadgets that require power when they are not in use, and use these things less often. Walk when possible, make do with less, avoid disposable and processed products, recycle or cut back on convenience items, grow at least some of your own food, and insulate your home. Consider doing something "freaky" like composting your organic wastes, using energy from the sun, or pursuing some other endeavor expressive of environmental respect. Living ecologically is a "no-lose" proposition. Even if you personally do not change the world, you will find that doing well with less helps to make you feel better by giving the satisfaction that comes from doing your part.

2. If you smoke, try extra hard to quit; if you do not, assert yourself around those who do.   Other than self-flagellation and successful suicide attempts, nothing seems more antiwellness and proworseness than smoking (pipes, cigars, cigarettes, anything). You know all this, of course, but for the record, be advised that smoking heats the tissues of the respiratory system, depletes the body of nutrients, and causes noxious gases inimical to people who breathe. The linkage with cancer, bronchitis, emphysema, and half a dozen other conditions is so evident it would bore you to recount the facts. Smoking blocks the transfer of oxygen from the lungs to the blood, causing an imbalance in blood gas and electrolytes. Since the tobacco is grown in fields usually drenched in pesticides, these poisons get into the lungs of those exposed to noxious fumes.

There are innumerable approaches to smoking abatement; one that seems especially promising is active involvement in developing your own wellness program. As others have discovered, those who get into exercise, thoughtful diet practices, stress-management activities, and environmental programs build up a momentum of satisfaction and strength of resolution that makes cessation of destructive habits easier.[4] And the rest of us can help those who want to quit, and ourselves, by safeguarding and defending our own rights not to be polluted by those who value their health so much less than we cherish our own.

3. Eat lower on the food chain.   It is in your interest to develop a taste for rice, beans, wheat, barley, oats, and all kinds

---

4. When you give up a destructive behavior such as smoking, it is important to have something better to add to your life, such as a wellness program of your own devising. Katie Baker of the New England Center told me that the best substitute, at first, is group support.

of things that grow from organic soils. They require less energy to produce and are better for you than meats, many experts tell us. They are certainly likely to be more readily available in the future at lower cost than pork, beef, and other animal products which currently constitute the staples of U.S. diet habits.

4. Living wisely is your best revenge.   Fuel costs are sky-rocketing, as power companies win one rate increase after another. One way to strike back is to use less of their products. Let the house get a bit chilly in winter, for example. Just dress warmly and have lots of blankets. Some believe our homes are too warm for our health in any case, causing colds and assorted upper respiratory problems. A temperature of 65°F. is quite comfortable when you get used to the idea of wearing a sweater, jacket, or other warm garment around the home. And, as I've mentioned, using less of a limited resource is a fine way to save money.

5. Boycott the fast-foods industry.   In addition to serving primarily junk food, the fast-food chains are energy hogs: the serving plates, utensils, wrappers, condiments, plates, cups, and all the rest are one-way products. Neither you nor the planet are likely to derive much benefit from this industry's continued success. Of course, you alone cannot hurt its business, but you might derive some personal satisfaction, as well as avoid empty calories, by virtue of dining elsewhere. And, of course, if enough people act as you do, such practices might change. But do not count on this in the near term (and in the long term, we will all be dead).

6. Consider participating in an environmentally oriented organization.   There is no shortage of worthy groups, wherever you may live. The list includes the Sierra Club, Zero Population Growth, Planned Parenthood, Friends of the Earth, and countless others. Do not expect to have much impact on the world situation; your purposes are to become better informed and to feel good by becoming involved. Rain dances did not have much effect on the weather, either, but they certainly lifted the Indians' morale.

7. Have fewer children—or more of someone else's.   We are
at or near zero population growth in this country for many
reasons. Among them are changed economic conditions, greater
freedom for women to pursue careers, birth-control advances
and acceptance, and a greater environmental consciousness than
previously existed.   Having children can be a beautiful
experience; I have two and there is no question but that they are
great joys. To love and be loved, to need them and know that
they depend upon me—these are among the fulfillments that ac-
company being an involved parent. But it is equally "right" not
to have children for whatever options you prefer. In my view, it
seems of special value to adopt or otherwise care for someone
else's child. The world, and this nation, are plentifully popu-
lated with unwanted infants, tots, older children, and particularly children having learning disabilities, handicaps, or other
disadvantages in getting started in life. To have or not to have
children is a very personal choice. One measure of a good choice
is that you feel good about whatever it is you do.

Principles for Personal
Environmental Sensitivity

1. Catalog the impact of your personal environment.   Do not
be oblivious to the obvious. We are shaped by our spaces from
birth to death, and we too seldom take time to identify, catego-
rize, and assess the impact of these images. Even less often do
we take time to deliberately design our office, home, and
leisure-place environments. Think about what upsets you in the
course of a day, what interrupts, distracts, or prevents you from
doing something constructive in one or more of the other wellness dimensions. Then make a list of things, events, sounds,
scents, opportunities (e.g., for recreation and relaxation) that
could be *added* to your daily routine. Evaluate the positive and
negative impact of that of which you had not been conscious,
and consider what you might want to do about these conditions
affecting your health. Consider that your goal in environmental
sensitivity is to structure spaces to enhance your well-being and
lead to continued progress toward self-actualization. In our

childhood we had to adapt to and cope with handed-down spaces, but as adults we have the opportunity to design and shape our spaces to a great extent. In a very real sense, it is a matter of shape or be shaped.

I'll give you a brief example of what I mean. There is convenient bus service from Mill Valley to the San Francisco financial district, two blocks from where I have an office. The bus is comfortably air-conditioned and makes the run to the city in less than 25 minutes. But I take a shuttle bus instead to Sausalito, then transfer to the Golden Gate ferry, which docks at the Ferry Building in San Francisco, an eight-block walk to my office. The trip takes over an hour, as compared with the 25-minute express bus. But I take the ferry every morning, and return on it every night. Why? Because of the psychic income I derive from the quality of that commuting. The sights, sounds, the cold and clean wind—so many things about that ride on the Bay contribute to a daily celebration of being alive and involved in the experience of high level wellness. This one space-shaping activity makes me better able to deal with any negative events that may face me, and helps make all the good things seem even richer. I have shaped this space, and it, in turn, shapes me for hours.

2. Upgrade your needs to preferences.   You are better off if you would *like* something to happen than if your well-being is *dependent* upon it. Try to psychologically upgrade while emotionally downgrading your needs, wants, desires, requirements, musts, and the like, to circumstances and events that are preferred. If you do this, you will more often be pleased with successes and less often disappointed by failures. As a planning agency director, I had this maxim as my guide in setting organizational objectives: "Better to promise a little less than I expect to accomplish; and thus pleasantly surprise people, than to promise more than is realistic and eventually disappoint." The same principle can be applied in your life: promise yourself a little less and place moderate emotional stock in passionate needs, and just see if you don't end up with a lot more in a context of diminished turmoil and wasted emotion. If you don't get something you prefer, it is not the end of the world; when you achieve a preference, on the other hand, you achieve more perspective and enjoy as much satisfaction as you would from realizing a need.

3. Become an "eco-space" engineer. You deserve a fancy title if you have the foresight to deliberately arrange your personal environment to enhance the positive and minimize the negative elements in your life. And there is so much that you can do for yourself in this way. By becoming sensitive to the possibilities which everyday elements of your personal environment have for potentiating or negating, it is possible to increase the enhancements and avoid the unpleasantries.

For example, Muzak hits me as an insidious banality—I cannot recall hearing sounds from this system which have not either distracted or annoyed me. Muzak ranks high among the elements in my personal environment that cause me stress, along with people who smoke up my airspace, shout, whistle, pass gas, and pick their noses in public. Since I cannot change the behavior of others, I simply arrange my work space and leisure times to minimize contact with Muzak or people who engage in behaviors that annoy me.

You can engineer your own spaces in order to minimize those things which annoy and negate you, and for the purpose of attracting an abundance of whatever environmental aspects (e.g., quiet, plants, sunlight) reinforce your sense of well-being.

4. Match your values and spaces. Take an inventory of what is important to you, and examine the extent to which your personal environment works to enable or to frustrate your priorities. To what extent are the following values representative of your choices, and how well is your life organized, structured, and shaped to bring them about?

- Opportunities for continued self-development and expression;
- Prospects for frequent "rewards" of good feedback on accomplishments;
- Roles to play that you judge as important;
- Plentiful chances to give and obtain affection;

- Freedom from threats (financial security, bodily harm, etc.);
- Opportunities to be with friends and support networks, to experience leisure, and to control your destiny;
- Exposure to beauty, nature, and poetry;
- Reinforcement of health-promotive behaviors; and
- Variety, change, risk, the acceptance of failure, and the strength to recover.

5. Don't stay bored or unhappy with your life.   You cannot expect that your life will, every day, be joyous, satisfying, or otherwise terrific, or even OK. There will be disappointments, sorrows, and unhappy periods. They are a part of life too, and you can accept that reality. However, our expectations for a full life can temper and soften such occasions, and help us recover and move on as we age to new satisfactions and personal rewards. Studies of long-lived people (e.g., the Abkhasians, Hunzas, and Vilcabambans) suggest that it is not what happens in life that determines happiness and well-being, but "how you take it" that really matters. An individual who thinks he is happy is a "success"; successful aging might be thought of as accepting the consequences of choices made, and believing of life as Erik Erickson did, that "it was the best it could have been."[5]

6. Stay current with yourself on the basic questions.   An essential ingredient in the maintenance of a high level wellness lifestyle is the constant self-nurturance of a fully alive mind. People with a sense of who they are, how they got that way, where they want to go, and similar indications of self-awareness and wholeness have access to well-being not possible to those unwilling to pause for introspections about basic questions and purposes.

An important part of this is always becoming a more effective person. No matter how "together" you are, there are ways of taking self-stock that will help you generate new images of possibilities for your life. By observing your own behavior or

---

5.   Grace Halsell, *Los Viejos: Secrets of Long Life from the Sacred Valley* (Emmaus, Pa.: Rodale Press, 1976) p. 173.

"profiling" yourself, you can gain an introspective view of who you are, how you feel, and what you think. For example, ask yourself the following questions to test the degree to which you are skilled at self-observation and self-awareness:

1. What are your three most important beliefs?
2. What are your most cherished goals today, how have these goals changed in the past few years, and what obstacles stand in the way of your realizing current goals?
3. Characterize your early childhood space.
4. Describe your strong and weak knowledge areas.
5. Identify three character-building experiences in your life.
6. Discuss the kind of person you would like to become.
7. What adjectives would you use to describe yourself?
8. What raises, and what depresses, your energy levels?
9. What changes would you like to make in yourself in the next few years?
10. What evidence can you furnish that you are happy?
11. What are you most and least likely to notice about another person?[6]

The energy and vision generated in confronting such "inner spaces" always converts into the kind of a person you will be in your "outer spaces" or behaviors. As this illustrative set of questions implies, there are many domains acting upon your personal effectiveness. It is essential to know who you are to decide how you want to be. Learning to be comfortable with introspective questions such as these will help you adapt to and cope with spaces that cannot be avoided, and to design and shape spaces that are under your control. Your spaces can constitute a prison, limiting what you expect of yourself, or they can be expansive, allowing you to transcend to ever-higher realms of experience. To be genuinely effective, you should be in touch with and aware of the manner in which you determine and manage your personal environment.

---

6. Leland R. Kaiser, "Guide to Personal Effectiveness" (See footnote 3.)

7. Learn to recognize a poor space fit.   A "bad" space can be sensed intuitively because it is an energy drain. The demand load will wear you out. In addition, a poor space fit evokes worseness behavior, and makes a wellness lifestyle much more difficult to pursue. When you have a good space condition, you can get more done in less time because of the "high" such a space provides. A space should trigger inherent possibilities and contribute to the emergence of your best potentialities. If what you are doing (e.g., smoking, drinking six cups of coffee daily) does not make you feel better and more effective, stop doing it and find substitutes that do.

8. Do more for your future than hang around waiting for it.
Like planning, for example, which is always better than just working with the results of unanticipated events, circumstances, and consequences. Your ability to plan for your own future, which is shaping the big spaces to come, is very much determined by the extent to which you believe the future is open (not determined), flexible (not dependent on factors outside your control), and promising. Having a vision helps to bring it about, just as gloomy or negative expectations have a way of fulfilling themselves. You probably know more than a few people who "make themselves right" by affirming negative realities (e.g., "I can't stop smoking"), which of course become self-fulfilling prophecies. One element that will serve you well in planning your future relationship to your personal environment is a "survival kit" containing a high degree of self-awareness, a philosophy of life, a sense of humor, and a perception of change as opportunity (rather than crisis). With such a "kit," you will shape your future more than it will shape you.

Some Space-
Shaping Techniques

Like expanding the other dimensions, building environmental sensitivity should be a fun and energizing endeavor that complements and becomes an integral part of an overall wellness lifestyle. My own approach to this dimension is to focus upon the personal environmental aspect, in part for strategic reasons and in considerable part because the physical and social components are reasonably attended simply by virtue of where I live. If I were now located in a city burdened with the recognized problems of urban blight, including overcrowding, ugliness, isolation from nature, pollution, a barren culture, and constant anxieties of a social and economic nature, I would get out. I know that seems impractical for many people because of investments in a nontransferable job, family roots, and all the rest. But the price, in my value framework, is too great. A wellness lifestyle is possible in a blighted city, but the energy required to deal with the negatives seems excessive to me. So, given my values and commitment to wellness in all five of its dimensions, I would sacrifice whatever I had to surrender to live in a compatible physical and social space. That way, I could, as I do, concentrate on shaping my personal spaces for affirmations. Free from gross physical and social environmental problems, I can concentrate on "getting my way" ethically and responsibly, which equates with finding and giving love, realizing self-expression and fulfillment, experiencing risk-taking and growth, and otherwise enjoying a high level of well-being and change as my life goes by.

Part of the way I shape space for these purposes involves arranging lots of little things that make each day a bit richer. For example, I carry a small tape recorder with the classical music I enjoy on trips out of town, and I pack nutritious foods rather than rely on restaurants that generally do not offer the kind of food I enjoy. I also arrange my home in a way that suits my lifestyle, insuring that my work place has none of the trappings that disturb or annoy me, developing work agreements with employers (and employees) which allow for an exercise period in the middle of each day, and being clear in relationships about expectations and feelings as they evolve.

I thought President Carter made a nice contribution to the national well-being when he instructed his cabinet and White House staff members to safeguard their family space and avoid the tendency to become workaholics. Soon after his inauguration, the President was reported to have advised his people to the effect that "you'll be so much more useful to me and to the country if you do have some recreation, get some exercise, see your children and your spouses." While President Carter may not get around to singling you out for such counsel, you know the validity of safeguarding family and other space-time from the temptations of job and career. Sometimes, it helps to be reminded.

Anyone can design his or her spaces to make life a bit pleasanter, more comfortable, more wellness-inducing, or to contribute to whatever outcome he or she desires. A friend of mine, Julia Kendall Lynn, who designed stress-reduction workshops specifically for typists based on her typing experience and study of kinesiology, told me she used to suffer shoulder and back pain at the end of nearly every day when her work required heavy typing duties. One day, she got the idea that instead of accommodating her body to the space somebody else had arranged, she would organize her own personal environment. To her amazement, at the end of the first day of experimenting with deliberate space designs, Julie discovered an improved attitude toward others, greater effectiveness at her work, and much better feelings toward and images of herself. For Julia, space design meant coordinating typewriter placement, particularly height from the floor, the height of her chair, the location of her back support, and the location of supplies "so that my body can remain in comfortable alignment. I balance evenly on my buttocks, my spine straight and flexible, my head balanced. If necessary, I place a box or telephone-book footrest under my feet so that my knees are directly over my ankles, my thighs parallel to the floor. As soon as I recognize strain in my body, usually under my shoulder blades, my lower back, my neck, I do whatever is necessary to let go of that tension. I take a short break, go to the restroom and stretch and shake. I pound my buttocks with my fists. I swivel my hips, slowly, sensuously. I become a belly danger, breathing deeply, breathing aliveness all over my body. I treat myself gently, respecting my physical ranges in my muscles and joints." Julia said she found it essential to recognize and release tension early.

You can make up your own techniques for releasing the tightness or other physical symptoms of a poor space fit. "Sometimes," Julia remarked, "I find that just by stopping for 30 seconds, closing my eyes, and taking a few long deep breaths, pushing all my breath out completely on the exhale and letting my body inhale at its own speed, I can avoid feeling trapped in a space that does not feel right." Julia then described another technique I had not heard about, but one which seems so well suited to her unique approach to work-space design: "I isolate my body movements. While my fingers type, the rest of my body is relaxed. Relaxing doesn't mean collapsing. Relaxing means using the appropriate set of muscles to perform a movement. Periodically, I mentally scan my body, consciously loosening. I stop and shake my hands and massage them. I thank them for typing so well. I appreciate myself."

I work with a physician in Chicago who has arranged a "stay well" space for his children that illustrates how in shaping our spaces they shape us. Bruce Flashner, the head of the Arthur Young and Company health-care practice, told me that his children (who range from preschool through high school ages) have always been given the responsibility to determine when they are too ill to go to school. If they decide to stay home, they are presumed to be ill, and Dr. Flashner considers quiet and rest the best remedies. Thus, the children remain in their room for a minimum of 24 hours. Juice, fruit, and similar foods are sparingly made available, but there are no books, TV, telephone, games, or other enjoyable activities or amusements allowed; nothing but quiet rest to speed the healing process. Sickness is not punished, of course, but it certainly is not rewarded or reinforced in any way.

The result? The children are rarely ill; the "Flashner Method" produces a strong will to stay well and recover quickly when sickness does occur. A Flashner child does not stay home when a difficult exam must be faced, or when difficulties occur between the child and the teacher or classmates, or when similar tensions arise that children face just as often as adults. In my view, Dr. Flashner has shaped a "stay well" space. When illness occurs, it is genuine and the seclusion treatment speeds recovery; when a child is not quite healthy but able to function, going to school and wanting to feel better is clearly the best option, and usually leads to an early recovery from incipient illness. The space design in this model shapes and reinforces a "will" to be well.[7]

I could go on with details of my own environmental sensitivity designs and more examples of how my friends go about it, but these illustrations should be enough to encourage you to think about ways to set up your own spaces.

Well, there it is—everything you need to know to put together your own, completely unique high level wellness lifestyle. Like me, I'm sure you'll discover that to experience wellness, to know the difference it makes, and to feel what it's like inside and out is the best reward for pursuing this treasured state of being. But working at developing a more positive image of health—which is what high level wellness represents—also can help you to set and realize greater expectations for yourself. And living a wellness philosophy can, in my view, help you to reduce dramatically your share of what Erich Fromm[8] has termed the "pathology of normalcy"—the patterned defects (e.g., smoking, junk-food consumption, conditions of tension and anxiety, inactivity) shared by so many in our society. Popular as they are, these habits *seem* normal, but in fact they are sickness-inducing. When you are well enough to "celebrate your life," you'll be unlikely to accept such pathologies as normal. One day you'll probably leave them behind, as just so much excess baggage slowing your ascent to the exhilarating heights of wellness.

---

7. Dr. Flashner insists that he did *not* get the idea for this approach to space design from Samuel Butler's Erewhon, the 1872 utopian satirical classic that describes a culture wherein illness and disease are punishable offenses, a custom having the effect of discouraging acquiescence in ills which might be avoided or remedied.

8. Erich Fromm, "Humanistic Planning," *Journal of the American Institute of Planners*, vol. 38, no. 2 (March 1972) p. 71.

Part 3

Toward A Healthier Nation

A Contemporary Fable: Upstream/Downstream

It's been many years since the first body was spotted in the river. Some old-timers remember how spartan were the facilities and procedures for managing that sort of thing. Sometimes, they say, it would take hours to pull 10 people from the river, and even then only a few would survive.

Though the number of victims in the river has increased greatly in recent years, the good folks of Downstream have responded admirably to the challenge. Their rescue system is clearly second to none: most people discovered in the swirling waters are reached within 20 minutes, many in less than 10. Only a small number drown each day before help arrives; a big improvement from the way it used to be.

Talk to the people of Downstream and they'll speak with pride about the new hospital by the edge of the waters, the flotilla of rescue boats ready for service at a moment's notice, the comprehensive health plans for coordinating all the manpower involved, and the large number of highly trained and dedicated swimmers always ready to risk their lives to save victims from the raging currents. Sure it costs a lot, but, say the Downstreamers, what else can decent people do except to provide whatever it takes when human lives are at stake.

Oh, a few people in Downstream have raised the question now and again, but most folks show little interest about what's happening Upstream. It seems there's so much to do to help those in the river, that nobody's got time to check how all those bodies are getting there in the first place. That's the way things are, sometimes.

There are uncountable lists of things you can do to help make this country a healthier land and reverse the patterns of low level worseness that contribute to illness and disease in our nation. Yet, everything that can be included in these lists essentially reduces into two kinds of action: what you can do for and by yourself, and what you can do for the country as a participant with others. The preceding section of this book has concentrated on you-for-and-by-yourself; my own belief is that we can do little for others if we neglect our own well-being: besides, a wellness philosophy and a worseness lifestyle could provoke a credibility gap. However, assuming that you have made a personal commitment to pursue a wellness lifestyle in a manner suited to your own preferences and values and are comfortable acting out that personalized approach to well-being, you can do much of benefit to the larger culture.

There are, as I've already noted, innumerable specific policies that ought to be changed and almost no end to the number of steps that should be taken to reduce the risks of illness and enable people who want greater health to have a better chance for it. Yet, I believe that two basic strategies are sufficient for most people who want to go beyond the recommended priority focus on oneself to some social action.

The first strategy involves practicing personal assertiveness and effective techniques in communicating with individuals, business firms, local elected and appointed officials, national leaders in the congress, the president, or anyone else who has real or potential influence on policy issues that affect your well-being and ability to pursue a wellness lifestyle. The second strategy is to learn about your local health-planning organization, and begin to develop ways to "take over" that operation.

Practicing the
Artful Complaint

The first strategy is a simple and yet remarkably effective approach to change. It is, quite simply, that if you do not like something you complain about it. In this case, the idea is that if enough people complain *properly* to the right people about practices not in the interests of their well-being, changes will eventually be made that will benefit us all.

It helps to know how to complain. A well-put complaint, or compliment, can be a persuasive thing. It is important to communicate your concern in a manner that clarifies the nature of the problem, what can and should be done about it, why it is in the other's interest to consider your suggestion, and your appreciation for the serious attention you anticipate being given to your presentation. Of course, maybe you already know how to do this and are therefore accustomed to getting results. If so, terrific, and please keep it up. If not, consider practicing ways to tell people of your commitment to a wellness lifestyle when they behave in ways that interfere with it, and particularly get in the habit of informing storekeepers, politicians, and others about ways they can maintain your support. Let's take some examples. Suppose, like me, you are either inconvenienced, annoyed, or fit-to-be-tied about one or more of the following conditions:

• Having to visit out-of-the-way health food stores to buy herbal teas, raw certified milk, yogurt without artificial colors, and ice cream made with honey and no stabilizers, preservatives, or sugar.

● Being forced either to wait for another plane or to accept a seat in the smoking section when the nonsmoking section is already reserved on busy flights.

● Being stuck in an office or work area where noise pollution (Muzak, jackhammers, buzz saws, anything that is tension-producing) leaves your nerves frazzled by day's end.

● Having to suffer slights from a dentist or physician (e.g., unwillingness to explain medical procedures, causes of illness, or prevention techniques) because the doctor seems so busy and you seem (to him/her) to have nothing else to do with your time.

● Finding yourself in a parental crisis because the dry-cleaning lady, the town shoemaker, the neighborhood barber, and the sales clerk at Macy's all have this "friendly" habit of giving lollipops and assorted candies to the children, without asking if it is okay (with me, it is not).

Some of these illustrations from personal experience are, of course, minor grievances which hardly seem worth mentioning; others are more serious. It just depends on how you see things, based on your experiences, attitudes, and values. A few of the examples just given are purely local matters which you can deal with right then and there; other cases (i.e., the airline smoking dilemma) involve complex bureaucracies, conflicting interest groups, and oftentimes years of effort before you get results, if you ever do. In either extreme, you'll feel better after advising the other person or a company representative of your concern about a practice which you consider unhealthy. If enough people politely make clear that their continued patronage depends on a reasonable consideration for their concerns, and if the people who are committing the offending "worseness" behaviors are given ego-preserving ways to meet the needs of wellness-oriented folks, then our prospects for changing big and little, local and national, concerns will increase dramatically.

The "power of the people" to effect change through both individual and group strategies is enormous, and has been demonstrated dramatically on numerous occasions. Recognize *your* potential to make a difference, and learn to use it to facilitate a wellness lifestyle for yourself and others. Learn to complain effectively. Don't bully, don't exaggerate, and don't emphasize the dire consequences to the individual or company if they do not do what you want them to do, or cease doing what you do not want them to do. They will know where you stand and what you would like if you explain your ideas in even-tempered, reasoned commentary. They will appreciate the importance of maintaining your patronage if you mention (matter-of-factly) the number of people in your club or group who feel as you do. And you can probably even manage to compliment the offending group or its representative for something already done or being done to make it easier to pursue a wellness lifestyle. Do not expect sudden, dramatic changes, of course, and do avoid allowing your happiness and well-being to depend entirely on someone else doing something for you. But do not be too surprised when changes are made as you and others who share your commitment to high level wellness begin to unite and speak out for the innumerable small and not-so-small changes that need to occur as we move toward a healthier nation. No doubt of it, there's a lot to be said for group action. But don't wait around for a mass movement or an organization of some kind before taking some personal action to let "them" know where you stand or how you feel about concerns relevant to your well-being.

In addition to a myriad of relatively minor annoyances, there are a good many serious matters that deserve attention. You will no doubt have your own list, but just for the fun of it I'll share mine with you. If you have not drawn up your list and written a few (effective) letters (or made phone calls, personal contacts, etc.), this might encourage you to get started.

Changing Medical Care

If you and I and a great many others begin to *expect* preventive medicine, if we *demand* that our doctors emphasize what it is we need to do to avoid future illnesses and gain greater well-being, if, in short, we all let our medical friends know that we *require* health education as a part of the healing process, then we will see a change in both the physician's self-concept and the role of American medicine. Naturally, we cannot expect kindly old Doc Jones to become a late-blooming John Travis or the local Medicaid mill to convert to a wellness resource center, but the health education contributions the average physician can make are substantial, nonetheless. I remember economist Dr. Kenneth Boulding's comment to the effect that 1910 was a great year marking the advancement of modern medicine to a creditable science. Because "for the first time in history an average patient displaying more or less standard symptoms presenting himself to a representative physician stood better than a 50/50 chance of benefiting from the experience." From the standpoint of health education, perhaps 1978 might come to represent an equally notable watershed.

One of the changes I would like to see made a part of every physician/client relationship is a contract, either a verbal or preferably an informal one-page written agreement wherein the physician acknowledges his secondary role and the client agrees that the major responsibility for his health rests with himself. This might shift the primary role in maintaining well-being on to the client, where it belongs, and do a lot more than the PR campaigns and dangerous practices of defensive medicine (prescribing dubious tests and procedures to "cover" against contingencies) to alleviate the malpractice insurance problem.

Physicians might do well to ask clients in the beginning about what kind of health they want. A doctor could say: "Tell me, Mr. Smith, do you want the 'el cheapo' variety—no work/sweat/discipline/special effort required, or the premium brand—which requires a great deal of attention on your part to fashion and secure?" Just by raising the issue of personal responsibility and the limits of medicine, the physician will have provided a valuable service.[1]

So whenever I talk to doctors, medical associations, or

---

1. At least one malpractice attorney knowledgeable about holistic approaches to well-being has spoken out in favor of the contract mechanism. For more information about this attorney, Jerry A. Green, see "A Novel Approach to Malpractice" in the *Sunday Scene* section of the *San Francisco Examiner and Chronicle* (30 May 1976) and a similar article in *Marin Sonoma Living*, the weekend magazine published by the *Independent Journal*, (19 June 1976). Or write Mr. Green at 273 Page St., San Francisco CA 94102.

other medical system interests, I raise these kinds of concerns. And while it has not created any revolutions, I suspect that when I do show up in a doctor's office or hospital someday, I'm going to have a contract laid on me!

In the meantime, you and I should expect more than pills from a physician. Ask him or her what areas of your lifestyle might need attention, whether biofeedback or other methods of getting in touch with your stress levels might be useful, or if there are alternatives to medications and medical procedures, particularly surgery. If the answer is an adamant no, or if you feel intimidated for so much as having asked, consider finding another physician. And suggest to your friends and associates that they do likewise. Then write to the local medical society, and let them know that you believe physicians should be more aware of health-enhancement concepts and approaches, and suggest that this be considered as part of continuing education programs. Medical interests can be just as responsive as other marketing groups to consumer demands, and this one could save you more than money.

Making the Work Place
a (Partial) Wellness Center

Employers overlook opportunities to encourage wellness behaviors amongst their employees. Many people need help in getting started on a fitness program, for example, and employers large and small could gain from encouraging them and providing incentives for them to do so.

Last year, General Motors Corporation spent more money on employee medical benefits than it spent on the steel required for the cars it built. And General Motors is not alone; a representative of the National Association of Manufacturers testified to the Congress last year that its member organizations spent 6 percent of their payrolls on medical insurance and related costs.[2] All indications are that these figures will rise dra-

---

2. "Statement of the National Association of Manufacturers on Health Care Costs" made before the Council on Wage and Price Stability, 20 July 1976. Available from NAM, 1776 F Street N.W., Washington, D.C. 20016.

matically; perhaps doubling by 1980. One result will be raised prices, making U.S. firms less competitive with foreign companies, and leading to lower profits and fewer jobs. And yet, no improvement in the health of the work force is either likely or expected.

Rather than throwing more money at treating disease, big and little businesses could probably increase productivity, lower absenteeism, improve morale, and otherwise decrease the extent of illness by promoting wellness at the company's expense. Just think of all the things that could be done. For example, companies could:

• Provide benefits at local YMCAs, such as special class times for company employees and testing/counseling/and monitoring programs.

• Subsidize quit-smoking clinics, and health screening with wellness inventories, diet-counseling lectures and wellness readings.

• Offer special incentives for employees to get started, such as posting activity charts in prominent places, giving publicity to the wellness programs (and participants) in company publications, making periodic awards, distributing big discount coupons for running shoes or other fitness equipment, and having longer lunch hours and one or two wellness days off a year (for those who are into wellness in a big way, and feel "too good" to come to work). It's better to give a free day or two than to lose a week or more when employees lose their health due to worseness lifestyles.

These are hypothetical examples, but there are several real-world "live" instances of corporations establishing attractive programs which make it easy for employees to exert active responsibility for their own well-being.

At Northern Natural Gas Company in Omaha, Nebraska,

about 800 of 1,500 employees belong to the company's Fitness Center. The center program, which is available for family members, is only $6 a month; facilities include a swimming pool, handball/squash/paddleball courts, running track, weight room, and a testing laboratory. Northern Natural Gas has three objectives for its Fitness Center program: (1) to encourage an awareness and appreciation of physical fitness among employees; (2) to provide employees with enjoyable and healthful recreation; and (3) to create a pleasant social-physical-recreational atmosphere for employees. The overall emphasis is upon aerobic conditioning, although the recreational nature of the program is a major motivator for participation. Employees with cardiovascular problems participate in endurance programs two to four times daily, also receiving careful diet counseling. For these employees, the benefits are measured in specific results, such as serum cholesterol and triglyceride levels, percent of body fat, resting heart rate, maximum oxygen uptakes, and lung functions. For the majority of employees, the anticipated results are those stated in the company brochure: "A physically fit person is better appearing, more alert, and has the capacity to produce over a sustained period . . . he is less susceptible to fatigue and sickness . . . he misses less work days and works at maximal capacity while on the job . . . . Fitness and health are vital both to the employer and the employee."

At Phillips Petroleum in Bartlesville, Oklahoma, about 5,000 of the company's 6,000 employees are members of the recreation program, which includes a fully equipped gymnasium, swimming pool, weight and exercise rooms, bowling lanes, softball fields, and more! The staff includes a full-time director of athletics and recreation and an administrator of recreation. Most employees, including the Chief Executive Officer and Chairman of the Board, participate in the company's Executive Fitness Program, which includes swimming, running, and exercising. The belief in a correlation between sound minds and bodies is strong at Phillips, where a company handout links fitness with greater health, efficiency, productivity, and morale. Both Mobil Oil and Exxon in New York City have had (nonrecreational) fitness programs for executive employees in their headquarters offices for several years. These efforts are much more than "fit kits for fat cats": the Mobil Oil Corporation sponsors a planned series of exercises tailored to the individual capabilities of employees under the close guidance of company staff. Exxon's program also involves about 200 executive-level employees on a three-times-per-week basis. Both companies report general benefits from their respective programs; a study of the Exxon endeavor revealed lower heart rates, improved grip strength, decreased body fats, and such subjective responses as an increased sense of well-being, reduced smoking and weight, and an improvement in employee morale.

But you don't have to work for a major gas or oil company to expect a wellness orientation from the managers of the work place; a small hospital in Redondo Beach, California has proven that. Employees at the South Bay Hospital are encouraged by time off to participate, plus other incentives, to enjoy a physical fitness and general body-conditioning program as an employee benefit. Exercises are designed to improve posture, body mechanics, joint flexibility, muscle tone, and general body conditioning. Administrator Jerry Greene says, "Our employees are all engaged in the business of health care for others. This exercise program will provide the opportunity for self-care and fitness." That makes a lot of sense to me, and I am going to be surprised if the leaders of organized labor do not begin to raise a new kind of demand at bargaining tables in the years to come. Imagine—a strike for high level wellness!

In addition to all the things a corporation can do to increase the opportunities for employees to accept responsibility for their own well-being, there are plenty of things companies ought *not* to do in order to make the work place a healthier setting. For example, it has been suggested that a great proportion of absenteeism and employee turnover is due to job boredom, stress, ugly surroundings, and a sense of hopeless routine rather than to general physical illness. An employer who cares enough to consider a range of positive wellness programs for employees will first want to examine and rectify any already existing negative, worseness conditions. And you, the employee, know far better than the top brass or expensive consultants what these sickness-inducing conditions are, if any. Let them hear from you.

Creating A Tax Shelter For Wellness

There is a growing recognition of the fact that this nation can neither afford nor be benefited by a continued reliance on the medical system as *the* way to improved national health status. Too many Americans suffer prematurely from degenerative diseases brought about by years of poor diet, inadequate exercise, high stress, boredom, unhappiness, and the general surrender of their sovereignty and commitment to enhancing their own minds and bodies. In my view, the U.S. Congress and the administration can nudge people toward healthier life patterns by providing incentives for wellness.

I think we should consider making it part of our national policy to use the income tax mechanism to promote the ethic of self-responsibility and to encourage citizens to learn more about what they can do for themselves.[3] If the congress were to provide a modest tax credit for authorized wellness expenses—a tax shelter of sorts for those who might want to resign from what Illich terms a "patient career," the government would make that possible. Elements of the proposal might include a tax credit for up to 1 percent of an individual's gross income for expenditures of a wellness nature.

Let's suppose that you earn $20,000, and that you choose to spend a moderate amount in the course of the year on wellness programs, courses, and seminars. You might attend an Erhard Seminars Training (EST) program (cost, $250), enroll in a series of lectures at the Wholistic Health and Nutrition Institute at a cost of $40, and go through the Wellness Inventory and evaluation at Travis's Wellness Resource Center at a cost of $150. Your total wellness investment would be $440; under the tax-shelter proposal, you could deduct $200 from your tax bill (or add it to the amount of your rebate). Of course, there are things of a wellness nature which you can do for yourself.

The range of such efforts, particularly in the dimensions of physical fitness, nutritional awareness, and stress management,

---

3. This would be quite a switch in policy for the IRS. On p. 167 of the 1976 edition of Lasser's *Your Income Tax*, the following can be found: "You may not deduct as a medical expense special foods and beverages unless they have no nutritional value to you and are taken only to alleviate or treat an illness."

is enormous. And your pursuit of such health enhancement efforts will require expenditures, which in the proposed tax shelter would be deductable to the 1 percent limit. In *Newsweek* (19 April 1976), national columnist George F. Will proposed that the IRS "allow people to deduct, as a cost of preventive medicine, the price of snappy double knit sweatsuits," noting that "the government subsidizes tobacco, so why not jogging?"

Depending upon the number of takers in each year, the proposal could cost the U.S. government up to $30 billion annually. Of course, it could save taxpayers dollars in other ways, such as by reducing the need and thus the expenditures for government-subsidized illness services which cost billions of dollars annually.

The tax shelter concept would encourage people to try a wellness program or two at government expense. Under such an approach, you and I would think (accurately) that we were actually losing out if we did not invest some time and effort in a health enrichment endeavor. The exposure to wellness philosophies and techniques would in turn strengthen our motivation to assume a more aggressive sense of control over our own destinies. This internal direction is the factor that can sustain the lifelong pursuit of high level wellness.

The U.S. government has long permitted the tax structure of this nation to be used in support of favored investments and industries. Most people are quite familiar with oil-depletion allowances, tax benefits related to capital gains and to mortgage interest costs, and countless other examples of tax policies designed to promote selected investments and developments. It does not seem inconsistent to me to expect that our government might give its support to investments that enhance the well-being of its people. The proposal for a tax shelter for wellness might deserve at least as much attention as national sick care.

So this is a third item on my own list, about which I'm quite willing to write, meet with, organize delegations to, and help elect sympathetic congressmen, senators, and presidents in order to promote specific strategies to help us move toward a healthier nation. Maybe if enough people do the same, we will get action and creative new directions.

Transforming Medical Institutions to Health Centers

We are all familiar with those great biomedical research bastions where you go in trauma and sickness, and to be certified dead. Many of these hospital complexes are termed "health centers" by the trustees and others who control them. Actually, that is really a fine idea, and I wish the term "health center" represented the way it is. There is, of course, nothing wrong with providing all the medical services in concert with wellness education. Unfortunately, despite the promising phrase "health center," the commitment to wellness education is nonexistent save in a very few remarkable places.[4]

Yet, these medical complexes have the facilities, resources, and opportunities for shifting the focus from treatment to health enhancement, education, and practice. If enough clients demand lifestyle education programs, nourishing foods, the elimination of cigarette, drug, and junk food vending machines from these centers, and insist on other wellness modalities, then the term "health center" might fit. And the patrons of these places will certainly be better off.

Imagine what would happen if the staff of a medical-center-type hospital were to take some training in health promotion practices and be exposed to the philosophies and approaches seen at such places as the Wellness Resource Center, or WHN. Or think of the benefits through changed attitudes and reorganized priorities that would occur in the traditional treatment-oriented hospitals if there were such an emphasis in medical and nursing programs and other provider training systems. Maybe what the medical institutions—and the people—really need is a new type of practitioner: a wellness resource guide trained in

---

4. The St. Helena Hospital and Health Center, a Seventh Day Adventist institution located about 30 miles north of San Francisco in Deer Park, California, is one such exception. Viewing lifestyle and environment as the prime determinants of illness, the center concentrates on ways to enable people to accept greater responsibility, to eliminate high-risk behaviors (special live-in programs are offered in smoking cessation, weight management, alcohol detoxification and rehabilitation, and executive health), and to teach wellness principles and approaches in the areas of nutrition, fitness, stress management, and environmental sensitivity. For more information write to the center in Deer Park CA 94576.

the basic medical approaches but aware of and attuned to the self-responsibility ethic of wellness. Such persons would be a blessing to encounter in most contemporary medical institutions.

Another dimension in the reform of the medical care system is the matter of encouraging medical self-care. Self-care can be taught at the school level and to adults; such skills are a universal attribute of all cultures and have historically accounted for the vast proportion of all health care. Self-care is a logical add-on to a wellness lifestyle, and a growing number of physicians are publishing books describing how we can, and when we should, be our own doctors.[5] Prior to World War II, families commonly made use of medical almanacs to diagnose and treat common ailments (e.g., high blood pressure and TB). However, the decades of medical "miracles" (vaccines, antibiotics, surgical techniques, complex diagnostic technologies) have undermined peoples' confidence in their abilities to learn to doctor themselves. We have lost sight of the fact that the treatment of many conditions has not been affected very much by all the medical marvels. In fact, the widespread abuse of prescription and over-the-counter drugs and the adverse effects of an increased dependency on doctors and diminished reliance on self have probably placed the average person in the late 1970s in a less-advantaged position in terms of health than a typical individual of thirty or forty years ago. In any event, you can enjoy the best of both eras by learning how to doctor yourself for most of what does or could ail you, avoiding the use of aspirin/drugs/all manner of pills save in extraordinary circumstances, and most of all by living a high level wellness lifestyle that vastly decreases your chances of needing either self-care *or* doctor care.

So, again, this kind of wide-reaching change is high on my

5. Such books include *How to Be Your Own Doctor (Sometimes); Take Care of Yourself: A Consumer's Guide to Medical Care; Self-Care: Lay Initiatives in Health; Managing Your Doctor; The Well-Body Book; Our Bodies, Ourselves: A Book by and for Women; A Barefoot Doctor's Manual;* and *An Everyday Guide to Your Health.* See review of *Our Bodies, Ourselves* in the Self-Responsibility section of the Wellness Resource Guide.

agenda for a healthier nation, and I am willing to communicate my suggestions to various officials, hospital administrators, and others. I want them to know I take the idea of a health center seriously. Maybe you will let them know what you think, also.

Influencing the Model for National Health Insurance

There are several bills for National Health Insurance before the congress, and most observers of the health system believe that the passage of such a program will occur in 1978 and 1979. NHI (which in fact is simply medical insurance) is focused on rising costs, poor access by some people to medical care, and inadequate distribution of services and programs—all serious problems, to be sure. Unfortunately, the Congressional proposals take for granted the assumptions that equate more medical care with better health. As a result, passage of NHI is likely to "lock in" everything that is wrong with today's medical system, particularly the hospital-centered, treatment-oriented, technology-weighted focus on disease, illness, and medical caregiving. No attention is to be given to incentives for self-care, personal responsibility, or education concerning any of the wellness dimensions. The opportunity to learn from the current "crisis" will be lost if the medical and public policy leaderships do not take a fresh look at foundation assumptions regarding the determinants of health.

The medical system is rife with inefficiencies that cost taxpayers and insurance purchasers dearly and encourage overtreatment, thus spreading iatrogenic (doctor-caused) illness. Further, the fear of malpractice suits does not automatically lead to higher quality care; in fact it often encourages procedures that make treatment more complicated and expensive, and testing more extensive than warranted. One doctor recently described how health insurers would not *allow* cost savings.[6] The doctor gave numerous examples wherein less expensive treatment (i.e., office surgery) was just as effective and safe as hospital

6. Andrew S. Markovits, "Health Insurers Won't *Let* Us Save Them Money," *Medical Economics* (10 January 1977), pp. 227–34.

care, yet the giant insurers would not cover the simplest procedures unless they were performed in a hospital operating room. Other examples have been cited to show how patients themselves sometimes find it easier and more logical to depend on the medical system for repairs than to live sensibly so as to stay well from the start. As one doctor reported, "A young mother I know recently insisted on rabies shots for her boy. He'd been bitten by a playful puppy under circumstances where the chances of his acquiring rabies were about one in a million. She insisted she didn't want to take any chances with her son's health, but when she drove away, the child was standing up in the front seat of the car, and she hadn't bothered with safety belts for either of them."[7]

If 10 percent of those of us concerned about the misdirected emphasis upon the medical model were to write to our newspapers and to our legislators, as well as raise the issue in church, social, and other organizations to which we belong, a lot of important people would surely take note. Eventually, such reappraisals could lead to a different kind of setup—one that truly deserves to be called a health system because of its incorporation of lifestyle and environment as legitimate dimensions of well-being.

Taking a Moderate Approach to Wellness Legislation

Nobody can or should be "forced" or "browbeaten" to adopt wellness behaviors or forego high risk habits and patterns, no matter how destructive such choices might be to individuals and how expensive they are to society. I agree with the Canadian Minister of Health and Welfare who wrote:

> While it is easy to convince a person in pain to see a physician, it is not easy to get someone not in pain to moderate insidious habits in the interests of future well-being. Nor is it easy to make environmental changes which

---

7.   George B. Markle, IV, " 'Perfect' Medical Care Just Costs Too Much," *Medical Economics* (24 January 1977), pp. 172–74.

cause social inconvenience when the benefits of those changes fall unevenly on the population and are only apparent over the long term. The view that Canadians have the right "to choose their own poison" is one that is strongly held.[8]

However, there are important steps of a regulatory and/or legislative nature that both can and should be taken to protect the rest of us who choose not to practice "worseness" patterns from those who do. Honor their right to poisons of their choice, yes; allow them to pollute or otherwise adversely affect us, no. So I am in favor of regulations, ordinances, rules, requirements, laws, and other mandated enactments that:

• Force restaurants to set aside at least half of all available space for nonsmokers through the enactment of federal legislation to this effect; by 1980, smoking in any public eating establishment should be totally barred.[9]

• Require employers covered by the Occupational Health and Safety Administration to provide optional physical fitness activities and/or stress management periods for all employees.

• Lead to the removal of junk food vending machines from public schools, hospitals, and long-term care facilities.

• Require managers of all office buildings to provide alternative food products (nonsugared, nonprocessed, nonrefined, etc.) if junk food machines are located on the premises.

---

8. Marc LaLonde, *A New Perspective on the Health of Canadians*, (Ottawa: Government of Canada, 1974), p. 6.

9. The rationale for federal rather than state or local laws to this or similar effect is to avoid uneven legislation in some places which would, of course, financially penalize restaurants in the nonbanning communities. Also, any federal effort in this direction would necessarily include an educational campaign on a far greater scale than the antismoking ads on TV a few years ago (which got very good smoking-reduction results). This in itself would be a major gain from such an endeavor.

• Encourage employers, particularly large manufacturing firms, to humanize the work place. Now I recognize that my view of a humane work place conducive to healthy employees is so subjective as to be of almost no use to the lawyer-types who draft laws, regulations, guidelines, and ordinances. However, there could be enactments by congress or a federal agency (e.g., OSHA) requiring employers of more than a minimal number of persons (10?) to prepare a plan with full participation by employees. The objective would be to make the work place a healthier setting within, say, a five-year time period. Such a participative process would almost certainly result in a plan that could contribute to reduced absenteeism and turnover, as the workers themselves become energized by the tasks of discovering ways to minimize conditions of boredom, stress, and ugliness.

• Lessen the health-denying impact of the media by inhibiting the child-directed promotion of foods high in saturated fats, cholesterol, sugar, and salt.

• Ban all advertisements of alcohol and tobacco products, including billboards, leaflets, free sample distributions, tournaments of athletic events carrying the names of such products, and other public displays of alcohol- and tobacco-related images or connotations.

• Increase taxes on alcohol, tobacco, and junk foods in proportion to the harmful substances within each (e.g., alcohol content, tar and nicotine, and refined sugar/preservatives), and direct the proceeds to research on them and treatment for their effects (cirrhosis of the liver, cancer, heart disease, etc.)

• Require that sugar-coated cereals, and all other products in which sugar comprises more than 20 percent of the item, be displayed in sections of supermarkets and other food stores clearly marked as "candies and other sweets." This will not prevent people from buying junk food if they really want it or believe they need it, but will help to make consumers conscious of what they are obtaining when they choose such products.

• Encourage the Federal Trade Commission to require networks to make prime time available for ads with wellness messages (in concert with the negative appeals, such as antismoking spots).

• Require the major health insurance companies (i.e., Blue Cross, Blue Shield) to pay for those things that in fact have to do with health, and not restrict payments to medical treatments. At a minimum, the health insurance giants ought to be experimenting in different locations with such matters as reimbursement for health education services (e.g., wellness evaluations such as are given at various centers) in order to estimate the impact over time on utilization of medical care.

• And, last, but not of least importance, require health impact statements on all new medical technologies and other policy actions by governments costing more than a certain amount (to be determined) or likely to affect large numbers of people. (Recall how few thought of the health effects when the speed limit was dropped to 55 mph, and yet this action, taken for energy conservation reasons, has been credited with saving thousands of lives through dramatic reductions in auto accidents.)

The underlying intent of this call for a moderate approach to wellness legislation is to encourage free and enlightened points of choice for everyone in this country regarding behaviors and habits for wellness or worseness. Given real choices, most people, in my opinion, will choose wellness.

In addition to supporting regulations, laws, ordinances, and other regulatory strategies that encourage wellness, you might want to do what you can to discourage legal efforts that poorly serve the public interest. A concern in this regard is the prospect of established powers promoting legislation that would make illegal, impractical, or otherwise inhibit new approaches that offer alternatives to treatment-centered medicine, particularly those modalities which promote self-care, personal responsibility, and/or remedies by nonphysicians. The practice of homeopathy, the delivery of babies at home by midwives, the use of meditation and nutritional approaches to disease avoidance and care, and a variety of other "holistic" and nontraditional approaches are all fair game for regulations that would try to lock in the prescribed approaches controlled by a select group of licensed healers. The problem with this kind of limitation is that it discourages new discoveries and keeps people dependent on a limited number of highly expensive, and not always appropriate, practitioners. Such regulations should be discouraged and resisted. Any major new health program, such as National Health Insurance, should have built into it some kind of technology-assessment provision, whereby the merits of various procedures and techniques, both old and new, are evaluated for effectiveness.

This, of course, does not complete my shopping list of changes which I would like to see evolve in order that I, and others who share my wellness orientation, can pursue high levels of health and well-being without distractions, nuisances, and outright affronts. Naturally, I have other things to do besides write letters, however much satisfaction doing so occasionally brings me. But if I were to devote a few days to raising the wellness consciousness level of society, I would have multiple targets for either positive reinforcement or the "concerned citizen" letter or phone call. You, too, might care to:

• Send a letter of appreciation to the Hyatt Corporation for its enlightened policy of setting aside 10 percent of rooms in all Hyatt Hotels exclusively for nonsmokers. (And you can send a second letter when that percentage is raised to the level reflective of the percent of nonsmokers in the population, about 70 percent).

• Register a complaint (with many courtesy copies) every time you travel on commercial airlines and have to breathe polluted air from the smoking sections (there is no escape from the nicotine and tar, carbon monoxide, ammonia, and benzopyrene of second-hand smoke in pressurized cabins).

• Make a suggestion to the managers of Wards, Sears, and other large department stores requesting that alternatives to hamburgers and hot dogs be made available in their lunchrooms. It would not take a great deal of training or expense for the department stores to offer such nutritious choices as high-protein milkshakes fortified with brewer's yeast and lecithin, avocado and other fresh vegetable sandwiches using whole grain breads, unpolluted yogurts, seasonal fruits, honey, and similar foods. Such practices have led to demonstrated profits in other stores; if enough people requested nutritional practices the stores would respond.[10]

• Wage a campaign to convince the local city or town council members to spend public funds to improve the community environment for wellness. There is so much that can be done at moderate cost to make it easier for citizens to practice wellness lifestyles. Paths could be built for safe jogging, biking, and hiking, and par courses could be established in every neighborhood. Careful monitoring against all forms of environmental contaminants seems as essential to community wellness as do good schools and policy and fire protection.

• Ask your local school board to phase junk foods out of school cafeterias, and to make education for living whole lives an integral part of the secondary school curriculum. Request that at a minimum, all youngsters are given a chance to thoroughly understand the nature of high level wellness, or very good health by whatever name, and that they are presented with interesting information on self-

10. See "Where Shoppers Refuel on Natural Foods," *Prevention*, (December 1976), pp. 89–94.

responsibility, nutrition, stress, fitness, and the environment.[11]

• Send a communication to your life insurance company to the effect that people (like yourself) who practice healthy life styles have fewer heart attacks, cancers, and all the other chronic diseases, and live longer—and therefore are entitled to lower rates. (At a minimum, health and life insurance premiums should be based in part on weight tables, with lower-than-standard rates for persons within their ideal weight ranges.)

• Suggest to your employer that the purchase of medical insurance beyond a minimal level is less advantageous than providing wellness education opportunities as part of the employee benefit package. It is becoming increasingly evident that we need fewer, not more, doctors in this country.[12] More doctors will lead to more "doctoring," higher costs, a larger medical system, greater depersonalization of care, less self-maintenance, and lowered personal acceptance of responsibility, all leading to poorer health. An employee benefit plan can cover less in the medical area and more of a health promotion nature by making wellness programs available to employees as part of the benefit package. This way, you do not have to become sick to gain from the company plan. But somebody has to be

11. For a description of a curriculum focusing on "self-enhancement for every child, an appreciation of the human body, an understanding of how it interacts with the environment and daily practices of the individual, knowledge of body systems and their relationship to the function of the whole being," write for information about the School Health Curriculum Project to Community Program Development Division, Bureau of Health Education, Center for Disease Control, Atlanta GA 30333. Also see: Anne Moyer, *Better Food For Public Places* (Emmaus, Pa.: Rodale Press, 1977).

12. This statement applies to the treatment-oriented doctors that predominate today. If the medical profession were to produce more holistic-oriented physicians interested in the whole person and committed to the promotion of client self-responsibility, then this statement would not apply. More doctors in this case would bring about not more "doctoring" in the perjorative sense, but rather more self-caring, guided autonomy, and attendant personal well-being.

informed that you, and many other workers, would welcome this kind of supplemental fringe benefit, and would give up some sickness insurance coverage to get it.

Naturally, I would not recommend that you make such "waves for wellness" if I were not willing to do a few turns myself. My avocation, to some extent, consists of finding ways to encourage people to not do things which interfere with my freedoms, and to get them to consider other possibilities that might actually do me, and others interested in healthy living, some moderate good.

The following is an example of the kind of letter I write. When I compose these communications, I try to remember that I'm doing it at least in part for my own benefit (it helps me let off steam), and I remind myself that my happiness or wellness lifestyle is not dependent on the recipient accepting my advice or granting my request. If I complain and the other person impolitely suggests that I go to hell, I'm not upset. I may not seek out that person's company, buy his or her product, or use the service involved, but I'm not going to allow the rejection to discourage me or devalue my preferences. With this attitude, I'm free to take on the Goliaths as well as the minor annoyances.

So it was only natural that I would notify a friend in the TWA hierarchy whom I knew to have some interest in wellness of my dissatisfaction with the airline's dining service. Here are some excerpts from that letter.

Mr. John O. Truex
Vice President, Western Division
Trans World Airlines, Inc.

Dear John:

As a once-a-month TWA traveler from San Francisco to Washington, D.C. and as a former classmate of the firm's most "wellness"-oriented executive, I want to take a moment to comment—and advise—on a recent in-flight incident . . . .

What was the incident? Just a lovely stewardess's comment at 9:15 A.M. PST at 38,000 feet over the Rocky Moun-

201

tains. Quote: "Would you like a chocolate or sugar donut?"

John, it's funny, but this innocent and well-intended question is symbolic of what is wrong with the American diet. Our food habits, and overall lifestyle, have led to an extraordinary state of unhealth throughout this country. No other people have ever suffered the death rate from atherosclerosis and other respiratory diseases, cancer, strokes, and diabetes that is the contemporary American condition. The U.S. Senate Select Committee on Nutrition and Disease recently released a massive report linking a diet overloaded with sugar, fat, low-fiber foods, preservatives and artificial coloring agents, and "enriched" white flours to the above-noted diseases of civilization—and stated that Americans are digging their graves with their teeth. I have been studying diet and disease since leaving the Stanford SEP program and I have come to believe that nutritional awareness, in concert with exercise, stress management, and an ethic of self-responsibility, represent the best alternative for citizens who want to avoid the inevitable senescence and debilitation pursuant to the "chocolate or sugar donut" lifestyle—and choose instead healthier lives. I believe a great many citizens—including air travelers—would choose to adopt richer lifestyles if more information about "high level wellness" were made available—in an interesting and nonthreatening way . . . .

The suggestion I want to put to you is that TWA adopt "high level wellness" as the basis for the company's approach to excellence in offering the best service and being the number one airline in quality and progressive thinking. Get rid of the "chocolate or sugar donut" mentality which neither sets you apart from the competition nor contributes to the nutritional benefit of your customers. Little things can mean a lot—offer fruit instead. Promote the ethic of "wellness"—the idea of health as more than just the absence of illness. Make sure every meal has adequate fiber or roughage. Offer vegetarian alternatives to those who might appreciate the thoughtfulness. Make bran available–also herbal teas, vitamin C tablets, varied fruit juices (e.g., papaya), and sweets made with honey or molasses instead of refined white sugar. Avoid artificial colors, preservatives, and other chemicals whenever possible. These are just off-the-top examples—there are countless little things you could do . . . .

I am enclosing a few items about wellness for your information. I would appreciate hearing from you as soon as convenient, John. There are many exciting possibilities inherent in this approach to the airline business.

My friend John wrote back a few months later. Here is an excerpt from his letter relating to my recommendations (the omitted sections were personal asides about job changes, travel, family, etc.):

> As you may note, my responsibilities now include In-Flight Services which comes to grips with the subject about which you wrote, even though the determination of menus and meal service is not in my specific responsibility. As one who fights the "battle of the bulge" constantly, I am sympathetic to the need for a good diet and am sure that the airlines can do a more expert job in this area—even though we have specific and unusual constraints which the normal food service activities do not have to contend with.
>
> In any event, I have forwarded your letter to our director of dining service, Mr. Dieter Buehler, and have asked that he correspond directly with you on this subject when he gets a few moments to review the file.

Mr. Buehler's response came shortly thereafter:

> Dear Mr. Ardell:
>
> John Truex has passed along your information on "wellness" and your views about what is wrong with the American diet and lifestyle.
>
> Being one that was reared in the old school of "you are what you eat," I understand what you are saying, and for the most part agree with your observations. While there is growing interest and concern in this country in what we eat, and its ultimate influence on our well-being, unhappily we Americans have a long way to go in our awareness, and follow-through in the marketplace . . . .
>
> Witness what is happening in the commercial food service marketplace, and the types of places that the public is supporting—fast food establishments and dinner houses, all pretty much serving foods that do not necessarily enhance our state of "wellness." In short, what the public

practices is different than what is being preached.

In our area of in-flight food service, we are faced with somewhat of a dilemma—recognizing views such as yours, giving the public what it wants and is accustomed to, and what is logistically practical, realistic, and feasible in a fairly complex feeding system. It becomes a matter of what is our primary role, which we interpret to be providing the public with an attractive, tasty, well-balanced meal during normal periods while they are enroute and unable to otherwise satisfy their needs. As you recognize, whatever effort TWA could initiate would be modest. As we view the situation, it could only be supportive of an overall effort, and at the same time, be responsive to the wants and needs of our customers. At this point, it doesn't seem that this entails more than being aware of "wellness" in our planning efforts and being alert to what opportunities may exist. Thank you for your interest . . . .

Naturally, I responded to Mr. Buehler's discouraging comments, suggesting that it would be in TWA's interest as well as to the public benefit if a more hopeful view of the human condition and possibilities were adopted by the company leadership, and that wellness in any event (as I thought I suggested in my first letter) encompassed more than food service. I then suggested other possibilities.[13]

This instance of letting somebody know that healthier practices would be appreciated did not result in any dramatic changes. I still get the "chocolate or sugar donut" routine on TWA flights. Complaint letters, no matter how grievous the perceived problem, seldom evoke visible returns. But they often enable the writer to feel better about whatever annoys him, and when expressed properly—by *many* people over

13. Apparently, I had little effect on TWA's image of or concern for the traveling public. In being "responsive to the wants and needs of its customers," the company in March of 1977 sent me notice of an "In-Flight Beverage Book" which offered a savings of $2.50 on every five alcoholic drinks consumed in flight. In declining the offer, I suggested that TWA was contributing to the excessive consumption of alcohol in this country, which the U.S. government has stated costs society $15 billion annually in lost work time, health and welfare services, and property damage. (Source: *Forward Plan for Health*, DHEW Publication No. (05) 76-50024, p. 101). While the company should not be required to adopt a wellness orientation, I wonder if it has to work so hard at promoting worseness?

time—can oftentimes lead to reforms and satisfactions. Someday, maybe sooner than later, a friendly flight attendant is going to come up to me, smile, and say, "Granola, herbal tea, or me, Big Boy?"[14]

Exploring the Social Possibilities of High Level Wellness

Individuals who practice health-enhancing lifestyles often find it difficult to meet others similarly inclined. To meet people, some wellness-oriented folks must endure smoke-filled bars where everyone, just by virtue of being there, is expected to drink toxic substances. Most of the patrons in these establishments are decidedly not into wellness. Couples fare little better: most parties and gatherings of friendship and business groups, relatives, and so forth, are organized around drinking, smoking, and eating foods not primarily selected for their nutritional qualities.

What is to be done about this? How can individuals and couples interested in sharing knowledge and ideas about wellness possibilities connect with each other?

One possibility, and there are undoubtedly other ways, is to form a high level wellness club in your community. Run an ad a few times in the local paper announcing a meeting to discuss wellness possibilities. See what kinds of folks show up and the variety of interests these people have. Perhaps there will be sufficient support to organize activities, such as tours of local wellness resources (e.g., natural foods restaurants, smoking abatement or alcoholism clinics, and holistic health centers). Maybe some people would be interested in nature walks, picnics, bicycle tours, and similar outings. If you like some of the well-

---

14. Even under the prevailing conditions of "worseness" associated with commercial air travel, there are wellness-promotive steps you can take to mitigate negative circumstances. Let me offer this hint: have your travel agent do more than make a reservation when you order tickets. Have the agent specify that you want a window or aisle seat in the nonsmoking section and that you want a special meal. You have lots of choices, including vegetarian, seafood, kosher, and more on some flights. Most of the airlines outdo themselves on the special meals. In fact, I have enjoyed United's seafood platter so much that I'm sometimes tempted to fly someplace just to have one. (Just kidding.)

ness-oriented folks sufficiently, perhaps you could party together—imagine the differences in atmosphere, dining patterns, and conversational topics.

Your new friends may want to go a little further after a period of time, perhaps by sponsoring a public meeting to hear someone like Dr. John Travis lecture on high level wellness. Or maybe you and a few friends would decide to invest in a health-conducive singles bar or restaurant catering to wellness-oriented people, or some other enterprise that would affect more than the group itself. Which suggests one other, perhaps most daring prospective endeavor for a high level wellness club: namely, social action. If enough individuals in a community began to form a constituency around wellness patterns and behaviors, you could marshall your influence to have health education programs revitalized in the schools, insuring that all students are socialized from grade school forward regarding elements and principles of well-being. Joining the PTA in order to help bring this about might be a good strategy. Your social action programs might also monitor other health-related customs and practices, such as the nutritional quality of foods served in schools, the kinds of vending machines found in public buildings, rights for nonsmokers, the quality of local air and water, and so on.

In concert with other wellness clubs throughout the nation, you and your lifestyle-conscious friends and associates could exert quite an impact on health levels. And meet nice people, in pleasant places, in the process.

For those of you who may want to do more than attend to your own well-being and write a fun hot letter now and then, I recommend involvement in the health planning system. I believe that if even a small fraction of the residents of a community were to become involved, the possibilities for converting the existing medically focused health planning agencies into wellness education forums would be overwhelmingly favorable.

Helping to Create a
New Kind of
Planning System

Health planning has not been taken seriously in this country. In the first place, health planning is, as you might have guessed, medical system planning. Second, health planning has only existed for about 15 years, and has not, until recent developments, had any "clout" or implementation authority. Third, the medical system has, at least before the advent of the financially disastrous Medicare and Medicaid programs, been largely the province of private enterprise and not-for-profit organizations—and the tenets of planning for the larger public interest have never been popular in these contexts. So officials in government and most of the people in this country generally paid little or no attention to the nature of the prospects for "health" planning. That is, until the congress enacted and the president signed P.L. 93-641, the National Health Planning and Resources Development Act of 1974.

To comprehend and evaluate the prospects for a wellness-promotion strategy, you'll need some background on P.L. 93-641 and an understanding of how it differs from the planning programs it superseded.

Before 1960, what passed for community health planning was conducted by private health and welfare councils, community chest organizations, and similar voluntary councils composed of blue-ribbon citizen committees. Such "planning" (which focused on certain problem areas of a health nature) carried no authority, was rarely comprehensive, related primarily to hospitals or treatment orientations, and was dominated by the providers of medical services. Programs instituted at the federal level in 1960 and later in 1966 attempted to establish more ambitious and effective planning mechanisms, but they had limited success. By late 1973, the popular consensus was that health planning remained medically centered, underfunded, controlled by the special health industry elements it should have coordinated and managed, and all-in-all worth approximately what was being spent on it (which was not very much). In some important respects, P.L. 93-641 promised to change the nature of the health-planning function and increase its impact.

The new program, signed into law on January 4, 1975, fed many new elements into the planning system in an effort to correct recognized deficiencies. In laying out the broad directives designed to make planning more effective, the congress:

• Made a finding that "large segments of the public are lacking in basic knowledge regarding proper personal health care."

• Directed the secretary of HEW to issue guidelines on national health-planning policy, and suggested that certain matters deserve "priority consideration" in the formulation of health-planning goals. Two of the recommended priorities are the promotion of activities for the prevention of disease, including studies of nutritional and environmental factors affecting health and the provision of preventive health care services, and the development of effective methods of educating the general public concerning proper personal (including preventive) health care and methods for effective use of available health services.

• Established a National Council on Health Planning and Development, and directed that not less than a third of the 15 voting members be "consumers" rather than "providers" or medical service personnel.

• Created a network of regional Health Systems Agencies (HSAs). At this writing, there are 213 such agencies in operation.[15] The membership of all HSAs must include a consumer majority.

15. *Health Planning in Transition*, the newsletter of the *American Health Planning Association* (21 October 1976), p. 3.

• Set up statewide Health Coordinating Councils to advise the HSAs, made available grants for state health planning and development, and provided funds for health research, technical assistance centers, and implementation of HSA plans.

• Established a clear-cut set of functions for health-planning agencies, the first of which is "improving the health of residents of a health service area." Another is to assemble and analyze data concerning the status (and its determinants) of the health of the residents of its health service area.

The legislation is long (52 pages) and technical, and has two titles, 10 parts, and 45 sections! Yet, the basic message is rather clear: health-planning agencies are expected to produce results in terms of population health levels, and the councils, agencies, grants, functions, and all the rest should contribute to that result.[16]

Unfortunately, this is not the way things have developed in the years since passage of the legislation. As was true of the agencies which they supplanted, the HSAs remain dominated by medical service and insurance interests, and the agendas are still almost entirely focused on utilization of hospital and long-term care and treatment facilities, review of medical equipment and program proposals, illness data collection and dissemination, and the maintenance of cozy relationships with local medical institutions and various provider interests.

But you can change that. You can become a participant in the HSA in your community. You can do this by advising the HSA director of your interest, going to one of the agency meetings, volunteering to serve on one of its committees, requesting placement of your name on the mailing list, and/or through personal contact with a member of the agency's Board of Directors.

---

16. For information about this law in particular or health planning in general, write the American Health Planning Association (AACHP), 801 N. Fairfax St., Alexandria VA 22314. Also, see *A Consumer's Guide to Taking Over Health Planning*, published by Ralph Nader's Public Citizen Health Research Group (2000 P Street, N.W., Washington DC 20036), $2.

Once you are part of the process, you can, in cooperation with others who share your commitment to a health promotion orientation, move the organization away from a medical focus. There are numerous ways in which this can be done; the objective in every case will be to direct the staff to look at issues which relate to improving the health status of area residents. This is quite different from the current emphasis upon examining the pros and cons of a few more beds for a hospital, or whether the community needs three or four of the latest technological gadgets (which the medical staffs want in order to facilitate their specialty practices).

One of the reasons I believe you can gain access to these planning agencies is the prevalence of "subarea councils" which many HSAs have created to increase local participation. These local councils are usually found in individual counties; their purpose is to advise the decision-making regional organization. While it may take a year or more to scheme, work, and otherwise advance your way to a seat on the HSA at the regional level where you will be able to promote wellness as part of a potentially influential organization, you'll find that participation and oftentimes membership in a local subarea group is, in most places, an easy and direct step. The reason for this is that despite the congressional initiative and mandate, the level of visibility of these medically oriented bodies is still low. Not exactly a vast wave of interest has engulfed the planning councils, and this makes it easier for you to move into the program and begin to exert an influence for new directions.

There's nothing wrong with using a Trojan horse in a good cause.

Once you gain your seat on the HSA or Subarea Council, you might want to look around for friends, acquaintances, wellness practitioners, and others interested in health promotion who can be encouraged to participate with you. Every vote helps. From personal experience, I can tell you that among the best candidates to carry the wellness message are the recent converts to self-responsibility for their own well-being. People who recently quit smoking or drinking, or who in some fashion decided they were ready to surrender worseness behaviors in favor of jogging, natural foods, meditation, and/or other wellness alternatives are prime prospects for becoming active and effective board members. Their fervor will be a big asset to you and others working at the HSA level on the wellness mission.

There is no shortage of wellness programs and activities which you can promote once you get yourself appointed to the HSA or Subarea Council Board of Directors. A beginning effort might be to sponsor a wellness conference or seminar, inviting some of the most interesting persons in the wellness movement to speak to the people of the area on the nature and the benefits of wellness. For the past two years, I have organized annual seminars at Asilomar in Pacific Grove, California for health planners on the subject of high level wellness. Over 100 planners, hospital administrators, physicians, nurses, and others interested in making health planning more than a coordinator and regulator of the medical system have attended—and returned home to promote wellness strategies in their HSAs.[17]

In addition to sponsoring local wellness conferences, you may want to organize meetings of people in your area who have knowledge about and interest in health promotion activities. These people can help when the HSA gets around to writing a health plan—it is essential that a section of that plan be written on the subject of wellness as an agency priority. The HSA can then begin promoting individual self-responsibility for health and outlining some principles and dimensions by which such responsibility might be exercised. The HSA newsletters and other public relations programs should carry wellness information to the citizens, and an ambitious education effort could be launched. The HSA should be encouraged to undertake research studies of a wellness nature and to give special assistance to hospital and long-term care officials in order that they might incorporate wellness into their institutions. The agency should also, as a minimum, gather information on the levels of positive health as well as traditional sickness indices (e.g., infant mortality rates, morbidity statistics, etc.). Finally, though this listing is just illustrative, the agency should insure that wellness

---

17. For a brochure on forthcoming high level wellness seminars, write Daman-Nelson, Inc. at 115 Mission Street, San Francisco CA 94105 (415-982-9860. In the next few years, conferences will be conducted in Aspen, Colorado; Sun Valley, Idaho; Tahiti, and Guadalupe.

criteria are brought to bear on all the review activities under its jurisdiction for federal, state, and private health-related grant applications.[18]

To help you get started I suggest you contact one of the following offices for the names, addresses, and telephone numbers of the HSA in your community:

Management Information Systems Branch
Office of Operations Monitoring BHPRD
Health Resources Administration
Public Health Service
Dept. of Health, Education, and Welfare
3700 East West Highway
Hyattsville MD 20782
301-436-6110

American Health Planning Association
801 N. Fairfax St. #212
Alexandria VA 22314
703-836-2501

A Parting Note

"Come on, Don! How much can I realistically undertake?"

At this point, you may be wondering: "How in the hell can I work toward a healthier nation, assume so much responsibility, clean up my diet, renew my body, design my personal spaces, and stay calm all at the same time? Will there be any time left for the family? Or earning a living? Will my friends call me a wellness freak, a nut who is a malcontent fugitive from the 'American way'? And must I live in a commune, an Ashram, or a tent?"

Good news. Wellness is not like that. High level wellness is a lifestyle to be enjoyed. Remember how I claimed that it is more fun to pursue wellness, that it leads to greater highs and fewer lows? I believe that, as I have experienced this reality myself, and I see it in so many of my friends. You don't have to spend any time at all writing letters or artfully complaining, and you certainly do not have to join a health planning agency to obtain good health and a lifestyle of high level wellness. Nor do you have to become an exercise nut (like me), a food faddist, a

---

18. If you want specifics on recommended wellness activities for an HSA or Subarea Council, you might want to examine an article I wrote in the *American Journal of Health Planning* in October of 1976. It's entitled "From Omnibus Tinkering to High Level Wellness: The Movement Toward Holistic Health Planning." The *Journal* is available in most libraries and all HSA offices, but if you have difficulty finding it, just write AHPA for a copy (801 North Fairfax St., Alexandria VA 22314).

mystic meditator, or a space engineer. You know that. When you consider everything that might be done, it does sound and appear overwhelming, but in fact you choose what you want to do. These choices are made one at a time, and you add new wellness behaviors only when they prove more rewarding than old worseness patterns.

One of the main points I have tried to emphasize throughout this book is that a little activity and wellness behavior in each of the five dimensions is much more beneficial than a lot of attention to any single area. This is the basis of an integrated lifestyle that will encourage you to evolve toward the plateau of high level wellness most appropriate for you. You will gain more satisfaction and fulfillment by pursuing wellness in your fashion, in your time, and in harmony with the other phases of your life, than you could ever realize by following someone else's wellness plan, goals, and targets for you.

So, do what you can when you are ready, and as you feel good about your choice of wellness activities. There's just nobody who knows you as well as you do, or has more reason to be concerned about your best interests.

A Wellness Resource Guide/The High Level Wellness Honor Roll of Books

There are vast possibilities for varied review criteria for wellness publications; I am sure you have your own and are using them to review this book! Having and applying your own is the best way to evaluate publications on this subject, but I do hope that some of my reviews encourage you to read a few of the books I have found most helpful in my own personal and professional evolution toward wellness.

Grouping publications under the wellness dimension they most advocate, I have listed more books than I have reviewed. (Books preceded by an asterisk are reviewed after the general listing.) This more inclusive listing will give you other interesting leads for learning more about each wellness dimension. I would be interested in your response to these books; if you are inclined, write me care of Rodale Press and let me know about your own honor roll—and why you like some approaches more than others.

Dimension of Self-Responsibility

A. Self-Responsibility in General

- ●*Browne, Harry. *How I Found Freedom in an Unfree World.*

- ● Frederick, Carol. *EST: Playing the Game the New Way.* New York: Delta, 1974.

- ●*James, Muriel and Jongeward, Dorothy. *Born to Win.*

- ● Greenwald, Jerry. *Be the Person You were Meant to Be.* New York: Dell, 1974.

- ● Maslow, A. H. *The Farther Reaches of Human Nature.* New York: Penguin, 1976.

- ● Newman, Mildred and Berkowitz. *How to Be Your Own Best Friend.* New York: Ballantine, 1974.

- ● Sobel, David Stuart and Hornbacher, Faith Louise. *An Everyday Guide to Your Health.* New York: Grossman, 1973.

- ● Williams, Roger J. *You Are Extraordinary.* New York: Pyramid, 1971.

- ● Zunin, Leonard. *Contact.* New York: Ballantine, 1973.

Browne, Harry. *How I Found Freedom in an Unfree World.* New York: Avon, 1973.

"Freedom is the opportunity to live your life as you want to live it." These words introduce and set the tone for a controversial and influential guide to the philosophy and practice of personal freedom and self-responsibility. Browne puts emphasis on self-reliance, happiness, personal identity, and ways to avoid fourteen traps which most often prevent people from enjoying freedom. These traps relate to identity, intellect, emotion, morality, unselfishness, groups, government, despair, rights, utopia, burning issues, previous investments, boxes, and certainty. The book is in three parts; all of the above are contained in part one.

In the second part, Browne describes how to be free; from government, social restrictions, bad relationships, marriage/jealousy/family/business problems, insecurity, exploitation, the treadmill, and pretense. The third part of *How I Found Freedom in an Unfree World* is addressed to discovering who you are, your morality, the kind of life you want, and how to make changes and a fresh start.

Browne's purpose is to get people to think about what they want from their lives, and to make conscious choices for direct alternatives leading to greater personal freedom or sovereignty.

A list of recommended readings is provided on eight of the major topics described in the text.

Strengths

Browne is a provocative writer with uncommon ideas on freedom. This book is a game plan for personal self-responsibility. The concepts described can lead to liberation, conflicts, and separation from spouse and/or friends, major job adjustments, or other new directions depending upon the resources of the reader. In addition to the basic strength to reinforce this self-reliant approach, Browne provides plenty of memorable quotes, definitions, and principles. Some examples are in order:

> ● [On the importance of doing things without encumbrances—marriage, partnership, etc.] "Down to Gehenna or up to the Throne, he travels the fastest who travels alone."
>
> Rudyard Kipling

> ● [On the value of forthright action as against procrastination] "Why do you have to postpone moving to a warmer climate where you can swim all year until you are so old that you're afraid of the water?"
>
> David S. Viscott

217

• [Some definitions]" 'Happiness' is a feeling of well-being, what you feel inside you as a result of the things that happen to you. 'Personal morality' is an attempt to consider all the relevant consequences of your acts."

Browne, properly in my view, cautions against making important decisions except when emotions are in control, and constantly promotes the importance of personal responsibility: "You are the sovereign authority for your life. You are the ruler who makes the decisions regarding how you will act, what information you will accept. You do it anyway—but if you recognize that you do it, you can gain much greater control over your future." I particularly like Browne's ideas on life's purpose and the value of self-disclosure.

> I believe that life is to be enjoyed, to be tasted—or there isn't any point to it. I've found ways to live freely and joyously—because I was convinced there was no other reason for living . . . . There's so much to be had from life. There's pleasure and satisfaction and love and entertainment and excitement. There are enjoyable ways of earning a living, and there are adventures, uncommitted hours, challenges, and happy surprises. Use your imagination. Look for alternatives. Don't settle for less than the kind of life you need to make it worth having lived.

> Honesty is displaying yourself to others as you really are. But, of course, you can't be truthful about something you don't know. And that's why it's so important to examine yourself, understand yourself, and accept yourself. Only when you know who you are can you honestly represent yourself to others.

Shortcomings
• Neither Harry Browne nor I would expect you to like or accept all of the principles and concepts in *How I Found Freedom in an Unfree World.* Some of my friends, in fact, were offended at Browne's ideas on marriage (don't do it; if you already have, get out of it), social action (forget it—unless it gives personal satisfaction), and/or government (an agency of coercion comparable to the Mafia). But that is

OK, for as I mentioned earlier, you do not have to agree with everything in order to enjoy and sometimes benefit from a good book.

Personally, I found this book a treasure and have gifted many of my friends with copies (some returned!). Highly recommended—as either a primer or clincher on the importance of self-responsibility. A breeze of ozone in an otherwise turgid sky.

James, Muriel and Jongeward, Dorothy. *Born to Win,* Menlo Park, Calif.: Addison-Wesley, 1971.

Born to Win interprets transactional analysis and Gestalt-oriented concepts in terms of everyday events and challenges in the lives of just plain folks. The book was written to provide a rational method for understanding behavior and for integrating one's personality. Its purpose is to help people take responsibility for their own lives and to develop an increased core of self-confidence. The authors describe the characteristics of "winners" (people who respond authentically) and "losers" (who do not) and introduce the four elements of transactional analysis. These are: (1) structural or individual personality analysis; (2) transactional analysis, which deals with what people do and say to each other; (3) game analysis, which focuses on the ulterior transactions leading to a "payoff"; and (4) script analysis of specific life dramas that people seem compelled to act out. James and Jongeward emphasize the importance of positive strokes in childhood, show how to change old transaction habits that do not work, and suggest ways to structure time so as to maximize positive stroking through activities and intimacy.

A key concept in *Born to Win* is that of scripts, which come in individual, cultural, subcultural, family, and psychological forms. These scripts are roles learned from early dramatic life events and acted out throughout our lives. Winners have one set of scripts, losers a quite different kind of program. These differences are described in detail. Most of us are more or less one or the other in large part due to our scripts, which we can change through transactional analysis techniques. If, for example, we are scripted for overeating, smoking, and other destructive behaviors, we need to learn how to acknowledge this patterning and its origins in order to develop effective "counterscripts." This concept originated with Eric Berne, whom the authors quote on the subject:

> Nearly all human activity is programmed by an ongoing script dating from early childhood, so that the feeling of autonomy is nearly always an illusion—an illusion which is the greatest affliction of the human race because it makes awareness, honesty, creativity, and intimacy possible for only a few fortunate individuals.

Other sections of *Born to Win* are devoted to the "ego states" (i.e., parenting, childhood, and adulthood), identity (personal and sexual), game playing, and the eventual achievement of autonomy as the "ultimate goal in transactional analysis. Being autonomous means being self-governing, determining one's own destiny, taking responsibility for one's own actions and feelings, and throwing off patterns that are irrelevant and inappropriate."

Strengths

• The concept of scripts, developed by Berne and refined and extended by James and Jongeward, has important implications for those who would pursue high level wellness. It suggests that behavior patterns or "scripts" can be understood and changed—that we are not programmed for life to act out lifestyles schemed toward chronic disease and premature death. The techniques of analysis presented in *Born to Win* will work for some people as a technique for comprehending and redesigning habits, which can then lead to a more "autonomous" existence. This process includes, according to the authors, "releasing" and/or "recovering" the capacity for "awareness, spontaneity, and intimacy," which seems like a fine idea to this writer.

•*Born to Win* is written and organized in a way that encourages self-study, testing, and easy comprehension of complex therapeutic approaches. The authors provide a summary of each chapter, and illustrations, diagrams, photographs, and questions for the reader to ask himself or herself—which often makes the study of transactional analysis both fun and challenging.

Shortcomings
•None, really. James and Jongeward wrote *Born to Win* in the hope that it would increase the reader's awareness of his power to direct his life, make decisions, develop an ethical system, enhance the lives of others, and understand that "he was born to win." For many, transactional analysis has had this effect and, for quite a few, *Born to Win* has provided a beginning.

B. Self-Responsibility in Relation to the Medical System

●*Blue Cross Association, The Rockefeller Foundation, and the Health Policy Program at the University of California, San Francisco. *Proceedings of the Conference on Future Directions in Health Care*.

●*Boston Women's Health Collective. *Our Bodies, Ourselves: A Book by and for Women*.

●*Carlson, Rick J. *The End of Medicine*.

● Freese, Arthur S. *Managing Your Doctor*. New York: Scarborough House, 1975.

●*Fuchs, Victor R. *Who Shall Live: Health, Economics, and Social Choice*.

●*Illich, Ivan. *Medical Nemesis*.

●*LaLonde, Marc. *A New Perspective on the Health of Canadians*.

221

•*Nolen, William A. *Healing: A Doctor in Search of a Miracle*.

• Samuels, Mike and Bennett, Hal. *The Well-Body Book*. New York: Random House, 1973.

• Sehnert, Keither W. *How to Be Your Own Doctor (Sometimes)*. New York: Grosset and Dunlap, 1975.

• U. S. Government Printing Office. *A Barefoot Doctor's Manual*. Washington, D.C., 1974.

Blue Cross Association, The Rockefeller Foundation, and The Health Policy Program at the University of California (San Francisco). *The Proceedings of the Conference on Future Directions in Health Care: The Dimensions of Medicine*. Chicago: Blue Cross Association.

Some people think that organized medicine is hostile to wellness and generally opposed to the idea that individuals can do more for themselves to stay well through healthier lifestyles. Not so, as was demonstrated in New York in December of 1975 at a medical meeting sponsored by Blue Cross Association, the Rockefeller Foundation, and the Health Policy Program of the University of California Medical School (SF). Fortunately for those of us not in attendance, the highlights of this important gathering have been assembled and published in a book-like publication by the Blue Cross Association.

The *Proceedings* contain highlights of presentations by 22 key figures in the U.S. medical establishment, most of whom have been in the forefront of change toward wellness or holistic health directions. The issues address concerns critical to an understanding of the limits of medicine. The applications of wellness to medical care are defined in highlights of five workshops dealing with (1) self-care possibilities and limits; (2) the nature, activities, and results of the Institute for the Study of Humanistic Medicine (San Francisco); (3) physiological effects of relaxation techniques and therapy; (4) holistic-oriented care for the elderly through Project Sage at Berkeley; and (5) the Menninger Foundation's report on investigations of voluntary control of "autonomic" (involuntary) functions. A concluding section of the *Proceedings* contains the summary observations and conclusions of each expert present on the lessons and policy implications of the conference.

Strengths

• Some of the individual presentations were outstanding, especially those by Thomas Boudreau (on a lifestyle strategy for improving population health levels), Thomas McKeown, M.D. (on the influences affecting health over time), Ernst Wynder, M.D. (on the effects of lifestyle and ways to modify destructive health habits), and Jerome Frank, M.D. (on approaches to healing and well-being).

• As noted, these *Proceedings* demonstrate that the ethic of high level wellness is shared by many representatives of prestigious and influential medical institutions.

• The record of the conference offers a wealth of information on many aspects of contemporary problems related to excessive reliance on medicine as a treatment and "cure" agent.

• The *Proceedings* contain many interesting quotes and a wealth of factual information. Examples include:

> - The suggestion that health workers have an obligation to go beyond their immediate professional responsibilities in order to play a full role in improving the quality of life (made by John Knowles, M.D.).
> - The statement by the president of Blue Cross Association that "we must stop throwing an array of technological processes and systems at lifestyle problems and stop equating more health services with better health."
> - McKeown's point that when people realize that the technical system of medicine cannot save them, that

they must moderate what they eat and drink, how they drive, and all the rest, we will have to be ready for a genuine socio-cultural revolution.

- The labeling of expensive, relatively ineffective treatment procedures requiring a steady expansion of hospital facilities, more technicians, and so forth, as "halfway technologies" (by Lewis Thomas, M.D.).

- The constant iteration of the theme that nearly all improvements in health in the nineteenth and twentieth centuries came from rising living standards, not medical care and that the contribution of the latter to life expectancy is small.

- The summary by McKeown, in which he "concludes that the major influences which have brought about modern improvements in health have been first, an enormous increase in food supply; second, a reduction in exposure to infection, critical in respect to the water- and food-borne diseases; third, a change in behavior which controlled population growth; and fourth and belatedly, the introduction of effective methods of immunization and therapy in the twentieth century . . . it has begun to be possible for an individual to influence his own health far more profoundly than can those measures which society is capable of introducing."

- The conclusion of Lowell Levin, M.D., that self-care education is the best way to better health outcomes at less risk, lower cost, and "less assault on the human spirit" for the diseases and illnesses of most concern to most people most of the time.

• Another strength of the *Proceedings* is that most speakers recognize the barriers to implementing changes in medicine and instituting a massive shift to self-care and high level wellness. These barriers include cultural and financial obstacles, professional resistance from organized medicine, the absence of incentives and a constituency for health promotion, the fact that "the system" is designed for

illness, and a host of other factors by now familiar to most
readers.

Shortcomings
• The publication was assembled in a hurry and therefore
contains errors and oversights no competent editor or
publisher would tolerate. For example, there is no date, no
publisher listed, and no information as to who produced the
Proceedings and where copies can be obtained.

• For me, the substantive problems relate to my simple
disagreement with statements by many speakers urging
more biomedical research to help cure diseases. Similar
points of view at variance with the wellness principles
enumerated in this book are found throughout the *Proceedings*; however, others support such opinions—and there is
always the possibility that those who disagree with me may
be right! But I do think a few remarks seem out of place and
inconsistent with the thrust of this interesting conference.

Overall, a nice booklet worth the effort of writing for it.

Boston Women's Health Collective. *Our Bodies, Ourselves: A
Book by and for Women.* New York: Simon and Schuster,
1971.

This book is the encyclopedia of self-responsibility for
women. Body education is considered core knowledge for
women; *Our Bodies, Ourselves* is designed to help women to
understand, accept, and be responsible for their own health and
well-being. *Our Bodies, Ourselves* was compiled by a committee
of twelve women; the contributions of over a hundred others are
acknowledged.

Major sections are devoted to changes in the self-concepts
and attendant expectations and values of women, the nature of
female relationships, and linkages (historical and emerging)
between women and the health care system. Chapters focus on

the major health problems of women, menopause, and sexuality. In addition, attention is given to issues focused on diverse concerns important to many women: lesbianism, feelings about relationships (with men/children/other women), and decisions about whether to bear children. Finally, separate chapters are given to nutritional awareness and physical fitness—for women, naturally.

Containing anecdotes and personal experience statements, the book is thoroughly illustrated with photographs, technical drawings, charts, and line figures. An extensive listing of "further readings" is provided after each chapter.

Strengths

• Barbara Brown, author of *New Mind, New Body*, has written that a woman cannot understand the world if she does not know her own body. No woman reading this work is likely to have this problem, or to overlook the central force in a wellness orientation; the recognition and acceptance of principal responsibility for her own well-being.

• The highlights of *Our Bodies, Ourselves* from a wellness perspective are the chapters on "nutrition and the food we eat," "women in motion," and "women and health care." The nutrition section is especially informative, with some provocative commentaries on "necessary nutrients," proteins, fats and oils, carbohydrates, and what to expect of the food and agricultural industries (not much).

Shortcomings

• In many respects, *Our Bodies, Ourselves* is an angry book which, depending upon your sex and attitude toward the women's movement, seems agreeable and appropriate or unnecessary and overdrawn. So, what might offend some is a source of affiliation and support for most—including sympathetic male readers.

• The book reads as one might expect a committee production to read—unevenly. The chapter on lesbianism does not fit, it's interesting but what's the point?

Overall, a splendid effort totally consistent with a wellness orientation, highly recommended reading for all *persons*. (A new edition has been published, with many content changes.)

Carlson, Rick J. *The End of Medicine*. New York: Wiley, 1975.

This book is presented as a lawyer's brief against medicine and the expectations which people have that medicine's capabilities will safeguard, restore, or promote health. The thesis is now a familiar one to informed wellness-oriented readers: medicine has very little to do with health, and people must learn to care for themselves, using providers as resources without becoming dependent. More medical care, such as that coming via national health insurance, will be worse than an ineffective and crippling expense: it will lead to greater health problems than we have today. Carlson writes that medicine will not change until the public's conceptions about health change.

Strengths
• Offering an overview of the issues, along with Illich's *Medical Nemesis*, Carlson's effort ranks near the top of the "limits of medicine" documentations. Among its major contributions are commentaries and analyses on:

> - iatrogenesis—the hazards of overutilization, or how people sometimes get more than they bargained for.
> - the dangers of the prescription and over-the-counter drug habits of Americans.
> - what medicine has contributed and remains good at, and what it does not do very well at all.
> - the cost/benefit calculations of medical versus other types of expenditures and the relative effects on health.

- lifestyle and environmental sensitivity as keys to well-being.
- the tendency of people to allow organized medicine to define "quality" of care without reference to patient outcomes.

• Carlson's prose is easy reading and, despite certain curious lapses provides many rewards of memorable quotes.

- "The efficient physician is the man who successfully amuses his patient while nature effects a cure."— Voltaire
- "Physicians think they are doing something for you by labeling what you have a disease."—Immanuel Kant
- "There is a great difference between a good physician and a bad one; yet very little between a good one and none at all."—Arthur Young
- "A diversified enriched diet will probably contribute to the health of the population . . . more than any other specific addition to medical resources, such as an increase in the number of doctors or the number of hospital beds."—Eli Ginzberg
- "I firmly believe that if the whole *materia medica*, as now used, could be sunk to the bottom of the sea, it would be all the better for mankind—and all the worse for the fishes."—Oliver Wendell Holmes
- "Americans have a peculiar illusion that life is a disease which has to be cured . . . . Everyone gets unpleasant diseases and everyone dies at one time. I guess they are trying to make life safe for senility."— Dr. Frances Crick

• The tables, charts, references, and bibliography are outstanding, and enable further study for those interested in related subjects.

Shortcomings

• Carlson occasionally tosses in terms that are Brobdingnagian (that is, unnecessarily long, like Brobdingnagian).
These seem tortured and a bit self-consciously scholastic.
Examples are *an emerging zeitgeist, paradigm shifts, re-
crudescence of the occult,* health as a *nonfungible good,* and
reference to its (health's) *transmogrification to a com-
modity.* With the aid of a dictionary, I understand. But was
it necessary?

• While recommendations are provided, they seem rather
skimpy and generalized. A follow-up action strategy would
be useful to help us sense how Carlson would have us establish sweeping institutional changes and other aspects of
his "design for the future."

Fuchs, Victor R. *Who Shall Live: Health, Economics, and Social
Choice.* New York: Basic Books, 1974.

Fuch's book provides a partial listing and discussion of
medical system problems and choices which face those responsible for making policy decisions. The nation has a limited supply
of dollars to allocate for health: how are these funds best distributed and for what purposes? Fuchs devotes entire chapters
to four major elements of the medical system: the doctors, the
hospitals, the drug industry, and the payment mechanisms.
Other chapters are devoted to analyses of the variables affecting
the "health" of the people (e.g., schooling, income, race,
medical care) and a brief listing of the author's choices (universal
and comprehensive health insurance, decentralized medical
systems, prepayment or health maintenance organizations
instead of the fee-for-service method of payment, competition,
elimination of doctor-protection laws, and better utilization of
hospitals).

Strengths

• I have used this book as a text in a graduate health planning course because it treats key medical system issues as choices, and thoroughly demonstrates that investments in one sector (e.g., more medical care) represent decisions to bypass opportunities in other areas (e.g., better housing, income maintenance). Within the health category, this means that a continued emphasis on research dollars for treatment and curing efforts will leave less money for programs that promote wellness and health enrichment.

• Fuchs does a good job of articulating the limitations-of-medicine theme: "Individual decisions about diet, exercise, and smoking are of critical importance, and collective decisions affecting pollution and other aspects of the environment are also relevant . . . . by changing institutions and creating new programs we can make medical care more accessible and deliver it more efficiently, but the greatest potential for improving health lies in what we do and don't do for and to ourselves. The choice is ours.

• The book documents the impact of lifestyle on morbidity and mortality patterns in a section entitled "A Tale of Two States." Fuchs shows that excess death rates in general and for cirrhosis of the liver and malignant neophasms of the respiratory system in particular vary markedly between Nevada and Utah, two states comparable in every major way (income, schooling, urbanization, climate, medical system) save one: lifestyle of the people.

Shortcomings

• The physician is billed as the "captain of the team" in the reformed "health" care system Fuchs advocates. Neither the client-provider relationship nor the treatment emphasis is singled out for change. The "omnibus tinkering" approach which Fuchs advocates is a major flaw, more serious than the accompanying imbroglios of incomplete alternatives, bias or narrow focus concerning economics, strained

230

choices, and unimaginative recommendations, though these don't help, either.

For its strengths and use as background, however, this is a worthy addition to the literature.

Illich, Ivan. *Medical Nemesis*. New York: Pantheon Books, 1976.

The theme (and first sentence) of *Medical Nemesis* is that "the medical establishment has become a major threat to health." The focus is the growth of iatrogenesis: doctor-induced illness. Illich examines what medicine does versus what it can do, the myths surrounding patient-provider relationships, the disabling dependence fostered by the profession, the effects of the resulting inability to cope, and the waste of human and material resources caused by the "expropriation" of autonomy. Among the perpetrators of these counterproductive conditions is our social order, which induces a maintenance mentality geared to the service of an industrial, technological, and basically inhumane system. A footnote buried at the bottom of a page might contain the leitmotif of the entire work: "The number of surgeons available was found to be the significant predictor in the incidence of surgery." Illich, however, provides his own best summary, and it warrants reproduction in part here:

> The level of public health corresponds to the degree to which the means and responsibility for coping with illness are distributed among the total population. This ability to cope can be enhanced but never replaced by medical intervention . . . . That society which can reduce . . . intervention to the minimum will provide the best conditions for health. The greater the potential for autonomous adaptation to self, to others, and to the environment, the less management of adaptation will be needed or tolerated . . . . The true miracle of modern medicine is diabolical. It consists in making not only individuals but whole populations survive on inhumanly low levels of personal health. Medical nemesis is the negative feedback of a social organization

that set out to improve and equalize the opportunity for each man to cope in autonomy and ended by destroying it.

Strengths

• *Medical Nemesis* is one of the two or three publications to have had an impact in affecting public attitudes toward the limits of medicine. The book is a library full of references, notes, and bibliographical treasures. The emphasis on what you can do for yourself without becoming dependent upon doctors is clear and forceful. The call for personal, autonomous behavior, assaults on technological myopia, and documentation of his theme of "a patient population scripted for illness" are all on target.

• Illich is angry, but one suspects there lurks within a sense of humor. His language is overkill to the point of satire. Phrases which provide recreational reading are dropped throughout the text. Some typical references are to:

> - doctors as "rash artery-plumbers" or "biological accountants";
> - medical spectator sports;
> - the U.S. as a world leader in "organized disease hunts";
> - medical Olympics;
> - hospitals as disease museums;
> - medicalized addictions.

• I am glad Illich addressed the issue of increased demands by poor people for greater access to medical care, particularly to costly therapies of questionable utility. Also, he describes the dynamics of union demands for more and more medical aspects in employee benefit packages. While the intent is greater access and equality, if not health, the results are, according to the author, "professional illusions and torts."

• Illich describes several controversial aspects of patient dependence. An example which he claims stands as an invisible barrier to greater personal autonomy and wellness behavior is the physician's role of exonerating the sick from moral accountability for their illness. Few other writers are willing to go near this political and ethical minefield.

Shortcomings
• Illich offers a fine framework for what's wrong but little in the way of policies, programs, strategies, or guides providing solutions. *How* one might go about strengthening himself for the task of self-responsibility is not addressed; neither does he suggest how society might move toward changing all those aspects of our medical system which are shown to be wrong.

• Illich wanders in places, to the extent that a reader wonders what point he is attempting to establish. For example, an entire chapter on death is interesting but largely superfluous, except when it notes that death under intensive care is another manifestation of the medicalization of all life stages, including the last.

Despite these quibbles (must everyone have solutions?— maybe defining a problem is enough), *Medical Nemesis* ranks high on the wellness publications list.

LaLonde, Marc. *A New Perspective on the Health of Canadians*. Ottawa: Government of Canada, 1974.

At the same time as improvements have been made in health care, in the general standard of living, in public health protection, and in medical science, ominous counter-forces have been at work to undo progress in raising the health status of Canadians. These counter-forces constitute the dark side of economic progress. They include environmental pollution, city living, habits of indolence, the abuse of alcohol, tobacco, and drugs, and eating patterns which put the pleasing of the senses above the needs of the human body.

For these environmental and behavioural threats to health, the organized health care system can do little more than serve as a catchment net for the victims. Physicians, surgeons, nurses, and hospitals together spend much of their time in treating ills caused by adverse environmental factors and behavioural risks.

It is evident now that further improvements in the environment, reductions in self-imposed risks, and a greater knowledge of human biology are necessary if more Canadians are to live a full, long, and illness-free life.

With these words, the Minister of National Health and Welfare introduces a "Working Paper" designed to stimulate interest and discussion on future health programs for Canada. The focus of the document, which is oriented to choices which must be made regarding health policy in that nation, is largely on the deadly implications of health-denying lifestyles. The book provides a wealth of information, with chapters addressed to: (1) the nature and limitations of the traditional medical view of health; (2) a review and analysis of major health problems (health status, organizational concerns, and delivery-system problems); (3) a discussion of high-risk populations; (4) options for the federal role; and (5) an assessment of research possibilities. Commentaries are devoted to mental health, the clash between the scientific method and intuitive approaches in health promotion endeavors, and the emphasis at present on the cure of chronic conditions to the neglect of care and prevention.

A conceptual framework developed by the Canadians for classifying the principal elements within the health field into manageable segments amenable to analysis and evaluation is presented. This framework, called the Health Field Concept, has four broad elements: (1) human biology (all aspects of health developed within the body based on the individual's organic makeup); (2) environment (all matters external to the body over which one has little or no control); (3) lifestyle (the aggregation of decisions by individuals over which they do have control); and (4) health care organization (all people and other resources given to the provision of medical care). Utilizing the Health Field

234

Concept as a universal frame for examining all health problems and for suggesting courses of action needed for their solution, the Canadians outline two broad objectives, five overall strategies, and 74 specific proposals. One basic objective is to reduce mental and physical health hazards for "obvious high-risk populations," such as drinking drivers, cigarette smokers, abusers of alcohol, very fat people, drivers who do not use seat belts, and people who live in remote areas.

Strengths
- Some of the best things in life are (still) free, as the Canadians have demonstrated by generously distributing 60,000 complimentary copies of this watershed document. Bureaucrats are not supposed to write clearly, and they certainly have no business waxing poetic, citing Corinthians and historians and, most significantly, assaulting sacred medical cows in a manner both entertaining and persuasive. The government of Canada has managed all of the above in *A New Perspective on the Health of Canadians* and, except to readers of the wellness literature, it is indeed a new perspective.

- This document has been extraordinarily influential in elevating a recognition of lifestyle as a major—in fact the *primary*—determinant of health and well-being. It has been used by the U.S. Department of Health, Education, and Welfare in its *Forward Plan for Health* and is probably the most quoted reference in holistic health and related conferences. When speakers address the myriad of issues relating to prospects for government intervention in the area of lifestyle and environment, the policy statements, research targets, and prose excerpts from *A New Perspective on the Health of Canadians* are often cited.

- As noted, the document is a pleasure to read. Here are some excerpts showing the literary style used to convey important ideas and explain why so many people choose to self-destruct through lifestyle behaviors:

The behaviour of many people also reflects their individual belief that statistical probability, when it is bad, applies only to others. This belief is the comfort of soldiers at war, criminals, and racing drivers, none of whom could sustain their activities did they not look on the sunny side of risk and probability. It is also the solace of those whose living habits increase the likelihood of sickness, accidents, and early death.

It is therefore necessary for Canadians themselves to be concerned with the gravity of environmental and behavioural risks before any real progress can be made. There are encouraging signs that this concern is growing; public interest in preserving a healthy environment, in better nutrition, and in increasing physical recreation has never been higher.

The government of Canada now intends to give to human biology, the environment, and lifestyle as much attention as it has to the financing of the health care organization so that all four avenues to improved health are pursued with equal vigour. Its goal will continue to be not only to add years to our life but life to our years, so that all can enjoy the opportunities offered by increased economic and social justice.

In most minds the health field and the personal medical care system are synonymous. This has been due in large part to the powerful image projected by medicine of its role in the control of infective and parasitic diseases, the advances in surgery, the lowered infant mortality rate, and the development of new drugs. This image is reinforced by drug advertising, by television series with the physician as hero, and by the faith bordering on awe by which many Canadians relate to their physicians.

When the full impact of environment and lifestyle has been assessed, and the foregoing is necessarily but

a partial statement of their effect, there can be no
doubt that the traditional view of equating the level of
health in Canada with the availability of physicians and
hospitals is inadequate. Marvelous though health care
services are in Canada in comparison with many other
countries, there is little doubt that future improvements in the level of health of Canadians lie mainly in
improving the environment, moderating self-imposed
risks, and adding to our knowledge of human biology.

Shortcomings

• There are no faults deserving of mention. As my extensive
attention to this document might suggest, I would recommend LaLonde's *A New Perspective on the Health of Canadians* to a busy person who felt he or she had time for
only one wellness-type publication. By now, my reasons for
this recommendation are obvious; one additional reason is
that I share LaLonde's belief that messages designed to influence the public must be "loud, clear, and unequivocal."
To quote LaLonde quoting I Cor. 14:8: "If the trumpet give
an uncertain sound, who shall prepare himself to the battle?"

Nolen, William, A. *Healing: A Doctor in Search of a Miracle.*
Greenwich, Conn.: Fawcett, 1974.

A first-person investigation of faith healing and psychic surgery, this account by an American surgeon studies three quite
different kinds of healers: the late Kathryn Kuhlman, faith
healer of the masses; Norbu Chen, healer and originator of the
"power of the way" concentrated-point-of-"hit" technique; and
assorted Filipino psychic surgeons. Nolen describes how he
learned about each healer investigated and how he conducted
his study. Also given in some detail are follow-up reports on
cases of "cures," as well as commentaries regarding those not
cured. Nolen includes descriptions of how healers work, how
they become healers, and who patronizes them. Most im-

portant, he presents an analysis of the findings and lessons of the experience.

Strengths

• William Nolen is a talented writer, a surgeon-author whose previous books (on more traditional medical subjects) have been best sellers. This time he has engaged in investigative reporting, scientific analysis, and story-telling.

• All of the healers are of interest, but one, Norbu Chen, is fascinating, humorously vulgar, and, like the others, a very controversial figure. If the entire book were on Chen, it would still be a worthy publication. However, the sections on Kuhlman and the psychic surgeons add depth and variety, and are themselves worthy illustrations of principles the author presents at the conclusion of the work.

• Though a physician himself, Nolen properly roasts organized medicine for contributing to the existence and attraction of bogus healers. These sins include failing to teach as well as attend, failing to cure or do much good in so many instances, and failing to provide as much warmth and compassion as the healers. Also faulted is the doctors' tactic of "putting down" healers and those who patronize them as idiots "beneath our contempt," which Nolen demonstrates is certainly not accurate. Nolen accurately assesses the AMA's public image as that of an uptight, conservative organization at war with progressive legislation.

• In acknowledging and expanding upon the theme that the body heals itself, Nolen contributes to a growing public recognition that the doctor can facilitate recovery, but that the cure must come from within.

• Other strengths of *Healing* include the manner in which Nolen:

    - restates the characteristics of the "true believer," the faith and psychic healers' best customer.

- demonstrates compassion and insight in the presence of the most flagrant instances of chicanery, as when describing a young girl's effort to claim a cure (based on Kathryn Kuhlman's power of hypnotic suggestion) for a polio-withered leg.

- raises complex ethical questions regarding whether bogus healers do little harm or great damage. The former possibility is seen in the following comment: "It is possible that 'healers,' by their machinations, their rituals, their sheer charisma, stimulate patients so that they heal more rapidly than they otherwise might; charismatic doctors do the same. In all probability, this is why doctors who have warm rapport with their patients seem to get better results than doctors who treat their patients briskly and impersonally." The possibility that faith healers do great harm, which I believe more likely, is also expressed: "When healers treat serious organic diseases they are responsible for untold anguish and unhappiness; this happens because they keep patients away from possibly effective and lifesaving help. The healers become killers. Search the literature, as I have, and you will find no documented cures by healers of gallstones, heart disease, cancer, or any other serious organic disease."

Shortcomings
● There are a few major problems and several less troublesome, but annoying, shortcomings in this book. The greatest problems, from a high level wellness perspective, are: (1) a total neglect of lifestyle or even prevention consciousness; (2) an emphasis on present and hoped-for future technological cures for illness in lieu of recommending or even recognizing self-care and/or health promotion activities; and (3) an apparent unawareness of holistic health or wellness principles—all of which could have related and added immeasurably to the utility of the book. Illustrations of each failing may be of interest:

[On lifestyle change to avoid need for the services of healers] It's often difficult, sometimes impossible, for a patient to make a radical shift in lifestyle; after all, most of us have to earn a living and it may be difficult to find a new job. Besides, we are what we are, and it's difficult to shift abruptly from being a highly competitive, driving individual to a relaxed "who cares?" sort of person.

[On reliance upon treatment and cures] Even though we don't yet know all we'd like to know about cancer, we are making strides. We have new x-ray equipment that now enables us to cure many patients who, ten years ago, we couldn't help . . . . If research continues as it has, we may in the not-too-distant future be able to cure or at least control most, possibly all, cancers.

[Unawareness or neglect of wellness principles—the principle of an acceptance of the eventuality of death, in this case] I don't want to die. Ever. As a minister friend of mine says, "Heaven is my home, but I'm not homesick." As far as I've been able to determine, after twenty years as a surgeon, no one else wants to die either.

• There are other annoying aspects of Nolen's approach.

- He sometimes writes silly sentences: "Mrs. Fisher is doing reasonably well. Multiple sclerosis is a cyclic disease (symptoms come and go) and at the moment, except for the fact that she drags one foot when she walks, there's not much evidence of the disease."
- His belief in God is foisted upon the reader at key points in the analysis; no one would deny him respect for his views, but he does not seem to reciprocate the same regard for non-God-oriented readers: "Frankly, and I don't want to get into an argument over this because my knowledge of theology is not deep, I find it difficult to comprehend how anyone cannot believe in God; it seems to me you have to be almost irrational to be an atheist . . . . What I've learned, and I hope I've been able to communicate something of this feeling, is that we don't need to seek out miracle workers if we're ill. To do so is, in a way, an insult to God."

- He is sometimes guilty of making sweeping generalizations without offering any evidence or reference support, after warning the reader to guard against healers who do likewise: "To be logical, the cancer patient should go to a healer only if the healer had a cure rate of 50 percent or better—the cure rate physicians can achieve . . . . Healers can't cure organic diseases. Physicians can.

These shortcomings are balanced by the strengths of the work. It is an especially useful publication to read after becoming acquainted with the basic wellness ethic. Think, for example, about the suggestive effects of the sometimes elaborate settings, the religious fervor of believers, the enthusiastic testimonials, the seeming expertness of the practitioners contrasted to the naivete of the participant, and the tales of wonderful results, and realize that it can be difficult at times *not* to believe in charlatan healers, physicians, or both. A well-developed skepticism toward the unfamiliar, whether you're dealing with faith healers, psychic surgeons, or M.D.'s, is highly advised, and amply supported by a reading of this book.

Dimension of Nutritional Awareness

● *Airola, Paavo. *Are You Confused?*

● *Davis, Adelle. *Let's Eat Right to Keep Fit.*

● Dufty, William. *Sugar Blues.* New York: Warner Books, 1975.

● Elwood, Catharyn. *Feel Like a Million.* New York: Pocket Books, 1965.

● Fredericks, Carlton. *Carlton Fredericks' High Fiber Way to Total Health.* New York: Pocket Books, 1976.

● Gerrard, Don. *One Bowl.* New York: Bookworks/Random House, 1974.

● *Jarvis, D.C., M.D. *Folk Medicine.*

● Leonard, Jon N., Hofer, J.L., and Pritkin, N. *Live Longer Now: The First One Hundred Years of Your Life.* New York: Grosset and Dunlap, 1976.

● *McGuire, Thomas, D.D.S. *The Tooth Trip: An Oral Experience.*

● Null, Gary and Null, Steve. *The Complete Handbook of Nutrition.* New York: Dell, 1973.

● Nutrition Search, Inc. *Nutrition Almanac.* New York: McGraw-Hill, 1975.

● Passwater, Richard A. *Super Nutrition.* New York: Pocket Books, 1976.

● Rodin, Marscell. *The Organic Gourmet: A Guide to Preparing Natural Foods.* Mill Valley, Calif: COFU, 1976.

● *Reuben, David. *The Save Your Life Diet.*

● *U.S. Senate (Select Committee on Nutrition and Human Needs). *Nutrition and Health: An Evaluation of Nutritional Surveillance in the United States.*

● *Williams, Roger J. *Nutrition against Disease.*

Airola, Paavo. *Are You Confused?* Phoenix, Ariz.: Health Plus Publishers, 1971.

Airola's lively book contains a review of nutritional controversies, an explanation of why the public is confused, and the author's program for "straightening out the most common myths, fallacies, misconceptions, and half-truths relative to nutrition and health." The author makes a case for his approach to superior well-being by citing the International Society for Research on Nutrition and Diseases of Civilization, his reading of the "empirical evidence of centuries and milleniums of actual application," personal experience, and data from research in various European countries.

Airola's nutrition-based approach is built upon the following basics:

● A high natural carbohydrate/low animal protein diet, which allows the eater to avoid toxic residues of metabolic waste products and eventual disease. For Airola, raw vegetable proteins have the highest biological value; raw vegetables, such as fruits, seeds, grains, and nuts, plus milk and cheese (i.e., lacto-vegetarian diet) supply an abundance of all needed proteins, vitamins, minerals, carbohydrates, fatty acids, enzymes, and trace elements.

● Seven basic "macrobiotic" diet rules for long life: (1) eat only natural foods—that is, foods grown on fertile soil under natural conditions and consumed in their natural state (e.g., fertile eggs, unpasteurized milk); (2) eat only whole foods—not those that are concentrated, fragmented, or refined (e.g., no white sugar or white, enriched flour); (3) eat fresh, raw "living" foods as much as possible ("cooked food is dead food"); (4) eat only "poison-free" foods (that is, cut down on residues and additives to the extent possible); (5) eat high natural carbohydrate/low animal protein foods; (6) systematically undereat in conjunction with periodic fasting (with enemas); and (7) practice correct eating habits (slow, calm, and complete mastication in combination with a food-mixing science).

In addition, Airola provides chapters on vitamins and food supplements, whole grains/seeds/nuts, milk, the hazards of rancid foods, facts and details about fasting, dry brush massage, and vitamin P, or bioflavonoids, as a healing substance. He also discusses hair loss and baldness and answers a large number of most frequently put questions about nutrition and health. Finally, Airola outlines his conception of the "healing science of tomorrow," which he calls "biological medicine."

Strengths
• This book is a warehouse of information, data, references, and explanations. It provides a perspective on the enormously complex subject of nutritional awareness that is understandable, clearly written, and supported by interesting references to European health centers and selected research findings. While you may not buy into 100 percent of Airola's diet and lifestyle regimen and may in fact come to dislike Airola himself, you are unlikely to deny the logic and benefits of most of the recommendations.

• A great deal of high level wellness thinking is evident in Airola's approach to nutritional awareness. Included in this framework, which he terms biological medicine, is an emphasis on prevention and health enhancement, avoidance of drugs and other synthetics which only suppress symptoms without eliminating the causes of disease, a call for new types of medical schools that integrate all the healing arts, a focus on natural systems and the body's own healing powers, and a special place for the influence of the mind and/or will in disease avoidance and the maintenance of health. He sees tomorrow's doctor as a teacher, helping people learn the correct ways of eating and living in order that sickness may be avoided.

● All the great hazards are reviewed and guides are provided for minimizing their effects. The hazards include chemicals in most foods and the guides include principles for reducing the adverse impact of processed toxins, ways to avoid rancid foods, and rules for fasting without doing more harm than good to yourself.

Shortcomings
● Airola footnotes himself and the availability of his other books at the bottom of fifteen separate pages; after a while, this constant hucksterism becomes annoying.

● Airola is not objective or open to other possibilities. Any evidence that is contrary to his findings is attributed to "scholastic dogmatism," "sentimental prejudice," or the dishonesty of researchers "bought by" food industries with a stake in the outcomes of nutritional research. While some of this, particularly the last point, is often true, Airola's attitude is that any factor or data inconsistent with his views is the result of "obsolete information and poor research methods."

● The author is often guilty of overkill through sweeping promises ("100 percent glowing health," "perfect" health, etc.) and unrealistic regimens (who can live fully the dietary and other health practices he advocates?). He claims, for example, that if we follow his approach into the future, "a new era of glorious, buoyant health and a total freedom from disease will emerge."

● At times, Airola gets plain nasty and mean-spirited in seeing conspiracies all about. The support of the American Dental Association for fluoridation, which he vigorously opposes, is attributed to dentists' wanting more tooth decay because this gives them more business and higher incomes. One need not be an apologist for the dental profession to object to this kind of reasoning. (Incidentally, no other provider group has been as consistently supportive and effective in advocating prevention rather than treatment as the dental profession.)

Despite these annoyances, *Are You Confused?* is outstanding as a reference resource and should be high on the list of readings in the area of nutritional awareness.

Davis, Adelle, *Let's Eat Right to Keep Fit*. New York: Signet, 1970.

The late Ms. Davis's best-selling books are known to nearly everyone who has studied nutrition. This classic in the field contains over thirty separate chapters, each of which stands independent of the rest.

Let's Eat Right to Keep Fit begins with the case for nutrition, which Davis suggests is not understood or given the emphasis it warrants because of food faddists, crackpots, advertising, "should not" admonitions (which eventually turn people off), inaccurate information, and our tendency to see physicians as guides to health. She says the latter are disease experts—that only a few recognize and have studied the importance of nutrition. Attention is devoted to the value of proteins, essential fatty acids, vitamins A/B/C/D/E, iron and iodine, magnesium, sodium, potassium, and calcium. The role of each element in the body is detailed, and the characteristics and disorders linked to each and its lack are described.

Davis devotes a substantial portion of this book to the cellular struction of the body and concludes that the almost "inconceivable synchronization" of it all underscores the perfection of the Divine. She comments on approaches to food selection and preparation, vitamin supplements (recommending them only when wholesome foods are unavailable), and the great "personal rewards of good nutrition." Concluding sections are devoted to the status of our national health (awful), the destructive propaganda machine of the food and drug industries, an action strategy, and lists of things people can do for themselves and their country in overcoming personal and national malnutrition.

Strengths
• Adelle Davis was perhaps the most influential nutritionist of recent times, and her books continue to attract a wide public. The Davis approach to physical and emotional well-being deserves a careful reading by all who seek to find their own patterns. In light of all the persuasive, but often contradictory expert advice from which to choose, this book serves an important moderating role.

• The book contains so much basic information about required vitamins, minerals, and food balances that three hours of college credit should be awarded all who read it from cover to cover. While the foreword to the first edition (1954) by the physician head of the American Academy of Nutrition may be wildly excessive ("If the principles set forth in this book were followed by most people, I believe a greater advancement in health would result than from any other occurrence in the history of mankind"), the book is good and well worth the hours required for complete digestion.

Shortcomings
• Many persons deeply committed to a given approach to nutritional awareness take great exception to Davis's ideas about food supplements, red meat (she highly recommends liver and kidneys), and the role of different minerals in combating illness. This, of course, is part of the game when the players in the nutritional-expert sweepstakes are all so highly attracted to their particular regimen.

•*Let's Eat Right to Keep Fit* has so many strengths that exceptions seem like quibbles. Enough said, except perhaps to note that I wish she had given some attention to the importance of other dimensions of high level wellness to go

247

with her approach to total health through proper diet.

Jarvis, D.C., M.D. *Folk Medicine*. Greenwich, Conn.: Fawcett, 1958.

Folk Medicine explores the beliefs, practices, and prescriptions of many generations of Vermont people, and contains theories and explanations of why Vermonters and others benefit from a variety of time-honored remedies. A physician, Dr. Jarvis describes in this classic publication his many reasons for preferring Vermont folk medicine to the out-of-touch-with-nature interventions which he learned in medical school. The principal areas of emphasis are: the Vermont people's philosophy and environment; animal laws and nature's ways; the instincts of youth toward healthful behavior; the medical or scientific basis of folk medicine; and the importance of selected substances (e.g., potassium, honey, kelp, iodine, apple cider vinegar, castor oil, and corn oil).

Strengths
● Dr. Jarvis's Vermont folk remedies are interesting to read about and I would be surprised if most of them did not actually work, especially if the user believed in the treatment method. But the real joy of the book from a wellness perspective is Jarvis's introductory forecast that may still come to pass: "I believe that the doctor of the future will be a teacher as well as physician. His real job will be to teach people how to be healthy. Doctors will be even busier than they are now because it is a lot harder to keep people well than it is just to get them over a sickness." That's pretty heady stuff—for 1958!

● Whether or not the remedies for high blood pressure, overweight, chronic headache or fatigue, dizziness, or whatever ails you actually do work cannot be assessed by this writer; however, certain Vermont and Jarvis principles certainly seem unimpeachable:

- The importance of food to the body and how we build and rebuild our "human house" by means of food we eat, liquid we drink, and air we breathe.
- The value in learning to live well by observing nature's laws and animal behaviors; practicing preventive medicine by sensible living; knowing the role of will in healing; and realizing the hazards of sugar/meats/preservatives/enriched flours, the benefits of high fiber eating patterns, and the interconnectedness of all living things.

• Dr. Jarvis writes in an agreeable, lucid, and sometimes profound communicative style, as seen in the following summary passage at the end of the book:

> We are all pretty much alike in that we wish for continuous good health and to have the energy and endurance which will make enjoyably productive both our work and play. I can assure you that if you follow the pathway outlined, you will come to the December of your life with good digestion, good eyesight, good hearing, good mental and physical vigor . . . . Sickness is the posing of a problem in restoring the balance when it has knowingly or unknowingly been interfered with. Sickness is the road sign telling that we have tried to wander cross-lots, off the main road Nature laid out for us.

Shortcomings
• Some readers might have trouble with certain "far out" folk remedy approaches and the somewhat dated theories regarding race and optimal diets.

McGuire, Thomas, D.D.S. *The Tooth Trip: An Oral Experience*. New York: Bookworks/Random House, 1972.

The Tooth Trip contains a detailed plan for dental self-care designed to prevent decay and degeneration of teeth and gums. It also represents a consumer guide to economical and effective use of dentists, an indictment of the dental profession, and a comprehensive accounting of the benefits of a prevention philosophy. The entire book is focused on personal responsibility for one's own oral good health, and it is written and illustrated in a manner designed to encourage easy reading and comprehension by just plain folks (particularly those in the "counterculture"). McGuire's thesis is that "no one should get tooth decay."

He comes down hard on the American diet of artificial and refined "garbage" foods as the first-ranking villain in the decay process; the antidote is natural, raw foods with vitamin supplements. Readers of this book will not be surprised to learn that fresh fruit and vegetables, nuts, juices, whole wheat and rice, raw milk and cheeses, honey and organic fertilized eggs provide substantial rewards before as well as after ingestion.

McGuire describes all the common (but "unnatural") diseases of the mouth and how preventive dentistry eliminates the causative factors. Sections are also addressed to problems which most people confront at some time—wisdom teeth, orthodontics, how much x-raying to allow, mouth sores, bridge work, and so forth. Home care and the use and misuse of assorted tools and appliances are described, as are issues of more general interest, such as women in dentistry (why so few?), preventive dentistry for infants and small children, and the potential relationships between M.D.'s and D.D.S.'s.

Strengths

• McGuire's opus is a high level wellness book for the mouth. Many of the basic principles of wellness discussed in this book are found in *The Tooth Trip*, including the overarching ethic of self-responsibility and the idea of gradually implementing a healthier (dental) lifestyle.

• Anyone who follows McGuire's path on *The Tooth Trip* will find himself well into a wellness regimen of nutritional awareness. The chapter on diet further reinforces the importance of "getting your food trip together." The importance of vitamin supplements is effectively explained, and the reading list and memorable maxims are helpful

("The best way to eat a lot is to eat good food and little of it; that way you'll live long enough to be able to eat a lot").

• Other features which I think distinguish *The Tooth Trip* are the illustrations by Amit Pieter, the polemic against the status quo in dentistry, the statistical summary of the national dental situation (98 percent of Americans have suffered or will suffer tooth/gum disease, 25 million have no teeth left, 42 million have never been to a dentist, 60 million teeth were pulled in 1970, and Americans have a lifetime average dental expenditure of around $30,000).

Shortcomings
• The "hippie" style of writing aimed at a drop-out type of reader is great for readability for that kind of audience, but may distract some others, which would be unfortunate. A more serious problem could occur if readers take to heart McGuire's advice to find another dentist if the one they have fails to meet McGuire's standards. His recommendations are certainly reasonable matters to expect of a dentist, but there is probably some action short of dismissal that could be taken to improve the doctor's performance. My concern is that McGuire-inspired consumers are going to run up big travel bills tripping about seeking a dentist sufficiently committed to the author's good principles. A little moderation seems in order.

• Another quarrel I have with McGuire is his failure to go all the way and counsel avoidance of aspirin, cigarettes, and various drugs. This could be written off as part of his "hang loose," nondirective manner except that he is quite directive in urging the elimination of white sugar/candy/soft drinks/preservatives/etc.

• One other minor cavil: I thought McGuire recommended *The Tooth Trip* about ten times too often. He has readers hustling copies to their dentists, State Health Departments, legislators, friends, and neighbors. It is a good book, but I would have preferred him to have left the selling to others.

Reuben, David. *The Save Your Life Diet*. New York: Ballantine, 1975.

Touting a high fiber approach, *The Save Your Life Diet* suggests that it can be the most effective preventive medicine available. To Reuben, bran is your best safeguard against elevated cholesterol, constipation, obesity, appendicitis, diverticular disease of the colon, ischemic heart disease, cancer of the colon and rectum, and phlebitis and resulting blood clots to the lungs. Most of the action in this book is set in the colon, the body's sewage plant. The villain is our modern diet, which causes a stagnation of fecal products in the colon, leading to a variety of disorders.

Strengths
• Reuben provides impressive evidence and references which document studies and reports supportive of his high fiber diet proposals.

• The book is readable: the author has an effective style and an interesting way of organizing material.

• In addition to the case for bran and a high fiber diet, Reuben has given us a basic reader on certain diseases; what they are and how they come about (e.g., diverticulosis).

• The book succeeds in making the digestive system high drama, and helps one respect the intricate machinery of the body and thus better maintain it through a sensible diet and the avoidance of destructive dining behaviors. Interesting menus are included.

• Of most consequence, this book simply disseminates a

considerable amount of very good advice:

> - eat bran, fruits, yogurt, and high fiber foods;
> - avoid refined white sugar, soft drinks, fats, meat, instant foods, imitation anythings, and convenience pastries;
> - keep the feces on the move, that is, feces which are soft, relatively odor-free, and plentiful are better than hard droppings that are putrid and scarce; and,
> - get rid of body "sludge" as soon as possible after the organism has extracted and digested the needed fuels (fats, proteins, carbohydrates, vitamins, and minerals) by eating the high fiber way.

Shortcomings

● I think that Reuben puts too much reliance on the physician and fails to acknowledge the importance of an integrated program of well-being. Hardly a word is written about exercise, stress control, or any other dimension of high level wellness.

U.S. Senate (Select Committee on Nutrition and Human Needs). *Nutrition and Health: An Evaluation of Nutritional Surveillance in the United States.* Washington, D.C.: Government Printing Office, 1975.

Nutrition and Health contains a report on the status of nutritional awareness in the United States, the progress (or lack thereof) toward a comprehensive national nutrition policy, and a critical analysis of the major causes of current nutritional ignorance and neglect. The Senate report is an outgrowth of a series of hearings and staff studies in 1974 intended to measure progress made in achieving goals originally set at a White House Conference on Food, Nutrition, and Health in 1969. The focus of the report is upon how much people know about nutritional health, the availability of nutritional guidance, and the adequacy of monitoring systems concerning national nutrition. Also addressed, in the form of bureaucratic letters, memoranda, documents, charts, tables, testimony, and summary statements, are all the problems that discourage sound nutritional practices. Included in these data are facts on the status of nutritional research and education and the quality and safety of foods. This is the fifth in a series of staff documents on various aspects of nutrition and the federal role; at least one additional report has been published in recent months.

Strengths
● This is an excellent source document, and contains an eloquent foreword by the committee chairman, Sen. George McGovern. In his remarks, McGovern notes the rise in food prices, the inadequate diet of millions of Americans, and the deadly temptations for rich and poor alike posed by a food system overloaded with fat, sugar, salt, and all the other items leading to obesity, high blood pressure, diabetes, and cancer.

● The language of the report and the facts that are provided in the appendices make this a valuable primer for comprehending the implications of continued neglect of this vital dimension of well-being. Five of the 10 leading causes of death are attributed to poor diet habits, and the levels of ill health and the misuse of human potential are judged incalculable. Excerpts seem in order:

> The American public is eating blind. Medical schools have underemphasized nutrition with the result that the typical physical examination does not involve thorough nutritional evaluation or counseling.

> The American people know more about what their cars need than what their own bodies need. The result is an American public tempted by unhealthy food on one hand and weight-reducing gimmicks on the other. The result is a physically unhealthy nation.

> Our hope as a nation rests now, as it always has, on the active, informed involvement of our citizenry, as much in

the area of food policy as any other. The public must have access, and it does have a right, to proper nutrition evaluation and counseling. The nation needs continuous monitoring of its nutritional health. All government nutrition activities must be given coordination and direction.

The strength of the nation is based on the health of its people. We must realize that the simple act of choosing our diet, day after day, determines our personal health and national health and may well affect the health of other nations. Americans eat on as they have at their peril.

Shortcomings
•Except for the chairman's foreword, most of the material is disconnected and not intended for a general audience. Thus, the content gets a little heavy in places, though certain sections are surprisingly well written as well as beneficial (e.g., chapter 1 on the question of access to individual nutrition assessments).

Overall, an important and authoritative source document.

Williams, Roger J. *Nutrition against Disease.* New York: Bantam, 1973.

Nutrition against Disease makes the case for nutrition as *the* independent variable in disease formation. Williams documents the neglect of nutrition by the medical profession and suggests that adequate nourishment of our body cells or microenvironment is crucially important to health and well-being. The focus is on poor nutrition as it relates to mental illness, heart disease, obesity, dental problems, arthritis, old age, alcoholism, cancer, and many other disorders.

Strengths
• This book focuses on how the average physician overlooks opportunities for effectiveness due to ignorance of specific nutrients needed by the cells in our bodies. Williams decries the fact that, due to medical training and payment

255

linked to illnesses, doctors are less interested in health than in disease.

• The book details the hazards of aspirin and all other drugs having no known connection with the disease process itself, asserting that aspirin and other drugs mask the roots of the illness without eliminating it, contaminate the internal environment, create dependence, and complicate the search for the genuine source of the problem. Rhetorically, Williams asks: "Do you really believe you have headaches as a result of your system's lack of aspirin?"

• Williams focuses attention on the human element in disease, that is, the state of host resistance and the influence of will in both healing and remaining well.

• He provides a comprehensive survey of the nutritional awareness literature and demonstrates conclusively that living creatures are greatly affected by the quality and balance, as well as the amount, of food they ingest. The reader is not likely to finish this book without a thorough appreciation of the importance of a balanced assortment of amino acids, minerals, and vitamins to high level wellness.

• Williams stresses the uniqueness of all people and describes how we need varying amounts of different nutrients, depending upon our individual constitutional requirements.

•*Nutrition against Disease* convincingly links the nutritional adequacy of a pregnant woman's diet to the health of her baby.

• Williams is one of the few nutrition experts who demonstrates an integrated appreciation of wellness by virtue of the attention he gives to stress management and exercise, as well as to the destructive effects of cigarette smoking and alcohol abuse.

Shortcomings
• While he may be completely accurate in every respect, Williams risks losing some readers with his suggestions and unsubstantiated speculations that nutritional deficiencies are at the root of most diseases and disorders, including mental illness! Plus infection, nasty personalities, alcoholism, and mental retardation. As I mentioned, he may be right, but it does seem simplistic and inconsistent with his comments in other places regarding the value of other wellness dimensions.

Dimension of Stress Management

● *Benson, Herbert, M.D. *The Relaxation Response*.

● Brown, Barbara. *New Mind, New Body: Biofeedback, New Directions for the Mind*. New York: Bantam, 1974.

● Denniston, Denise, and McWilliams, Peter. *The TM Book*. New York: Warner, 1975.

● *Downing, George. *The Massage Book*.

● Friedman, Meyer and Rosenman, Ray H. *Type A Behavior and Your Heart*. Greenwich, Conn: Fawcett-Crest, 1974.

● Halsell, Grace. *Los Viejos: Secrets of Long Life from the Sacred Valley*. Emmaus, Pa.: Rodale Press, 1976.

● Karlins, Marvin and Andrews, Lewis M. *Biofeedback: Turning the Power of Your Mind*. New York: Warner, 1973.

● Maharishi, Mahesh Yogi. *Transcendental Meditation: Serenity without Drugs*. New York: Signet, 1968.

● *McQuade, Walter and Aikman, Ann. *Stress*.

● Pelletier, Kenneth R. *Mind as Healer, Mind as Slayer: A Holistic Approach to Preventing Stress Disorders*. New York: Delta, 1977.

● *Samuels, Mike and Bennett, Hal Z. *Be Well*.

● *Selye, Hans. *Stress without Distress*.

Benson, Herbert, M.D. *The Relaxation Response*. New York: Avon, 1975.

The Relaxation Response provides a synthesis of modern discoveries and religious/philosophic literature regarding the effects of meditation techniques in coming to terms with and adapting to environmental and other stresses. Dr. Benson manages to identify a method by which modern man (and woman) can deal constructively with the increased pressures of contemporary society, namely, through the use of a meditation technique he terms the relaxation response.

Prior to describing the technique of the relaxation response in the next-to-last chapter of the book, Dr. Benson explains in considerable detail the physiological nature of stress, the concept of the fight-or-flight response, the dangers of hypertension (high blood pressure), and the four elements that must be part of the relaxation response if it is to be effective (a quiet environment, an object to dwell upon, a passive attitude, and a comfortable position).

Along the way, Benson quotes the teachings of Buddha, William James, an anonymous Christian mystic, St. Augustine, Fray Francisco de Osuna, St. Teresa, the monks on Mt. Athos in Greece, Judaism, H. Saddhatissa, Lao Tzu, and Confucius, among others, to demonstrate "certain common elements in almost all cultures which enable individuals to periodically change their everyday mode of thinking." (If all these folks are for the relaxation response, it can't be all bad.)

Benson defines stress as "environmental conditions that require behavioral adjustment." Hypertension is described as the "hidden epidemic" of our time leading to atherosclerosis; the fight or flight response (which precipitates increased blood flow and blood pressure, and higher heart, breathing, and metabolism rates) is identified as the key factor in hypertension. The relaxation response is the "natural and innate protective mechanism against overstress" which protects against the harmful effects of the fight or flight response.

The Relaxation Response contains interesting figures and diagrams, including a few sixteenth century anatomical drawings by Vesalius, and a bibliography of articles and books on varied aspects of stress management.

Strengths

● This is another of those books which could have a positive influence on your lifestyle. It is hard to think about the test results and effects of the constant fight or flight syndrome our bodies experience and not appreciate the importance of including some stress management activity in your daily wellness regimen.

● The review of varied experiments on meditative states and bodily changes done with the leadership and adherents of Transcendental Meditation is of considerable interest. I found the objectivity and level of moderation which the author brings to the laboratory and the recording of his interpretations and conclusions especially impressive.

● Dr. Benson, unlike the writer(s) of the book's jacket cover, is careful not to raise excessive and unsupported claims for the relaxation response. For this, the reader can be grateful. Also admirable is the idea that meditation need not be done in any given way (e.g., Transcendental Meditation), and that we are all unique and have to find the time/style/technique that best suits our individualistic needs and preferences.

Shortcomings

● I found the lengthy selections alleging an age-old universality connecting altered states of consciousness and the relaxation response a bit of a distraction and rather tenuously linked. The citations intended to demonstrate the presence of selected elements of such a response throughout time simply do not seem convincing or necessary for purposes of this book.

● The writing style is clear but dull, and Dr. Benson ignores almost completely the policy implications of his work. If the relaxation response is such a good thing—and it certainly seems to be a breakthrough—why not outline how it might come to pass for more people and how society might change if it did? The only comment in this regard occurs on the next to last page: "We need the Relaxation Response even more today because our world is changing at an ever-increasing pace. Society should sanction the time for the Relaxation Response."

• Like other physician-authors, Benson is overly tied, in my view, to the old notion of patients dependent on doctors and the use of drugs, even when meditation itself is providing stress-reduction results. Excerpts demonstrate this problem:

> If the reader decides to use the Relaxation Response for the purpose of medical treatment, he or she should do so only with the approval and subsequent supervision of his or her physician.

> Standard medical therapy means taking antihypertension drugs, which often act by interrupting the activity of the sympathetic nervous system, thus lowering blood pressure.

> In the case of mild hypertension, the regular evocation of the Relaxation Response may be of great value, since it has none of the pharmacologic side effects often present with drugs and might possibly supplant their use. But no matter how encouraging these initial results, no person should treat himself for high blood pressure by regularly eliciting the Relaxation Response. You should always do so under the care of your physician, who will routinely monitor your blood pressure to make sure it is adequately controlled.

———————

Downing, George. *The Massage Book*. New York: Bookworks/Random House, 1972.

The Massage Book is about a form of communication without words. It is designed to explain all one needs to know to do a massage and to appreciate the meaning and purpose of this much distorted art form.

Much of the book is addressed to preparations for massage, including details about oils and powders, massage tables, organization, expectations, and the proper use of the hands. The major portion contains descriptions of the 80 key strokes for each part of the body, beginning with the head and neck and proceeding to everything in reach. A third section treats additional possibilities: how to do a ten-minute massage, massage for lovers, massage and meditation, and generally more than you ever wanted to know or would have asked about massage. *The Massage Book* has illustrations of nearly every stroke and posture, an entire chapter on anatomy (skeletal and muscular drawings), a bibliography of further readings, and an explanation of how the book came about.

Strengths
• Downing recognizes that massage is an important stress-reduction approach useful for getting in touch (no pun intended) with your body and the bodies of others whom you care about. It is also good fun and a special way of showing affection for another person. The brief chapter on body tension, which emphasizes the living tissues of the body as an interconnected whole, is outstanding for purposes of stress-management education.

• The major strength of this book is that it reinforces your awareness of your anatomy, which in turn encourages a wellness-enhancement lifestyle to "lubricate" this marvelous machinery.

• *The Massage Book* is well written, easy to read and follow, and as comprehensive as one could expect.

Shortcomings
• Downing does an excellent job of keeping the discussion on a nonflippant, straight forward, and sincere basis without being dull or overly elementary. However, some folks will still find certain sections to be a bit much. An example might be the brief chapters on massage for animals

("Do the right thing and they will sprawl in a heap on the floor. Do the wrong thing and they will snap at you") or "massage for lovers." Personally, I found the latter to be a bit dull and the former hilarious, but I suspect Downing did not intend to be funny. (My favorite humor is in the conclusion to the animal section: "I'm pretty much a dog and cat man myself. I've never really gotten into horses and buffaloes, or for that matter mice and canaries, all of which I'm sure are whole massage worlds unto themselves.")

In any event, neither *The Massage Book* nor massage is for everybody but, then, neither is anything else.

McQuade, Walter and Aikman, Ann. *Stress.* New York: Bantam, 1975.

The authors describe stress as the basic cause of contemporary degenerative or chronic diseases, noting that it has become a "shadow darkening our lives." They devote a considerable amount of attention to explaining the physiology of stress as it affects the mind and body, and they note in the process three basic sources of stress which humans have experienced through history (threat of mortal combat, worry of not getting enough to eat, and fear of death).

Stress is organized in four parts. Part one of the book deals with stress in our "take-society," definitions of the term, citations of varied studies, and an explanation of what Selye called the *general adaptation syndrome* in referring to the "wearing down" effect of prolonged stress. The impact of coffee and other drugs on adaptation energy is also described.

Part two contains an accounting of what unattended stress can do to you, with chapters on each of the major body systems and the diseases that result from prolonged tensions and anxieties. In the chapter on the cardiovascular system, heart attacks are recognized as a modern affliction; a relationship is established between the rise in the gross national product and coronary heart disease. As in their descriptions of all systems,

McQuade and Aikman cite numerous studies and research reports for nearly all statements put forth on the effects of stress. In this section on the cardiovascular system, focus is placed on the role of personality as the major predisposing factor or highest risk characteristic of coronary candidates. Special emphasis is given to tracing the links between stress and other cardiovascular system disorders, particularly hypertension, angina and arrhythmia and migraine.

Treated in a similar manner (i.e., linkages described between disease types and stress) in part two of *Stress* are the digestive system and related organs (involved in ulcers, colitis, diabetes, constipation, diarrhea, and diabetes); the body's immunity screens (involved in infections, allergies, rheumatoid arthritis, and cancer); and the skeletal-muscular system and what stress does to it (backache, tension headaches, arthritis, and the "accident-prone" syndrome).

Part three, the briefest section of the book, is devoted to the "pathways of stress," an accounting of how the mind and the body each deal with stress, and how the former sometimes "betrays" the latter. McQuade and Aikman emphasize the "mind rules the body as the most fundamental fact we know about the process of life" (quoting Franz Alexander).

Part four, the lengthiest section of *Stress*, is addressed to a shopping list of personal solutions for stress problems. The authors prescribe diet and exercise, and devote much attention to each dimension. In addition, they review other ways for altering the response to stress. Some of these are psychotherapy, drugs, encounter groups, meditation, biofeedback, and hypnotism.

A list of further readings is provided, with a sentence or two about each book.

Strengths
• McQuade and Aikman have translated a great many studies and research reports on stress into a readable book that is never dull and always informative. It is an excellent work on the stress management dimension for you if you think you have time for only one book on stress, which of

course would suggest that you are under too much of it.

• I especially appreciated the way the authors emphasize the linkage between stress and exercise and diet, a crossing of dimensional boundaries not often found in books on one dimension. Also of note were the descriptions tying stress to cancer and accidents.

Stress helps to cause cancer because it depresses the immune response, the body's only real means of defending itself against malignant cells.

Twenty percent of all fatal car accidents involve drivers who have suffered an upsetting experience within six hours before the crash, and one out of three accident victims was depressed.

• As I've noted, each of the major parts outlined above is well written and packed with data and conclusions from the major stress research findings. One section deserving special note is the authors' summary of how our needs, if met, can best safeguard us from damaging stress:

People in their daily lives all need such things as food, drink, shelter, rest, success and power, communion with other people, sex, intellectual and physical growth, a sense of good and evil, a sense of beauty, a little fun, and a sense of self, a sense of the meaning of one's life. A person will lead a satisfying life if he can more or less fill all these needs.

Shortcomings
A few minor quarrels I had with this work included:

• Excessive reliance on medical authorities, and warnings to the reader not to do one thing or another without a doctor's permission. While consultation is advised in some circumstances, the authors go too far, in my opinion.

• Occasional failures to go beyond the pros and cons of an issue or to provide us with a clear statement of what they believe to be true. Noting the pros and cons of a controversy is not always sufficient, I personally expect "experts" to tell us what they think.

• The personal wellness regimen of the authors leaves something to be desired in the area of diet. For example, McQuade is discussing personal solutions regarding diet when he tells us the following about his own approach:

> There are many trim people who deliberately keep so busy at the office that they skip lunch. I frequently cross the street to a good hamburger place and have one with a lot of pickles (and no roll) and two black coffees, and am amazed by how much work I get done in the afternoon.

• The self-responsibility dimension is lightly regarded at times. In describing ways to break habits, reference is made to the "average patient" in a way that suggests he has to make the best of what he has regarding medical resources. For example:

> Actually, in recent years it has been discovered that some people can deliberately lower their own blood pressure, or reduce their gastric secretions, if they are trained to do so . . . but the technique is not readily available to the average patient.

Why settle for being an "average patient?" If biofeedback and other nontraditional modalities are not available, why not find another provider who will see that such approaches are a part of the resources available to facilitate a client's well-being?

All of these concerns are of minor impact in relation to the overall value of this good book—highly recommended on the subject of stress management.

Samuels, Mike, M.D. and Bennett, Hal Z. *Be Well*. New York: Random House, 1974.

Be Well describes the manner in which the body heals itself and what a person can do to increase healing by an attitude that centers on well-being. Feelings are isolated as guides to health or its absence, and approaches for getting in touch with feelings that result in ease are outlined. Samuels and Bennett use the terms *universal self* and *individual self* to describe that part of us in touch with the universal law (which personifies inborn healing abilities) and one's uniqueness, which sets us all apart. The idea of a "feeling pause" is developed as a tool to shape the experience of feeling good. A check list to assist in the process of developing "feeling pause" capability is provided, as are exercises, cases, resources for further study, and a glossary of terms.

Strengths

• *Be Well* is fast and easy reading; the drawings illustrating forms "manifest in the universe" support the thesis of the interrelationships of small and large forms. (You probably did not know a gorgonocepholus is a very lovely creature; a tungsten atom's kind of cute, too, claim Samuels and Bennett.)

• The authors demonstrate how we create our own levels of wellness or dis-ease, and how through the "feeling pause" we can acquire an awareness of and control over changes taking place within.

• The book contains an interesting outline of the specific regulatory processes or "inborn healing abilities" (the antibody system and the body's other processes for maintaining optimum heart beat, blood pressure, respiration rate, blood flow, acid-base balance, electromagnetic properties, and body temperature). This tends to encourage us in our quests for higher levels of well-being.

• Samuels and Bennett make the important point that you can exert a positive influence on the growth of new cells by virtue of lifestyle patterns conducive to well-being. In making such statements, the authors make reference to almost all of the wellness dimensions.

Shortcomings
- Samuels and Bennett, unfortunately, shamelessly promote *The Well Body Book*, their first and best known publication. A little of this might have been OK, but it is cited to excess, in my opinion.

- Another shortcoming is that *Be Well* seems not to have been edited; it is ungrammatical to the point of distraction.

Selye, Hans, M.D. *Stress Without Distress*. New York: Signet, 1974.

Selye distinguishes between stress as pleasure, challenge, and fulfillment, and stress as frustration, anxiety, fear, hate (i.e. dis-stress). Good stress enables creativity, idealism, and harmony; dis-stress leads to ulcers, hypertension, and the eventual destruction of the organism. In his design for living with and learning to enjoy and utilize the positive aspects of stress while avoiding the negative damages of uncontrolled dis-stress, Selye explains the nature of stress, describes what it is and is not, and discusses at length the relationships between stress and "aims in life." He also comments on the meaning of work and leisure, optimal stress levels, goals, critical or discerning love, purpose, and the elements of a full life.

Strengths
- *Stress without Distress* synthesizes most effectively a great deal of information on the stress control dimension and provides a philosophical framework to facilitate the examination and refinement of your own sense of purpose.

- The book reinforces notions of self-responsibility and individual uniqueness; Selye notes at one point that you must analyze your own situation to find the stress level at which you are most comfortable.

- *Stress without Distress* offers an attractive prescription for constructively managing stress: this is to collect as much "love" (gratitude, respect, trust, and admiration) as possible via the excellence of your efforts. As far as science can tell, this collection and attendant enjoyment is the ultimate aim in life, claims Selye. And the greatest dissatisfactions—and thus negative stresses—come from your own disrespect for your individual accomplishments.

• Correctly, in my view, Selye claims that the "lack of hunger for achievement" or the absence of "work that fulfills" constitutes the major source of distress. The fatal enemy of all utopias, writes Selye, is boredom. The antidote is to work on "perfecting your own self." A search for higher levels of wellness is, of course, one way in which you might approach this work.

Shortcomings
• This book is a classic and contains no flaws which deserve mention. In promoting self-responsibility, sense of purpose, a theoretical framework for stress control, and an appreciation of aspects of personal environmental sensitivity, it has few rivals.

Dimension of Physical Fitness

- Cooper, Kenneth H. *Aerobics*. New York: Bantam, 1968.

- Cooper, Kenneth H. *The New Aerobics*. New York: Bantam, 1970.

- *Glasser, William, M.D. *Positive Addiction*.

- *Gomez, Joan, M.D. *How Not to Die Young*.

- *Gore, Irene. *Add Years to Your Life and Life to Your Years*.

- *Leonard, George. *The Ultimate Athlete*.

- *Morehouse, Lawrence E. and Gross, Leonard. *Total Fitness: In 30 Minutes a Week*.

- *Proxmire, William. *You Can Do It! Senator Proxmire's Exercise, Diet, and Relaxation Plan*.

- Reichman, Stanley. *Instant Fitness for Total Health*. New York: Dell, 1976.

Glasser, William, M.D. *Positive Addiction*. New York: Harper and Row, 1976.

Positive Addiction is about behaviors that strengthen us and make our lives more rewarding. Glasser, a psychiatrist, describes these behaviors as positive addictions, and tells how to cultivate them in order to overcome destructive lifestyle habits in favor of more satisfying and integrated life patterns. An analogy is drawn between the withdrawal effects from a negative addiction (e.g. drugs, alcohol) and the milder but nonetheless self-reinforcing sense that comes from ignoring a positive addiction, if one is *lucky* enough to have such. A program for cultivating a positive addiction is set out and case studies are provided.

Strengths

• By demonstrating how one becomes positively addicted to jogging, meditation, or other behavior that strengthens, Glasser indirectly describes how one can become addicted to a high level wellness lifestyle.

• Glasser conveys important points about the psychology of personal behavior and keys to its modification in clear, nontechnical language. Some insights are:

> - that some people give up trying in life or develop disease or illness symptoms as substitutes for the love and worth they feel unable to obtain.
> - that illness is a choice sometimes made as a way of coping with and disguising feelings of inadequacy.
> - that the essences of life—for the strong—are fulfillment, pleasure, recognition, a sense of personal value/worth/purpose, and the enjoyment of loving and being loved.

• Glasser's listing of the benefits of having a positive addiction serves as a catalog of the rewards of a wellness lifestyle—the pursuit of which is exactly what Glasser would term a positive addiction.

Shortcomings

• Methodologically, Glasser's survey methods are pretty shaky, his data are incomplete, and the selection of positive addiction forms (jogging and meditation) seems limited. In addition, I'm afraid he underestimates the difficulty some readers may experience in moving from acceptance of the idea of cultivating an addiction to the reality of managing to do so.

The above criticism is picking nits in relation to the value of the book. Glasser has well described an important concept; *Positive Addiction* deserves a high priority on your wellness reading list.

Gomez, Joan, M.D. *How Not to Die Young*. New York: Pocket Books, 1973.

Dr. Gomez describes the human machinery (heart and arteries, lungs and breathing apparatus, kidneys and bladder, digestive system and liver, etc.) and how your lifestyle makes it run smoothly or obsolesce prematurely. In *How Not To Die Young*, she provides a summary of the risks of nutritional ignorance, obesity, long-term tension, and the hit parade of destructive behaviors—smoking and alcohol abuse. The author suggests a set of remedies for whatever ailment you care to avoid, after describing the miseries attendant upon continuing your errant ways. In addition, Dr. Gomez has a mini-plan for most of the major wellness dimensions.

Essentially, she is telling you to take stock through a wellness inventory, and learn what you need to know about your body in order to respect it and avoid premature obsolescence. Menus for how to eat right (i.e., use high fiber foods and, of course, avoid white sugar, refined flour, etc.), advice on how to keep fit, suggestions on ways to control stress, and approaches to developing a sense of purpose round out the message of *How Not to Die Young*.

Strengths
• The style of this book is both understandable and witty. Examples:
    - [On sex] This remains almost the only pleasure that isn't harmful so long as you are reasonably fit. In fact, it is a form of exercise and a first-class release from every kind of tension: the one green thing in our artificial world.
    - [On the limits of exhortation] A moral veto is no good against an instinctual drive.

- [On humor as an antidote for stress] If you can occasionally laugh at yourself you have reached the highest achievement of civilized man, and have attained the complete safeguard against inner arrogance.

• Gomez has written a comprehensive guidebook which gives substantial advice on most of the dimensions of high level wellness.

• The book contains an entertaining, provocative, and insightful 243-question inventory and a self-scoring analysis.

• *How Not to Die Young* also contains two chapters of special interest—one on the health problems and needs of women in particular, the other on a sense of purpose, entitled "Survival—For What?"

• I especially applauded her portrayal of smoking as the single greatest avoidable menace to good health—and the risks smokers run are convincingly articulated.

Shortcomings
• Dr. Gomez writes hundreds of sensible sentences and page after page of descriptive prose on the basic knowledge people need in order to take responsibility for their lives. One should not be too upset in finding a foolish pronouncement here and there, though when Gomez is bad she is very bad indeed. Examples:
- "If you have a kidney disorder, do get advice from one of the top 10 renal experts in your country." Nonsense! Why the top 10? Why not the number one provider—or the top 100? Is cost no factor? How does the consumer judge the field to define the top 10? What criteria should we use in such a situation?
- [On not hesitating to have checks for breast cancer] "Removal of part, or more likely the whole of one or both breasts? Don't let this dismay you. What else are

falsies for?" That's a rather casual dismissal—and damn small comfort.

- [On guarding against stress] "Antidepressants work miraculously for some kinds of miseries, and there is always some sort of help for other kinds."

Despite the above, all is forgiven. A wonderful book—do read it.

Gore, Irene. *Add Years to Your Life and Life to Your Years.* New York: Stein and Day, 1975.

Dr. Gore defines the importance of physical fitness, nutritional awareness, stress management, and environmental sensitivity to aging with vitality and grace. The book provides inspiration and understanding and demonstrates that getting "old" is as much a state of mind as of body. Dr. Gore provides a treasury of tips for maintaining vitality, improving vigor, and generally avoiding senescence and decline.

Strengths
• I liked the distinctions which the author made between pathological and physiological old age, showing the first as a condition of bodily disuse and misuse which is avoidable.

• Dr. Gore provides a persuasive array of evidence linking premature decline to asking too little of ourselves physically and mentally, and effectively establishes the idea that it is normal to feel healthy; that sickness, dissolution, and all the rest are not inevitable concomitants of aging.

• The book is written in understated British prose, with many a fine turn of phrase:

[On getting set in one's ways] There are also many people who live according to patterns hallowed by time and custom, and who run the risk of developing what may be termed "mental arthritis."

[On keeping an open, vital mind alert to change] A mind set in its ways is not necessarily a treasure house. There may be some priceless things in it, but there may also be a good deal of lesser value, which could with profit be cleared out from time to time, to admit some fresh light and air. Who knows how many priceless new things may drift into it on this current of fresh air?

[On fear as a motivator] Most of us need a jolt to spur us into revising our views and habits. If we take a good, long look at the worst features of a prolonged senility we shall get just such a jolt. We would, I believe, emerge from such an exercise determined to do everything possible to promote our own fitness and vitality to form a bulwark against dissolution, dependence, and decay.

•*Add Years to Your Life and Life to Your Years* also provides interesting and sensible exercise suggestions, dietary counsel, social policy ideas, a chart on the functions and sources of vitamins, and a catalog of the "immortals" who practiced wellness into distant old age.

Shortcomings
•Unfortunately, Dr. Gore, too, is unnecessarily and I believe mistakenly deferential to the role of the physician, to the point that she almost slights consumer self-responsibility. The book does, I'm afraid, follow too closely the outmoded model of doctor as controller and order-giver, which in turn denies the sovereignty of the client.

Leonard, George. *The Ultimate Athlete*. New York: Viking Press, 1974.

The Ultimate Athlete is an exploration of the life-giving, even transcendental possibilities within the realms of the "larger games," new dimensions, and changing philosophy of physical fitness. Leonard describes his concepts of an ideal athlete while drawing heavily on current and historical events and personal examples to illustrate what is wrong, misdirected, and a "turn off" about contemporary sports. Targets are winner-take-all,

competition-focused, specialized, inhumane, elitist, institutionalized, and winning-obsessed attitudes that split mind and
body and impose limits and restricted definitions on human
functioning. But Leonard suggests that we all have unsuspected
potentials that can lead to a rebirth of ourselves and the "unfold-
ing of a new world" of enjoyments and celebrations in fitness. To
help us get there, the author explains his ideas about old and
new games, transcendence via sport(s) of one's choosing, and the
characteristics of the "ultimate athlete." This person plays the
game of life intensely through the sport or game of his/her
choice, enjoying a full awareness of life and death with acceptance of both joy and pain. He or she transcends boundaries,
and joins mind and body in a "dance of existence" on an "evolutionary journey." *Ultimate Athlete* contains copious personal
examples, a review of new games and energy exercises, a design
for a changed approach to physical education in the schools, and
commentaries on running/flying/diving/risking and more.

Strengths
• There are many. Heading the list might be Leonard's
insight into physical fitness, lifestyle, and wellness:

> We have no way of knowing how much of our current
> sickness and malaise could be eliminated if people of all
> ages were turned on to "the vibrant, dynamic feeling that
> comes from being more than just well." But a number of
> scientists, notably Dr. Rene Dubos, have marshaled evi-
> dence to show that way-of-life is a major factor in the inci-
> dence of sickness. The degenerative diseases—ulcers,
> colitis, asthma, arteriosclerosis, hypertension, obesity, and
> the like—are clearly associated with the lifestyle of the
> technologically advanced nations, and could undoubtedly
> be greatly reduced by a change in that lifestyle, as could the
> current abuse of tobacco, alcohol, and other drugs. The vi-
> brant, fully active physical body provides the foundation for
> such a change.

• Leonard is a marvelous phrasemaker (e.g., Aikido as "a
lifelong journey with no fixed destination"), aware of the

new medicine and concepts of holistic health, and fully capable of working such ideas into *The Ultimate Athlete* (e.g., the connectedness with nature, the ideal unity of body and mind and spirit, etc.). The description of new games, the emphasis on personal reform as a prerequisite to the realization of social action, and the idea of an athlete that dwells within us all are certainly highlights of a consistently "healthy" look for those open to new directions.

• *The Ultimate Athlete* is an "up" book with a hopeful view of a better society—a view encompassing physical fitness—and beyond:

> There is a growing army of American joggers, hikers, swimmers, and bicyclists of all ages pursuing the joys of fine physical conditioning. And there are signs . . . that increasing numbers of athletes are beginning to find words to express those magical values in sports that make mere "winning out" seem empty indeed. We stand, in fact, on the edge of the most exciting period in the history of athletics, a period of newly awakened physical awareness, of creation and change.

Shortcomings
• There might be a bit too much of George Leonard, his buddies, and his Aikido in the examples and discussions for some readers, besides this one. Others, particularly those outside the Bay Area, may have trouble with some of the consciousness rhetoric (e.g., "re-visioning" sports, "moments of oneness," "energy bodies," and so forth) and feel suspicious about the psychic examples of "transcendental possibilities" suggested by disgruntled and/or far-out jocks.

Overall, a fine and important book.

Morehouse, Lawrence, E., and Gross, Leonard. *Total Fitness: In 30 Minutes a Week.* New York: Pocket Books, 1976.

Total Fitness: In 30 Minutes a Week presents a philosophy

of fitness and an original approach to exercise. The authors demonstrate that the right kind of exercise "buys years" by slowing the aging process and increasing the capacity for living. Morehouse and Gross advocate a fitness philosophy, originally developed for the U.S. space program, that is based upon physiological effort indicated by heart rate in lieu of the usual measures of time, distance, and load. The emphasis is upon developing good skeletal-muscle and circulo-respiratory endurance.

The authors introduce a concept termed *functional wellness*, which they define as the ability to cope with your environment. According to them, not everyone needs to be an athlete to be fit; the 30-minute routine is for the individual who seeks "minimum maintenance" and wants to do no more than is necessary to achieve a reasonable period of survival. Supplemental programs that go well beyond the 30-minute-a-week gimmick are provided for those who expect more from their bodies, a "reserve for fitness," or specific conditioning.

Total Fitness provides a guide to weight loss and control without the need for withdrawal pains or life-long calorie-counting. The diet plan uses the same principles as the pulse-count fitness program targeted for muscular and cardiovascular endurance. Morehouse and Gross include a review of what was good and not so good about all the popularized fitness programs over the years and explain how to take a pulse count, the basic tool in their theory of heart-rated exercise. The book concludes with drawings and explanations of "three short steps to fitness," a consideration of special problems, and extra things you can do to supplement the basic three-times-per-week routine.

Strengths

• Morehouse (Gross's contribution is not apparent, as the narrative in the first person is about Morehouse's background and experiences) takes on fifteen exercise myths which he claims are unfounded "old wives' tales" which interfere with enjoying exercise. Who amongst us has not heard, if not believed, that you:

    - should not drink while exercising;

- can increase your energy level by taking sugar before a workout;
- cannot safely eat before swimming;
- should avoid sex before an athletic contest for optimal performance.

These and other myths are convincingly, and often humorously, put to rest.

• This book reinforces the idea of a multiplier effect in a high level wellness routine. For example, the authors cite instances wherein many people showed dramatic changes in their behaviors in other dimensions (smoked less, ate better, reduced risk behaviors, and stopped drinking) when they became involved in a fitness program.

•*Total Fitness: In 30 Minutes a Week* provides a number of insights in a memorable fashion:

Sweating *does* burn calories, but it's a dangerous way to reduce. You could have the best figure in the morgue.

If I have learned one thing in my years of study, it is that the fountain of youth for which Ponce de Leon searched in vain was right inside his body. Exercise is the means to an alert, vigorous, and lengthy life. Inactivity will kill you.

As Noel Coward put it in a song, only "mad dogs and Englishmen" go out in the noonday sun. Actually, it's the safest time to exercise on a sunny day. With the sun overhead, all you need to shield yourself is a hat. In mid-morning or mid-afternoon, however, there is no way to shield your body from direct exposure to the sun's rays coming in at an angle.

• Perhaps the most important benefit of this book is that it can help you to realize that exercise need not be a grind to be beneficial and can, in fact, be a joy in your life that complements other health-enhancing activities.

Shortcomings
• An overwhelming negative impression that I had when I saw the jacket and that remained as I read through the text,

was a sense of "What's the hurry?" Except for the attention-grabbing lure of getting something (i.e., total fitness) for almost nothing (i.e. 30 minutes a week), the text does not support either the desirability or the feasibility of such an approach. But for all the other strengths described, *Total Fitness: In 30 Minutes a Week* is a fine publication which I recommend you read.

Proxmire, William. *You Can Do It! Senator Proxmire's Exercise, Diet, and Relaxation Plan.* New York: Simon and Schuster, 1973.

This book presents a United States senator's case for health and self-responsibility as a patriotic duty! The emphasis is on nutritional awareness (diet), physical fitness (exercise), and stress management (relaxation); the senator's recommended pathways to "human ecology" include walking, running, swimming, a weight-conscious diet, and biofeedback and/or meditation.

The good senator states in the introduction ("Your Patriotic Duty") that "a country's no better or worse than its people," and that Americans, in part due to our material wealth, are physical wrecks. Senator Proxmire pulls no punches:

> We are too fat, too soft, too tense. We are prone to alcoholism and increasingly to drug addiction. We are lazy. We are thoughtlessly self-indulgent, and unless we get a grip on ourselves, unless we straighten out, we are not long for leadership. We are going to fail and we will deserve to lose what we have. And this soft, fat, tense physical condition of ours is why in spite of all our blessings the world looks so grim, so sad, so boring, so empty to so many of us. A people that relies on booze for a pickup, on cigarettes or a tranquilizer for relaxation, on aspirin to relieve tensions, on sleeping pills for sleep—such a people is not only physically sick but bound to be sad and depressed, to feel that the world—even a good and happy world—is out of joint.

You Can Do It! is illustrated, written in a highly personal fashion (almost autobiographically), and contains frequent references to the wellness characteristics (or lack thereof) of American presidents, other notables, and Winston Churchill!

Strengths

• The book is easy reading, contains interesting personal anecdotes, and represents an integrated approach to health and well-being. In his unique manner, Senator Proxmire effectively expresses some of the key principles and concepts of high level wellness.

• The strengths of the book are found in key messages which stress that vitality is more relevant than age, that health is a duty to oneself as well as family in a free society, that a wellness lifestyle is hard work but fun, and that no laws or federal policies will ever substitute for self-responsibility in efforts to promote a healthier society.

• I especially enjoyed the senator's critique of various sports as exercise, his focus on the joys of eating, and his outspoken assessments of the typical citizen's lifestyle. Witness the following as an example:

> We are a fat, degenerated people. We are compelled to spend literally billions and billions of dollars a year in both private and public drains on our resources to provide the doctors, the nurses, the hospitals to correct the endless illnesses caused by obesity and overeating.
>
> I have been a critic of waste in defense. But I am certain that America has wasted far more of its substance, many, many times more, at the dinner table than it has even in the appalling extravagance of the Pentagon.

• As you can see by the above excerpts, Senator Proxmire does not tread lightly when pointing the finger at health hazards. One of his favorite targets is ethyl alcohol ("In my view this cocktail hour is the single most destructive habit in the civilized world, destructive of health for millions of people because it becomes compulsive. It can also destroy jobs and families, and it leads to tens of thousands of deaths

281

on the highways"); another is restaurants ("Many a restaurant serves nothing but steak, baked potato, booze, and
pastry. This formula for a living death is the backbone of the
restaurant industry").

• The senator decries wasteful government support of sickness and disease-oriented Medicare and expresses concern
about expensive new federal programs which provide little
or no incentive for self-responsibility.

Shortcomings
• Some readers may be intimidated by the senator's enthusiasm (how many of us do 250 pushups every morning—
and then run to work?), and feel rather hopeless by comparison. Of course, this is not the senator's fault or intention, and he is cautious to emphasize that each reader
should develop his or her own unique "you can do it"
program.

• I would take issue with his diet plan that allows an occasional refined sugar binge (I say the trick is to learn not to
even *like* junk food), his collegial corn (e.g., a half page on
Senator Humphrey's ability to be fat, not exercise, shun relaxation, and eat anything—with impunity), and his doctor-
dependency (get your physician's OK for this and that). But
these are minor quarrels; overall, the book is an outstanding resource in the wellness literature.

Dimension of Environmental Sensitivity

• Ashcraft, N. and Scheflen, A. E. *People Space.* New York: Anchor Books, 1976.

• Bakker, Cornelius, *No Trespassing: Explorations in Human Territorality.* Corte Madera, Calif.: Chandler and Sharp, 1973.

• Barker, R. G. *Ecological Psychology.* Stanford, Calif.: Stanford University Press, 1968.

• *Dunn, Halbert, L. *High Level Wellness.*

• Ittelson, W. H. et al., *An Introduction to Environmental Psychology.* New York: Holt, Rinehart, & Winston, 1974.

• *Lappé, Frances Moore, *Diet For A Small Planet.*

• *McCamy, John M.D., and Presley, James, *Human Life Styling: Keeping Whole In the Twentieth Century.*

• Moos, Rudolf H. and Insel, Paul M., eds. *Issues in Social Ecology: Human Milieus.* Palo Alto, Calif.: Mayfield Pub., 1974.

• Schumacher, E. F., *Small Is Beautiful.* New York: Harper and Row, 1973.

• Sommer, B. *Personal Space.* Englewood Cliffs, N.J.: Prentice Hall, 1969.

Dunn, Halbert L., M.D. *High Level Wellness.* Arlington, Va.: R. W. Beatty, 1961.

As seminarians read the Bible, so future students of high level wellness will seek the original publication on wellness written by the founding father, the late Halbert L. Dunn. *High*

Level Wellness is a collection of 29 short talks on key aspects of wellness. Beginning with his definition of wellness as "an integrated method of functioning which is oriented to maximizing the potential of which an individual is capable, within the environment where he is functioning," Dunn goes on to relate a wellness philosophy to the individual, family, and community. In fact, he addresses nearly all the major wellness components pertinent to "a dynamic state of full and effective living," and most of all that dealing with environmental sensivitity.

Strengths

• Nearly two decades before the resurrection of high level wellness, holistic health, and the "new" focus on health enhancement and enrichment, Dr. Dunn set forth many of the principles now associated with these concepts. At the foundation of his work was the goal of "forward progress" of the individual toward his unique potentials focused on the integration of mind, body, and spirit. The doctor emphasized the importance of nature and the ethic of self-responsibility, elaborated on cellular unity and wholeness, stressed the importance of will in healing, and recognized the body's own restorative capacities as the noblest ally in well-being.

• Also discussed in this classic series of talks are a concern for the nature of man, energy as the universal force to treasure and husband, aging as a revered and dignified life stage ("healthy maturity"), and the vital necessity to know oneself (and how, if necessary, to become acquainted). Self-disclosure, a balance between work and leisure, and his idea of a "maturity in wholeness" are the favored themes which Dunn also believed were ingredients of the wellness lifestyle. Over and over, the talks published in this little book show a commitment to effective communications, imagination, and the cultivation of the creative spirit, which he defined as "an expression of self-adventuring into the unknown in search of truth."

• Dr. Dunn placed a high premium on love, personal

dignity, family, the brotherhood/sisterhood of all people, humane environments, the sanctity of nature and the "beasties," and the inseparable interdependence of individual/social/environmental wellness. He was idealistic; you can choose whether hopefully or hopelessly so.

• Dunn was aware of the works of major writers who have contributed so much to the composite that is still becoming the wellness lifestyle, and he was able to relate his wellness concepts to their thinking. His book contains references to the writings and ideas of Abraham Maslow, Hans Selye, Carl Rogers, Gordon Allport, Erich Fromm, S. I. Hayakawa, and Sidney Jourard, among others.

• *High Level Wellness* contains chapters on directions for future wellness research, and Dunn's prescription for a personal discipline for wellness. His own philosophy addressed a synthesis of man's achievements, aspirations, and potential future. He was pleased to compress these thoughts into two sentences of less than a hundred words, which he titled "Our World:"

> You, I, and our fellow men are emerging into a new world, our world. In this new world, science, faith, and the destiny of man blend with the oneness of life in the alchemy of man's never-ending search for truth, as this search is carried on throughout society in an energy field of responsive awareness, love, and trust, and is directed toward improving the world for mankind as a whole.

• In addition to being a teacher, physician, statistician, public administrator, and wellness advocate, Dunn was a planner. He saw the planning process as an opportunity "to combat the social ills that afflict us," and he had a nine-point plan for raising public levels of wellness. When asked if U.S. planners should be "foolish enough" to try to plan 100 years ahead, he replied, "Yes, if we expect to be a great nation at that time."

Shortcomings

• Unfortunately, the original *High Level Wellness* seems to be available only in libraries. To get a personal copy you almost need to know someone who knew the author. My contact was one of my mentors, who generously loaned me his copy containing this inscription from Halbert L. Dunn himself: "To Henrik L. Blum, in appreciation of your trailblazing work on 'multiservice' centers." To me, possession of such a treasure seems the ultimate status symbol.

Copies of a revised 1973 edition (the 9th printing) are available, however, from the publisher (R. W. Beatty Ltd., P.O. Box 26, Arlington VA 22210).

Lappé, Frances Moore. *Diet For a Small Planet*. New York: Ballantine, 1975.

This book is divided into four parts. The first is a critique of our food production, distribution, and consumption patterns; the second deals with protein and human needs; the third details nonmeat sources of protein; and the fourth part consists of recipes which result in maximum protein utilization without reliance on unecological and unsafe meat sources.

Lappé describes a way to minimize the amount of concentrated pesticides and heavy metals ingested from meat protein. She presents eight basic "myths" about the body's need for protein and how it is obtained, and summarizes the facts with respect to each myth. Two important "mythological" examples bear noting: (1) Meat contains more protein than other foods! FACT—meat is in the middle of the protein *quantity* scale, and considerably below eggs, milk, fish, and cheese in terms of protein the body can use; (2) The only way to get enough protein is to eat lots of meat! FACT—the average person in this country eats almost twice what his body can use, and most of us could eliminate not only meat but also fish and poultry and *still* get the grams needed from other protein-rich foods.

"*Diet For a Small Planet*" contains a catalog of tables, charts, illustrations, references, formulas, and comparison calculations, and a cookbook of recipes for complementary-protein delights.

Strengths

• There are so many positive features in this book that it is hard to isolate highlights: each of the four divisions contains much information that is usable and directive in charting your own path to nutritional awareness in a high level wellness context. In addition to an appreciation for the clear writing, social consciousness, objective and low-key presentation of what she believes, I gained a considerable amount of new understanding from four fundamental concepts which Lappé describes. These deal with net protein utilization, protein complementarity, amino acid balancing, and the psychology of successfully moving away from meats to other protein sources.

• Of recipes attempted, I recommend as another "strength" a scrumptious concoction which Lappé calls "cheese-fruit crepes." For those who might wish to try complementing their nonmeat proteins, here is the recipe. It provides from 35 percent to 42 percent of one's daily protein allowance, or 15 grams of usable protein per serving.

> Have ready: Whole wheat-sesame crepes (Can be made in advance. Recipe makes approximately 15 crepes, or 4 to 5 servings.)

Sift together:
⅔ cup whole wheat flour
½ teaspoon salt

Beat separately:
2 cups milk
2 eggs
2 tablespoons oil

Combine wet and dry and add:
2 tablespoons ground
sesame seeds (toasted or raw)

> Fry crepes in a lightly oiled heavy frying pan—a heavy

287

iron omelet pan is best. Make one crepe at a time, using approximately ¼ cup of batter each. After pouring the batter into a hot pan, tilt the pan to spread the batter into a thin, round layer. Wait until the crepe is fully solidified and browned on one side before turning it. (With a spatula I loosen all edges before turning.) Cook on the other side until browned. Once you have started frying the crepes, you may not need to add more oil to the pan. If you do, add only a little, enough to barely cover. Also, the batter will tend to separate, so merely stir and scoop from the bottom each time.

Topping: 2 cups your choice of stewed or fresh fruit: berries, peaches, rhubarb, etc.

Filling: ½ cup yogurt
1½ cups cottage cheese (or ricotta cheese)
1 tablespoon honey
nuts (optional)

Mix filling ingredients, then spread several teaspoons of filling in each crepe. Roll crepes and place in pan. Cover with topping of your choice. Heat and serve.

Shortcomings
• None worthy of note. *Diet For a Small Planet* is in part a nutrition book but even more an exposition of our responsibilities to the rest of the planet, as well as to ourselves. The concern for energy conservation, for wise allocation of our natural resources, and for living better lower on the food chain mark *Diet For a Small Planet* as superb reading in the area of environmental sensitivity.

———————————

McCamy, John, M.D. and Presley, James. *Human Life Styling: Keeping Whole in the Twentieth Century.* New York: Harper and Row, 1975.

The author (Presley) defines "normal" health as being perfectly well (as opposed to "average" health) and describes a four-part lifestyle approach for remaining that way while eliminating susceptibility factors and increasing resistance to illness and disease. The four parts—ecology, nutrition, exercise, and stress reduction—are both complementary and synergistic.

In an introductory section entitled "The Four Horsemen of Health," McCamy and Presley summarize the causes of heart disease, stroke, and cancer, and attendant lifestyle strategies for avoiding these major killers. Attention is given to the commonality of risk factors found in each disease and the key to avoidance is presented as methodically changing one's lifestyle. The lifestyle pattern of the "average" American is analyzed and is judged "abnormal" relative to health. *Human Life Styling* is introduced as a life-long design for "normal" optimal health.

The chapter on ecology or environmental sensitivity centers on slowing down material growth, conserving resources, eliminating pollution, and stabilizing population. Use is made of the "J-curve" concept to demonstrate the doubling-time effect of population growth. The authors develop a strong case for personal involvement, and provide an environmental checklist to further stimulate concern and action.

Emphasizing "simplicity" in their approach to nutrition, McCamy and Presley in effect advocate major changes in diet for many readers. Entire sections are given to the hazards of sugar, white starches, additives and "poisons", smoking, saturated fats, and drugs. Also included in the chapter on nutrition are discussions on optimal use of various liquids, protein requirements, meals, food freshness, supplements, and weight control. The key elements in the human-life-styling approach to nutrition are summarized at the end of the chapter. Here are some abbreviated highlights.

POINTS

    1. No refined carbohydrates (sugar, sweets, white
[flour] starches).   15
    2. No smoking.   10
    3. Alcohol is an unnecessary caloric. Drink none
unless in good health and at your proper weight, then
only one drink per day.   5

4. Use unsaturated fats. Safflower oil is best, corn oil is fair.   2

5. Eat raw fruits or vegetables at every meal.   5

6. Have a large breakfast, like a king; a medium lunch, like a prince; a small dinner, like a pauper.   2

7. No coffee, tea, colas, chocolate, or other caffeinated beverages.   5

8. Nutritional supplements. Medium requirements are: 5

> (a) A general vitamin, preferably from natural sources;
>
> (b) A stress complex formula, including equal portions of vitamin B_2 and B_6 (5 to 10 milligrams), pantothenic acid (10 to 20 milligrams) and vitamin C (100 to 600 milligrams).

9. Increase the quality of protein . . . Eat no junk meats such as bologna, frankfurters, or salami.   5

10. Drink hard spring water, if available. Use no iced drinks.   2

The point system is included after each of the four lifestyle areas "for those who wish to measure their progress numerically." A weekly or monthly total of 30 is minimal; readers are urged to set an ultimate goal of a "perfect score—56 points.")

McCamy and Presley recommend an exercise regimen that is essentially aerobic workouts requiring sustained effort and high oxygen consumption. Exercise is considered the most important of the lifestyle areas, absolutely critical in maintaining body balance and warding off disease.

The chapter on stress reduction also includes a section on the importance of relaxation and methods for achieving it. The physiology of stress, the mind-body link, the variables of our response to or our definitions of stress are all emphasized. Twelve mental clues or "sets" are listed and described as guidelines in improving one's emotional lifestyle, and the brain states of alpha/beta/theta are defined in relation to the importance of stress management.

Finally, the authors offer case histories showing the practicalities and results of human life styling and a series of suggestions for promoting nutritional, ecological, stress reduction, and exercise initiatives on a national scale.

Strengths

• Few other books on the wellness honor roll are as explicitly targeted to an integrated-lifestyle route to well-being as this readable guidebook. Many of the fundamental principles of high level wellness are emphasized or recognized in *Human Life Styling*, including the wellness dimensions, the connections between mind/body/spirit, the focus on prevention rather than treatment, and the ethic of self-responsibility. One criterion I use to assess my own response to a book is the extent to which I deface it with underlinings, margin notes, "Xs", and exclamation points: on this basis, the book ranks high in utility (but low in resale value).

• I appreciated the ecology and nutritional sections more than the rest, largely because I share so many of the authors' judgments about population control, the pathology of smoking, and the dangers of additives, preservatives, and drugs. I also especially liked the emphasis on personally modeling that which one "preaches" and the sense of commitment to a better environment in which to enjoy a richer lifestyle. Also appreciated was the creative suggestion that clergymen have a special role to play: "It may be that more God-awareness and alpha-state sessions, with less verbalizing, will help more people *know* the cosmic power, rather than know *about* it. A clergyman could start his own human life styling groups, to help people build their body temples."

Shortcomings

• There is far too much emphasis on physician-guidance, physician-direction, and continued physician-dependence, in my view. The fact that the (silent) author is a physician is undoubtedly a factor in such statements as:

- Each patient needs primarily a health physician.
- The need today is obviously great for disease-treatment doctors, and they will always be needed.
- Although he is not God, the doctor remains a very important figure to the patient. [A generous concession!]

While the book acknowledges ultimate responsibility as resting with the patient in a partnership with the doctor, it seems to reinforce the dependence aspect. The individual, though pursuing a wellness or human life styling approach, still remains a patient.

• The recommendations are not always realistic, and the expectations sometimes seem to promise too much too soon. For example, a healthy person "should feel good all the time. He should wake up feeling good and go to bed feeling good, with a happy, productive day in between . . . . The normal person is one who lives his or her entire life without a symptom." As to realism, I suspect that many people will have difficulty, as I do, following these pointers on nutrition:

- Commit yourself to eating no empty calories for the rest of your life.
- Eat from a predetermined schedule.
- Never take seconds. Put what you need on your plate and limit your meal to that.
- There are no special occasions for gorging. Your heart and brain and the rest of your body have the same needs on holidays as on other days.
- When eating out, never look at the menu. Just place your order, such as steak and salad, and forget about all the other things they serve. If bread and crackers are on the table, ask the waitress to remove them; if your companion wants them, employ will power.

Overall, however, the book is quite good, and I recommend it—when it comes out in paperback.

Parting
Thoughts

Writing this book has been an extraordinary experience for me. At times, I wondered if it were good for my health. Now it is over. I'm "weller" than ever.

Though we may not have met, we have shared a lot. I told you my ideas and how I live; you gave hours of your time in reading my work. We are no longer strangers.

You and I share an awareness of the wellness resource and holistic health centers, the ethic of high level wellness, and the vital dimensions of wellness for an integrated lifestyle. Now we are both aware of ways to shape a healthier society and where to look for more information as we evolve toward our best potentials.

Enlightenment or endarkenment, wellness or worseness, life as a garden of Eden or a descent into hell—these are the choices. Muddling through or just being not sick will not suffice anymore. This may be the path for most people, but we want more. We know that we grow better or we diminish—turn on to being and becoming or degenerate to oblivion.

There is excitement, adventure, enjoyment, and fulfillment for us on this earth. A wellness lifestyle will not guarantee or assure that you experience these states, but it will certainly bend the odds your way. At a minimum, you can expect that a healthy body, emotional equilibrium, and an alive mind will give you one hell of a good start.

I'm on your side—I want you to know that.

Be well, drink deep, and go for it.

PART ONE

Reflections on . . .

Getting Clear of Worseness

Introduction: The Tyrant's Birthday

I still like the dictatorship analogy. We are all guided by rules, pages 1–2 norms, customs, and habits that affect the way in which we perceive our capacities and opportunities for health. In growing up, some of us have had the good fortune to receive reinforcement or encouragement to think about (and, if appropriate, change) the rules in order to realize better outcomes. But that is the exception; most people never get help in questioning the rules that imprison or limit their prospects for wellness.

Americans take freedom for granted, though it is a blessing desired in many countries far removed from the totalitarian reality. Yet so many Americans who are free in a political sense are captives to rules that imprison their health. As a consequence, they engage in lifestyle practices that produce the same results I described in that bizarre analogy: They choose not to condition the only body they're going to get, they feed it junk more often than not, and they allow stressors and other contaminants to run amok through their days. And they do this not because of the whims of a dictator but because they are numbed by expectations and early training that such health-limiting constraints are normal.

In a wellness-oriented environment, such constraints are nothing of the kind.

Maybe we need a wellness czar or emperor to draw the attention of the wellness somnambulates to the conscious joys of living fully, every day. (Which is, in fact, our birthright.)

295

Reflections on . . .

Why Not Wellness?

pages
3–48 The modern medicine that in 1976 cost Americans $140 billion annually now costs $400 billion. So in that sense, my book was a failure! But I hope I'm not entirely to blame, especially since the forecasts are for continued rises to $750 billion by 1990. Yes, costs rose exponentially despite *High Level Wellness*, and right in the face of the attendant but barely noticed wellness movement.

As for everything else I wrote in this chapter concerning the true nature of what we call the "health care system"—in my opinion, it's right on target. And my "roots in wellness," like my birthday, will never change.

Surprisingly, my initial four conclusions about wellness (see pages 6–7) remain part of my current belief system. Not only that, but they still seem to be four of the most important aspects of the wellness philosophy.

Reflections on . . .

The Wellness Centers

pages
8–48 In 1976, you could count the number of wellness centers on one hand. I did—and then wrote about them. My major focus was Dr. John Travis's Wellness Resource Center. The center had an interesting history, which I won't restate here, since it has been extensively documented and analyzed elsewhere. But I will comment a bit on Travis, as his ideas and the nature of his Wellness Center were the best part of the story at the time.

John Travis and I were friends when I wrote this book, and our association has grown a lot in the intervening years. He has gone through many changes, as you might expect, given the passage of years and the fact that the man seems to thrive on the cutting edge. As his books and lectures clearly demonstrate, John has reshaped many if not most of the concepts and practices, preferences and stylistic tendencies highlighted in my description of his original Wellness Resource Center. If the center were in operation today, it would inevitably have a different orientation. The same is true for nearly all the other (holistic) centers described.

Only two of the centers described in 1976 exist today in a pages 20–24, 42–48 recognizable sense. The rest seemed to fade away soon after my book was published (although no connection between these events has ever been established). The "survivors" are Meadowlark and Esalen, both of which were much older and better funded than Travis's Wellness Center. Dr. Loomis's retreat center and Esalen's seminar headquarters for "new age" studies and reflections have both grown, flourished, and prospered. If you check them out, I'm sure you will find them to be the "whole person"–oriented educational and healing places they were ten years ago. Of more consequence than the fate of the sample centers is the fact that my 1976 prediction that it would be easier to name cities *without* wellness or holistic centers in the future than to single out places *with* them has nearly come to pass. I hope this doesn't make me the Jean Dixon of wellness.

Travis's "Well Medicine/Traditional Medicine Continuum" pages 8–20 on page 10 heads the hit parade of popular wellness illustrations. The continuum was both simple and profound, and was suitable for expansion and variations. John himself has made major modifications to the original version. In fact, he started making changes *before* my book was published; I just did not know of them.

Therein rests a little historical aside. Once upon a time, way back in 1973 in a little corner of the Baltimore Public Health Service building, after regular business hours and at a time when no one was watching, young John Travis, M.D., was doodling with a typewriter. In no time at all, he discovered that he had created the world's first, absolutely original version of the Illness/Wellness Continuum. This was published shortly thereafter in the Wellness Inventory. In 1977, he "fancied up" the graphics and made the big change: the "medical model" became the "treatment model," and "wellness medicine" became the "wellness model." Naturally, given his current level of enlightenment, he regrets ever using the dreaded term "medical" in the same breath as the sainted word "well." Each clearly represents a mutually exclusive though complementary model. But this initial blunder, he has since admitted, actually served a useful purpose: "It showed that even Travis makes mistakes." Nevertheless, he still grimaces every time he comes across the phrase "well medicine" or "wellness medicine," as I do when I see or hear "total wellness." (Can you imagine a program for "partial wellness"?) Why does Travis grimace? Not only because "well medicine" is an oxymoron, but mainly because he knows that he was the first to make the error of joining these terms before his thinking got straightened out. Countless physicians have challenged him for rejecting this association, but he remains dauntless and resolute in affirming the revised nomenclature. Doing so preserves the uniqueness of the wellness model and highlights the need to keep the two valued but fundamentally different areas apart. They are separate and equal aspects, as portrayed in Dr. Travis's most recent recent version of the continuum, as follows.

Illness/Wellness Continuum

Moving from the center to the left shows a progressively worsening state of health. Moving to the right of center indicates increasing levels of health and well-being. The treatment model can bring you to the neutral point, where the symptoms of disease have been alleviated. The wellness model, which can be utilized at any point, directs you beyond neutral, and encourages you to move as far to the right as possible. It is not meant to replace the treatment model on the left side of the continuum, but to work in harmony with it. If you are ill, then treatment is important, but don't stop there.

Used with permission. *Wellness Workbook* (Berkeley, CA: Ten Speed Press, 1981), p. 2.

In 1981, he joined with Regina Ryan to produce the *Wellness Workbook*. This featured his newly developed "wellness energy model," which focused on twelve dimensions of health. In addition, a companion *Wellness Workbook for Helping Professionals* was published (Ten Speed Press) along with a resource kit of materials to support other professionals in various transitions, personal and professional.

But John did more than write books and give lectures. He went to Costa Rica and spent a couple of years working on a model of intentional communities "for people who share like visions, value clear communications, and honor norms which allow them to address basic needs." He found that many people could benefit from reinforcing and practicing the beliefs they thought they alone held. While living in Costa Rica, John and his wife, Meryn, began publishing the "Wellness Community Newsletter" which explores voluntary simplicity and the role of community support in personal and societal well being. Recently, he developed a video tape about his energy model, as well as interactive computer programs for his Wellness Inventory.

In a recent *Wellness Report,* I interviewed John. Since the motto of the *Report* is that "wellness is too important to be presented grimly," I had a little fun with the lead-in to the feature story:

> We are in the mid-1980s and wellness is fast becoming a household word and nearly everybody is wildly well and some people have forgotten the early days when not everybody jogged to work and ate only fruits/vegetables/and whole grains and meditated daily for an hour on company time.
>
> But it is good to look back on occasions and ponder the words of the prophets of wellness. But "looking back" is not enough! We must *go back,* search as necessary for the surviving legends in locations exotic and remote, and bring back the truth as they see it, distanced as they are from the commercialization, hype, consensual validation, and me-too-ism of contemporary enthusiasts for the wellness revolution.
>
> And that, my friends, is what I have done to inaugurate this new feature of the *Wellness Report.* At incredible expense/great danger/ and huge determination, I have located that one individual who more than any other shaped the frontiers of the movement—ten years ago! Is his name on billboards wearing Nikes? No. Is he seen as a member of Coach John Madden's "fun bunch" of beer-drinking good old boys on the commercials? No. Is he ever on the cover of *Time, People,* or *Ms.* magazines? No. Why has fame eluded this man? For that matter, of whom do I ramble so?
>
> Here's a hint.
>
> In an age when all others believed that only darkness and evil lay beyond the health system as it then existed, one bold, young and idealistic physician dared to challenge the unknown but possible future. In the course of his journey to deliver wellness unto the masses through The Wellness Resource Center and *The Wellness Workbook* and "The Wellness Inventory" and wellness seminars for those who dared risk imprisonment/banishment/torture/and death for the apostasy of enrollment (OK, so attendees were a little paranoid), this "doctor of well-being" pursued his intellectual/political/and theo-

logical odyssey. He learned courage from fearless warlords deep in the jungles of Central America. He learned passion from forbidden women in Mill Valley (though he denies this, claiming that he is still working on learning passion).

Finally, he learned a few exotic secrets so long hidden from the rest of civilization (God only knows where he learned the exotic secrets). Thus, for many years he ventured into an alien medical system—until at last he brought the ends of the wellness concept together—for all time.

Have you recognized the identity of this man of men, humanist of the species, and parent of that which we hold dear?

I refer to none other than "The Legend," the "Adventurer of the Attainable Spirit," the "Jacques Cousteau of Wellness," the "Man of Men"—JOHN W. TRAVIS, M.D. Extraordinaire.

This summer, I traveled to the mountain to seek out "The Master." (Of all those who aided me in my own search—humble by comparison—in 1975, none so inspired this student as Dr. Travis.) It has been ten years since *Prevention Magazine* published my first wellness article entitled "Meet John Travis, Doctor of WellBeing" (April 1975, 62–69).

I wanted to know what he thought of wellness in 1985. Was he surprised at the extent of the use of the word wellness. What words would he offer to express his feelings, thoughts, attitudes, hopes, fears, and other states occasioned by the manner in which the concept as espoused by himself, Dr. Halbert L. Dunn, and others has been interpreted and put into practice throughout the land. And so, seeking answers to all these questions, I did the logical thing.

I asked him.

I am sure you will be interested in his replies. Unfortunately, I have taken so much space to introduce this feature that the responses will have to be omitted.

Ha Ha—just kidding.

You should not settle for the brief quotations that follow. Go to the source. Subscribe to the *Wellness Newsletter*. Order Travis's videotape. Read the *Wellness Workbook*. Ask about the wonderful interactive Wellness Inventory computer software. Invite Travis to speak at a conference near you. Sponsor a Travis workshop. Rent him for an elegant sea cruise to Los Angeles or other glamour spot.

But be aware of one thing. He is not pleased at the manner in which wellness is being marketed. Here are teasers—after perusing these remarks, read or listen—or otherwise observe the message in context by taking one or more of the actions suggested above. Or, if you are ready to meet The Master, go to the mountain yourself!

> Halbert Dunn would turn in his grave if he knew what was happening to the concept he promoted in the 50s and 60s.
>
> Most hospital and company-based programs consist of warmed-over health education. A focus on don'ts (e.g., don't

smoke, overeat, and so on) is just pablum, a preachy diet that did not work before, does not work now, and will not work in the future. These appeals do not help people get at underlying issues.

The psychological, emotional, and spiritual dimensions of wellness are often ignored or at best given lip service.

Most wellness promoters sell people short—they do not think people are ready or willing to deal with spiritual/emotional values and concerns. This assumption about client beliefs limits the quality of the interaction and the attendant value of the exchange. They do not encourage clients to talk about what life means. Few would dare invite discussion about why we are here on the planet—and this is what wellness seekers want and need.

Most diet programs focus on food and sometimes exercise, but neither of these is the key variable in weight problems. Consciousness is.

Many Western people have adrenalin addictions. If basic needs are unmet and positive substitutes are unavailable, these addictions will take one or more negative forms.

Interactive computer video is a potent form of wellness education. Some people will open up to a computer more readily than they will to a person. If this high-tech approach can be merged with a caring touch dimension, wellness can more successfully compete with the simplicity and attractiveness of TV and movies.

What's it about? Life is about experiencing love for ourselves, others, and the planet. It is about accepting ourselves, connecting with the spirit within us, and knowing God in a generic sense.

For most people, love is the missing nutrient.

A disaster, setback, or mistake also represents an opportunity to strengthen values and focus on what is real and meaningful.

A key to greater wellness is accepting responsibility for your feelings. If you're feeling angry, sad, or otherwise imbalanced, try to be aware if and how you project negativity.

Those who grow and evolve nearly always do so out of personal pain and crisis. This may at times seem threatening to those who are not in a crisis.

Smoking, weight problems, substance abuse and other negative behaviors clear up when basic human needs are met. Self-destructive behavior is a poor substitute for basic human needs such as recognition, a sense of purpose, and personal fulfillment.

People generally require only a supportive environment to attain their needs. Openness and transparency are qualities to be sought on the path to wellness.

There you have it—a Travis primer, to stimulate your wellness pondering and shaping of the artful possible. To contact Dr. John, write or call:

John W. Travis, M.D.
22 Huckleberry Heights
Cazadero, CA 95421
(707) 632-5398

With that, I'll bring to a close this review of wellness centers. Centers are just fine as embellishments to your own initiatives and as an occasional source for coaching and support; but your own commitment to live wisely, according to a clear set of wellness principles, is what really makes the difference.

It just so happens that wellness principles are the subject of the next chapter. Developing a "wellness ethic" was one of the most challenging and satisfying tasks in writing *High Level Wellness*, and it is a pleasure to critique it ten years after inventing it out of whole cloth.

Reflections on . . .

Exploring the Wellness Ethic

pages
49–62 I view this chapter as the best part of the book. In fact, I was so enthusiastic about the material that I wanted to *be* the book when I wrote the ten principles in 1976. I was convinced that the best course was not to keep the world waiting for this information. Many others had written about nutrition, fitness, and stress management, but this was virgin turf, as well as hot stuff. Consequently, I wanted the publisher to feature and otherwise promote these reflections, declarations, and proclamations—and citizens throughout the Cosmos to act upon them, posthaste. Fortunately, calmer heads at Rodale prevailed, and I added all the other chapters. A really good idea.

Yet these principles remain true and succinct, and represent the wellness ethic as much as anything I have written or heard about since. What's more, I'm also convinced that our $400 billion medical care system would cost America less than a fraction of that amount (maybe five billion, max) if people believed and

302

acted in accord with the ten principles. Even a paltry five billion would enable the medical establishment to maintain its accustomed standards of chicanery, waste, and boondoggling in order that a transition to a wellness ethic not be painfully wrenching.

Would I change any of the principles? Not in any consequential way—only a word here and there in all cases, save one. I know the suspense must be terrible: What would I change in a big way?

The principle about not heeding the advice of the adipose physician, or "examine your doctor before you allow him or her to examine you." My reasoning was that a doctor who is careless about his/her own health habits or lifestyle will not contribute a lot of reinforcement or support for you to be conscientious about your own.

But I overlooked something: Why just pick on fat doctors? I think you ought to examine *everybody*, including doctors and other health-care types, who wants to sell you something/provide a service/get involved in any important way in your life who gives loud and clear evidence that he or she is an "Obviously Deranged Worseness-Oriented Weird Sicko" or ODWOWS!

Sharpen your focus, I say. You have more to guard against than the overweight doctor. He or she may, in fact, be the least of your problems. Look at it this way: Do you want to fly with a crazed airline captain? have your teeth cleaned by a suicidal dental hygienist? allow a zonked out, looney tunes to fix your brakes, perm your hair, pack your parachute, or run your local or (Lord forbid) federal government? I should hope not!

You may be thinking: "This guy has really mellowed over the years."

Even if not, you probably are asking yourself this question: "How can I determine just when I am in danger of being connected with a potential ODWOWS?"

That's a good question. In fact, I anticipated it. (You can do that when writing the questions.) Here is the answer: You can't, for sure. However, there is one particular tell-tale clue to look for. Being an overweight doctor (or other professional) is not it by a long shot. *The* clue to "smoking out" the likely presence of an ODWOWS is that:

> ●*The person smokes cigarettes.* This is not infallible, but it's close. In fairness, it must be noted that eleven confirmed exceptions have been documented since

1922, when testing for ODWOWSism began at the Engelbert L. Dunn Academy in Transylvania. (Engelbert was a distant cousin of Halbert L. Dunn, the first known promoter of high level wellness.) Usually, however, no testing is necessary. Is not the very fact of repeated ingestion of yellow-brown scum containing 34 chemicals known to cause cells to multiply uncontrollably, lungs to lose oxygen transfer capacity, and babies of those who smoke to be born deformed or stunted absolute, prima facie evidence that the offender is a near-certified ODWOWS?

Don't you agree? Of course you do—except that you have been too kind to put it so or even think it up to this time. But the situation is changing and the problem is getting worse. The time has come to play hardball. This smoke nonsense is serious! So, don't hire, promote, or buy a used car from an ODWOWS, or anyone who behaves suspiciously like one!

There are other indicators, nowhere near as reliable but still useful. They include such worseness practices as the following:

●The person rarely or never exercises if it can be avoided.

●The person sustains his/her life with a variety of industrial chemicals, salts, fats, and sugars.

●The person relies upon drugs and/or alcohol for "a good time."

●The person does not care for dogs, Mozart, Woody Allen, John Irving, seat belts, or the Statue of Liberty.

There are still more clues under study. Unfortunately, they cannot be released at this time as they are considered slightly subjective and personal!

That, boys and girls, is the extent of the change in this chapter. You be on the alert for ODWOWS, and when you have an opportunity to avoid one, leap on it. Other than that, I stand on my (old) principles.

Well, one more slight change. I think I may have understated the case for wellness in the tenth and concluding principle, "High Level Wellness Is More Rewarding than Low Level Worseness." It's ever so much better than I indicated. Wait no longer. Begin, or escalate, your wellness lifestyle now.

Especially if *you* are an ODWOWS.

Reflections on . . .

Other Wellness-Related Concepts

This section was a mistake! No question about it—I should have rested while I was ahead. The state of the wellness art in 1976 was so poorly developed that the tests and measures I described were truly primitive—or worse. One section, "Speaking Up for Wellness," is all right if you like testimonials. But personally, I think testimonials have lost a lot of credibility. Haven't you seen enough of Bill Cosby pushing Jell-O? O. J. Simpson pushing Hertz? Mary Lou hawking everything else? Anyone can find someone to testify for money, loyalty, or even genuine conviction on nearly anything most of the time, while others would have little difficulty locating a crowd ready to testify to the opposite. True, the persons I described getting their jollies on wellness behaviors were not paid to sing the praises of this or that technique; nevertheless, they were (are) friends and thus not completely objective. Besides, just because something works for one person does not mean it will work for you.

pages 54–58

pages 58–62

Since you have to make up your own mind as to what is sensible and good for you, given your unique situation, why muddy the waters with personal details that usually have no bearing on your situation? I added the testimonials because that was the style favored by Rodale Books and required by their editors. If I had it to do over, I wouldn't.*

---

*There may be another reason for my dislike of testimonials. One person quoted in the first edition (whose name, of course, cannot be given) turned out to be a drunk and a crook. He ran up a string of bad debts and broken promises and ended up a bankrupt. He still talks a good line about wellness, holistic health, and new paradigms. And he's probably still giving testimonials on topics of virtuous and healthy import. So, words to the wise: Be more attuned to what a person lives than what he or she proclaims. This approach will help you be suspicious of testimonials, as I should have been—and am now. No need for you to learn the hard way.

Reflections on . . .

Measuring Your Wellness

pages
63–91

You should not be at all surprised to learn that in every case the tests and instruments available in 1976 have long been replaced by more sophisticated and otherwise improved testing protocols.

Reflections on . . .

THE WELLNESS/WORSENESS CONTINUUM

pages
66–82

This chapter was organized in two parts. The first contained a set of definitions about health beyond the margins of non-sickness and my Wellness/Worseness test. By taking the test, you could estimate where your lifestyle practices placed you on the mythical continuum from one extreme to another. Of course, the test was not (nor intended to be) scientifically accurate. Enough that it be fun and that it provide a few insights on key issues in each of the five dimensions. This I believe it did, and did well. I have received large numbers of requests for the rights to the test from various authors and from representatives of nursing and other professional schools (always cheerfully granted). I have also updated the test on several occasions.*

Reflections on . . .

OTHER MEASURES OF WELL-BEING

pages
82–91

The second part of this chapter provided a listing of a few "other measures of well-being." Have you ever mailed a letter—and regretted it immediately? If so, you know how I felt right after this book first came out. Those measures sounded good to me at the time, but I soon had second thoughts. Soon after publication, "second thoughts" became heartfelt regrets.

pages
82–85

For the record, let it be known that I now have no use for the Voice Stress Analysis (a gimmick of dubious validity, at best—and

*See *14 Days to a Wellness Lifestyle* (Mill Valley, CA: Whatever Press, 1982), pp. 16 and 20.

maybe much worse), the Health Hazard Appraisal (another gim- pages 87–88 mick focused on reducing risks in order to live longer—an appeal that is neither effective nor wellness oriented), this particular Nu- trition, Health, and Activity Profile (much better versions are pages 88–89 now on the market), or the Maximum Heart Rate Test Profile (see pages 89–91 the critique of this approach in the fitness chapter on page 334).

And as for the Life Change Index, the Holmes scale is so odious that I saved discussion of it for last. That I quoted this ab- erration in the Rodale edition is a source of personal dismay sec- ond to none other. This turkey is truly an antiwellness instru- ment, a Draculalike bloodsucker that cries out for a wooden stake through the heart, or a silver bullet, or a crucifix—or whatever it takes to slay a fiend. If you will bear with me for a few pages, I shall proceed at this point to do just that. (Or lose my precious bodily fluids in the process.)*

OK, you are probably asking: "What's so bad about the Holmes Life Change Index?"

Reflections on . . .

THE HOLMES LIFE CHANGE INDEX —A DISASTER

The first thing anybody learns about stress management is the pages 85–87 Holmes "Life Change Index," or LCI for short. It has been around forever, or so it seems, having been hyped to death in newspapers, magazines, and endless health books. Worst of all, I included it in the first edition of this book.

There's just one problem with it: It's bunk! Especially if you believe in the value of a wellness lifestyle. It sounds good and looks scientific—but a closer look reveals that it's not what it's cracked up to be. In fact, it does more harm than good.

The theory of the Index is that the more life changes you have to deal with in a condensed period, the more stress you have and the more likely you are to get sick or croak.

This theory is unreasonable, negative, distracting, and dis- couraging of a healthy outlook. Here is a quick summary of the

---

*Naturally, all this is an exercise in wildly excessive rhetoric. Writers have to have fun, too. Besides, *wellness is too important to be presented grimly.*

case against the Index, followed by an alternative wellness version.

● *It's unreasonable to assign point values to life events.* Who's to say that divorce is a 73-point event? Holmes? Balderdash. *Not* getting a divorce could be a 73-point event, day after day after day! It just depends on who is divorcing you, or vice versa. Or who determines that a mortgage of more than $10,000 is a 31-point event? (There hasn't been a mortgage in California for *less* than $10,000 for about 127 years.) In short, which events deserve how many points (negative or positive) depends on the individual.

● *It's negative.* It is not the infrequent downer that freaks people out, but the everyday hassles they have to contend with. I doubt if it's any different for little kids and pets, for that matter. Deaths, mortgages, job loss, jail terms, divorce, and all those things happen infrequently if at all. But *every day* there are time pressures, frustrations with others, demands, and so on. Then there are the occasional traffic jams, TV commercials, dental appointments, broken dates, burned soufflés, etc. Now we're talking *real* stress.

● *It's distracting.* It emphasizes the events or changes, rather than the way we choose to respond to them. Some people seem able to deal with *anything*; others come apart over nothing. The latter would look at the Holmes scale and say: "No wonder I'm so screwed up. I scored 300 points. I ought to be in bed! I need a drink."

● *It discourages a healthy outlook.* It does not fit with being responsible for your own life. You don't have to be a health nut to realize that it pays to accept accountability for as much as possible—or plausible. The Index gives those who are unwilling to face this responsibility a convenient out; this way they don't have to be accountable for what goes well or poorly. In summary, the Index is not a tool for managing stress or other life issues—it is a power drain.

● *It does not reflect the special dynamic of modern life.*
Hey, where are the questions about the environment,
leisure time, stocks and bonds, Perrier supplies, con-
frontations with smokers, athletic injuries, alimony and
child-support payments, and viruses run amok in hot
tubs? The inventor of the Index, Dr. Thomas Holmes,
was obviously very narrow-minded and parochial.

Lately I've Been Thinking About . . .

THE ARDELL WELLNESS STRESS TEST

So just forget or ignore the LCI. Here is a better test, in part because it avoids the problems just listed and in part because it is
relevant to the interests of individuals pursuing optimal health.

Use the results of this test to understand your current reactions to everything! Once you know *how* you respond to everyday,
genuine, real-life events and circumstances, then you can start to
get your act together. In no time at all, based on the good things
you will learn about a stress-controlled, life-centered way of
being, you will have no trouble with stress. You will be the very
model of a modern health enhancer, and a credit to your ethnic
group (whatever it is).

Here is an example of how to score the Ardell Wellness
Stress Test. Let's say you just learned that your dearest friend is
getting married. There are seven possible points you can assign
to this event.

> +3 You are beside yourself with joy.
> +2 This is very good news.
> +1 That's nice.
> 0 Who cares? Not you.
> −1 You disapprove.
> −2 This is most unfortunate.
> −3 You are beside yourself with anger, fear, a sense of
> betrayal, etc.

THE ARDELL WELLNESS STRESS TEST

Rate your satisfaction with each of the following life areas:

1. Choice of career.   ____
2. Present job/business.   ____
3. Marital status.   ____
4. Primary relationships.   ____
5. Capacity to have fun.   ____
6. Amount of fun experienced in the last month.   ____
7. Financial prospects.   ____
8. Current income level.   ____
9. Spirituality.   ____
10. Level of self-esteem.   ____
11. Prospects for having a positive impact on those who know you—and possibly others.   ____
12. Sex life.   ____
13. Body—how it looks and performs (in ways unrelated to the preceding question).   ____
14. Home life.   ____
15. Life skills and knowledge of issues and facts unrelated to your job or profession.   ____
16. Learned stress-management capacities.   ____
17. Nutritional knowledge, attitudes, and choices.   ____
18. Ability to recover from disappointments, hurts, set-backs, and tragedies.   ____
19. Confidence that you are now at, or will in the future come reasonably close to, your highest potentials.   ____
20. Achievement of a rounded or balanced quality in your life.   ____
21. Sense that life for you is on an upward curve, getting better and fuller all the time.   ____
22. Level of participation in issues and concerns beyond your immediate interests.   ____

23. Choice whether to parent or not, with the conse- ____
    quences or results of that choice.

24. Role in some kind of "network" of friends, relatives, ____
    and/or others about whom you care deeply, and who
    reciprocate that commitment to you.

25. Emotional acceptance of the inescapable reality of ag- ____
    ing (though you are well aware that a wellness lifestyle
    will enable a dramatic "compression of senescence").

SCORE ____

0 to −24 = *A CANDIDATE FOR ADDITIONAL TRAINING IN HOW TO BE A HEALTHY PERSON.* In your case, the Holmes Index *does* apply. A sudden increase in events and circumstances of potential negativity could set you back severely. Participate actively in programs relevant to the kinds of questions on this stress test.

−25 to −50 = *A CANDIDATE FOR MEDICAL CARE.* Either you were too pessimistic and underrated your true level of satisfactions, or you are in a very hazardous place, inconsistent with getting the most from a quest for joyful wellness. Seek counseling—and know that you *can* make a comeback. When you do, life will seem even better for you than it does for others currently in "weller" categories. This is because you will have travelled a greater distance than they, and thus can better appreciate and glory in the contrasts between the bliss of wellness and the sorrows and perditions of worseness.

−51 to −75 = *A CANDIDATE FOR EMERGENCY HIGH-TECH PSYCHOLOGICAL RESUSCITATION.* You are still with us, since you have read this far; so it is clear that the fire within, though very much threatened, still burns. Know that a reversal of the ill tides to date is both possible and extraordinarily worthwhile. It is not too late—yet. But don't push your luck.

In conclusion, let's recognize that the old Index is the pits. Also, that stress is good or bad, depending on how you react to it. The key is to choose and pursue a wellness lifestyle, use some simple stress skills, and smile a lot.

Lately I've Been Thinking About . . .

A WELLNESS CULTURE TEST

Do you ever wonder, "Why doesn't everybody live a wellness lifestyle?" There are three good reasons why everyone *should*, even though everyone doesn't.

1. *Illness is inconvenient, medical care for illness is expensive, and skilled care under the best circumstances is painful and dangerous.* Furthermore, most illnesses can be delayed or avoided altogether via wellness.

2. *Aging is negotiable.* You can strengthen your bargaining position with Mother Nature by following an appropriate wellness lifestyle. The benefits in this regard need not be spelled out; suffice to note that they are substantial.

3. *People who choose wellness can have more fun and joy in life.* They look better, feel younger, enjoy high self-esteem, and so on.

OK. Granted this is true. But if wellness is so rational and attractive from a personal, business, and societal standpoint, how come everybody doesn't live that way? Why don't all the rest of them work out and take great care of their bodies and psychological well being, as you do?

The answer is quite simple, but its ramifications are complex. It is not because people are dumb, lazy, or less virtuous or "holy" than those who live healthy lives. It is all a matter of reinforcement. Or "the rules" of the culture(s).

For reasons of good fortune, fate, divine plan, personal ingenuity, or just accident, *you* were reinforced in varied ways to live sensibly and satisfyingly, consistent with Nature's laws, human-performance discoveries, and assorted principles for what Satchel Paige called "right livin." In short, chances are that you did not have to be heroic to pull off a wellness lifestyle. And, if you are a well-educated, reasonably affluent professional with boundless amenities conducive to healthful living, you have more opportunities than most people to sustain your good intentions. You have created or at least "planted yourself" in an environment that supports you in becoming and staying the whole, vital person you choose to be. Congratulations.

Unfortunately, the vast majority of people have not had such reinforcement.

Here's a little test you can use with your friends, relatives, co-workers, fellow fitness enthusiasts, and perfect strangers to generate discussion about whether or not their reinforcements, cultures, and environments are making them sick. It is a lot better than any of the tests I stuck you with in the first edition. Of course, one reason I favor it is that I made it up. But, never mind—it may be helpful anyway.

To add interest to the test, make up an interpretive scoring system. For example, the Ardell Culture Test has 14 questions. Suggest to your friends that there is overwhelming scientific evidence that, sure as smoking causes hair on the palms, you are in big trouble if you answer, "Yes, it is normal around here" to *five* or more of these statements. Then, cross your fingers and tell them that affirmative responses to *eight* or more of the statements represents Undertaker City. You don't want to carry this too far, but if you think your target can handle it and might benefit from a good fright, mention that *ten* or more guarantees everlasting spiritual hangnail and tooth decay. By this point, they should realize that you are full of it but have considerable interest in taking the test anyway.

Enough introduction. Here is the test. Good luck.

THE ARDELL WELLNESS CULTURE TEST

IT'S NORMAL AROUND HERE FOR PEOPLE:

	Yes	No
1. To celebrate special occasions with sweets, alcohol, or both.	—	—
2. To drink coffee throughout the day because it's so readily available.	—	—
3. To not wear seat belts, to not exercise daily, and to eat junk food.	—	—
4. To ignore the 55-mph speed limit, stop signs, and traffic lights—if it looks like they can get away with it.	—	—

5. To tolerate tobacco odors and smoke, because __ __
   smokers have rights too, and you don't want to be
   pushy or a crank.

6. To think you're weird if you take time out to close __ __
   your eyes and relax several times throughout the
   day to balance or calm youself.

7. To take pills or go to a doctor when you are not feel- __ __
   ing well, or to pass out aspirins and other medications to each other.

8. To avoid expressing feelings because that makes __ __
   you seem strange.

9. To get positive reinforcement for being rushed, __ __
   harried, or drawn in appearance—because the
   more harried you appear, the harder you must be
   working.

10. To complain a lot—about the job, the boss, the __ __
    weather, the president, the economy, each other,
    the food, local teams, and/or parts of your body.

11. To get feedback only when you have screwed up. __ __

12. To receive more attention when you are down, ill, __ __
    discouraged, saddened, and otherwise mired in
    the "Slough of Despond" than when you arrive at
    work ready to take on the world, jumping up and
    down with enthusiasm, urging fellow employees to
    "soar with the eagles" and to accomplish great
    things.

13. To tolerate or even ignore the potential harm of ad- __ __
    vertising during sports programming that pro-
    motes youthful drinking (e.g., Miller's and Bud-
    weiser's use of athletic heroes exuberantly guzzling
    the sponsors' products in bars).

14. To not give priority to quality-of-life issues, such as __ __
    protecting the environment, having fun in life, en-
    joying and taking pride in work, experiencing.

                                        SCORE __ __

So now that you have their attention, they will want to know what the test *really* indicates. Simply smile and explain that it exemplifies how so many things we take for granted are truly inimical to even our best efforts to live healthy lifestyles. Mention that recognizing these factors is an important first step toward improving one's well-being. But don't try to cover everything. Stop before you become a nuisance. Suggest to your friends and associates that they can promote *their* chances of sustaining healthier lifestyles by redesigning habits and customs in concert with others. Then switch to another topic before you wear out your welcome.

Lately I've Been Thinking About . . .

A TEST OF SUPPORT FOR WELLNESS AT THE WORKPLACE

The growing popularity of health-promotion programs at the workplace is traceable to two basic factors. One is the expectation that such initiatives will help moderate rising medical-care or health-insurance costs by encouraging healthier lifestyles, which in turn will mean less sickness (absenteeism) and use of expensive medical resources. The other is the fact that employees usually welcome health promotion (fringes) as a valued benefit. ("If the boss or company is willing to sport for a spiffy gym, aerobics classes, membership in the Y, and so on, hey, let's go for it.")

As a result, all the Fortune 500 companies and several thousand smaller enterprises have some form of workplace wellness program. However, they are the exceptions, not the rule. America has millions of small businesses, and most of them do not provide fitness, health-promotion, or other health-oriented opportunities for their employees. Despite the reality of rising medical insurance costs (from $33 billion in 1978 to $88 billion in 1985), increased pressures from employees to start wellness activities at the office or plant, and all the evidence that such endeavors *do* work, wellness at the workplace has not taken hold at all levels throughout the U.S. There are still companies that almost believe these words, observed on the wall of a meat-packing firm in Sioux Falls:

> This organization needs no wellness or physical fitness program: Everyone gets plenty of exercise jumping to conclusions, flying off the handle, running down the boss, knifing their friends in the back, dodging responsibility, and pushing their luck.

However, there is a new development on the horizon that could change things dramatically, even for rough workplace environments like this. This situation concerns a different perspective on what to expect. According to the latest studies on health-promotion benefits, investments in wellness programming offer not only reduced medical costs, sickness rates, turnover expenses, absenteeism, and other hoped-for gains, but also greater productivity. How can wellness at the workplace be tied to productivity? Through the generation and nurturance of a climate for *breakthrough performance.*

"Breakthrough performance" is an ethic, set of attitudes, and cultural support at the office or plant that reinforces excellence. It is a climate that encourages people to develop and practice the kinds of traits (e.g., a bias for action, autonomy, pride, etc.) being promoted in popular business books.* In short, breakthrough performance connects wellness to the kinds of issues all managers care about, even if they smoke, abuse alcohol, don't exercise, eat too much salt and sugar, kick their dogs, and otherwise ignore the value of health habits.

You will appreciate the potential of this growing aspect of the wellness movement for involving all segments of the workforce in health-promotion activities better if you take the following breakthrough performance test. Determine how well your company is doing in the nine vital areas essential to a wellness worksite.

Ask yourself the question: "How well is my company doing?" in each of the areas noted. Total the number of times you checked that your company is doing well or OK, and then read the analysis of your score.

This will give you a sense of how responsive your boss is likely to be to the idea of starting a wellness program at your business site. (Or you might discover that it's time to start looking for another way to make a living!)

---

*Including but not limited to *In Search of Excellence, Megatrends, Supermanaging, The Wall Street Journal on Management, The Changemasters, High-Output Management, Letitia Baldrige's Complete Guide to Executive Manners,* and *The One Minute Manager.*

The instructions are simple: Simply place a check next to those items that match your experience at work each day. If you find all or most of the following statements to be foreign to the reality of your daily work life, major changes are in order. Failing that, it may be time to update your resume.

Score on a scale of zero to three: three points if the statement strongly fits the way it is for you on the job; zero points if your response is "No way, my job does not come close to this standard." (One or two points, naturally, if "in some ways, more or less," the statement seems to fit.)

This wellness variation of your standards for excellence has nine performance categories and twenty-seven questions. Thus, the highest possible score is 81; the lowest is, of course, nothing. (Pray that no one has this problem.) If you credit your organization with 70 or more points, you are either self-employed and prospering or working for a company that knows how to support excellence in its employees. If you score between 50 and 69 points, the prospects for personal and corporate excellence are very good. If, however, the workplace gets fewer than 27 performance points, take heed. As Plato observed: You are in jeopardy if, to do what is right, you must be a hero or a fool.

THE ARDELL
WELLNESS-AT-THE-WORKPLACE TEST

Change and Innovation

1. People feel free to take risks and experiment in their work.   ____

2. Creativity is affirmed daily.   ____

3. A few key advisors take the responsibility for projects   ____
   as opposed to the assignment of projects to committees.

Motivation

4. People feel that they make a powerful difference and   ____
   are involved in experiences that prove it.

High Level Wellness

5. Salaries meet basic needs and also provide incentives. ____
6. People are rewarded and recognized for excellent performance. ____

Conflict Resolution

7. Conflicts are resolved with win/win solutions or are mediated by nonaffected third parties. ____
8. People constructively confront negative behavior when it occurs. ____
9. People avoid blame placing and finger pointing as a method of problem solving. ____

Participative Management

10. The decision-making process is highly participatory. ____
11. People emphasize cooperation over competition among members of the organization. ____
12. People help set their own work objectives and work methods. ____

Communication

13. People's beliefs are congruent with their actions. ____
14. People understand how their work relates to the goals or values of the organization. ____
15. People actively seek out the ideas and opinions of others. ____

Leadership

16. Leaders follow up on problems and new ideas in a swift way. ____
17. Leaders show a balanced concern between the quality work that has to be done and the people who are doing it. ____

18. Leaders are actively involved in providing quality service, and they model the behavior they expect of others. ____

Team Building

19. Some meetings focus on nothing but individual and/or group achievements. ____

20. Support for and caring of associates is strongly emphasized. ____

21. People are concerned about the success of the work group. ____

Stress Management

22. The work environment is relaxing, and families are included in some of the organization's programs. ____

23. Fitness facilities and programs are available, and their use is encouraged. ____

24. The organization provides the necessary staff, programs, or other resources to assist people under stress or having personal problems. ____

Follow-through/Results Orientation

25. Change efforts focus on measurable results. ____

26. Quality is something upper management not only talks about but also does something about. ____

27. Management acts quickly and decisively on quality improvement suggestions. ____

SCORE ____

+ 23 to + 27 = *A wellness environment of the highest order.* You should pay them to let you work there! It will be hard for you *not* to be healthy, happy, and positive about your prospects for continued satisfactions and fulfillments. Congratulations. I am pleased that you have such a favorable situation. Let me know if there are any openings!

+19 to +22 = *An environment of great promise.* Chances are that your workplace already has a wellness program and that everybody is excited about it and actively participating in it. You, too, are a fortunate person. Good wishes for continued progress.

+14 to +18 = *Your workplace is OK, it is not a serious problem, but it is not a big help, either.* You are ripe for a wellness program—the payoffs will be considerable.

+9 to +13 = *You are in a high-risk situation.* There is not much to be said in favor of maintaining the status quo. The good news is that improvements brought about by a wellness program will seem so wonderful and be appreciated, because the contrasts between how things are and should (will) be are so dramatic.

+5 to +8 = *The opposite of high level wellness is low level worseness!* You are close to the latter. Update your resume or your life insurance. Retire early.

0 to +4 = *Well, you're still alive.* Take the same action as above, but do it today!

Wellness activities, like this test, must be enjoyable as well as substantive. Please view the quiz as a guide, not as a conclusive statement about your work environment. Excellence is not impossible to build into the job as a "normal" expectation, but it requires management support and employee acceptance and leadership.

OTHER CHANGES/COMMENTS ON "MEASURING YOUR WELLNESS"

In addition to the Life Change Index, a number of other shibboleths cry out for commentary. These include notions such as that we should "pay the doctor when we are well," exercise and do other things "in moderation," and that "the good life is killing us." I believe this is an appropriate place to look closer at some of these misconceptions. I addressed these "dragons" that inhibit wellness practices in the *Wellness Report*.

First, there's the matter of paying the doctor when you are well rather than when ill.

Watch Out for Chinese Proverbs!

Chinese proverbs are like Motherhood and apple pie. Few pause to consider whether some Chinese Proverbs (CPs) might be a bit dated. The usual response to CPs is deference, reverence, and acceptance, a hazardous situation in one, maybe more, situations. The current situation wherein only a whale-killer Commie Pinko on bad terms with God would knock a CP must end. Thus, in the spirit of risking perdition for universal enlightenment, this bold publication shall be the first to slay yet another Illusory Unwarranted Dragon (IUD) restraining wellness truth-seekers from exploring frontiers beyond the confines of ancient superstitions.

False prophets of aerobic point systems, doctors of demagoguery, and nonsensical nabobs of myths and balderdash—beware: You may be next. The ever-vigilant, ever-pure investigative journalists of the *Wellness Report* never sleep. (Well, that's not literally true, but you get the idea.)

And what, pray, is the CP that Americans quote most often with the highest levels of approbation and genuflection? That's easy. It's the CP regarding the Ancient Chinese medical reimbursement system. It goes like this: "Golly, I understand the Ancient Chinese had the right idea. They paid the doctor when they were well!" (As opposed to when sick, for sickness care, as in America today.)

When that is said, the CP-quoter usually smiles and feels as if he/she has just struck a blow for wellness. The implication is always the same: That if we had as much sense as the Ancient Chinese, we would do the same—pay doctors when we did not get sick.

Which is one of the dumbest ideas I ever heard! Why in Hades do that? Who, after all, is responsible for your good health? Not the doctor, Dummy. *You.* You are the one who decides what to eat, how and how often to exercise and manage stress, to wear or disdain seat belts, and in other ways to do or not do what adds or takes away from your prospects for wellness. So why pay the doctor if you stay well?

Instead, pay the good doctor for quality medical care—if and when you really need it. And if you do not need it as a consequence of wise living, take all the money you saved and go on a vacation. Maybe to China. Or, treat yourself to a banana split—with bran!

Meanwhile, stay alert and ever on guard against cute-sounding but ludicrous CPs.

Think of this process as a search for a dragon to slay in the interests of making the Earth safe for all who would live healthy lifestyles. Here's how I handled the topics of "moderation" and "the good life":

A Dragon Hunt

Look! Over there! It's another one of those worseness dragons that roam all over the place frightening people away from wellness. No, wait! There are two of those suckers. What a day! What a chapter this is going to be. I recognize them both. One is the beast called "Moderation" by the natives; the other looks like that brute called "The Good Life." Make room—I'll soon take care of this. First, an attack on "Moderation" will be mounted.

You have heard the fearsome, intimidating sound of "Moderation" before, no doubt many times. Its most common form of threat to dwellers in the House of Wellness is as follows:

"You should exercise in Moderation."

Isn't that awful? If that fearsome dragon were not lurking about, would anyone be interested in moderation? Look at Webster: "Moderation" is defined as "within limits, away from extremes." Now consider this:

Is the choice really between obsessiveness and the holy state of "Moderation?" Obviously not. Further, who sets the limits? For how long? Standards of limits and norms for extremes are changing rapidly as America becomes fitter and more health conscious. If not, Toufexis would still be writing about pill potencies and heart transplants and other medical matters, just as *Time* would not be highlighting the new "shape-up" awareness with a special section. Women who exercised at all were certainly not considered moderate just a few years ago. In short, moderate is not a highly useful term anymore, as applied for fitness purposes or health in general. Why approach something as wonderful as wellness in namby-pamby fashion? It is a life-long pursuit of vast consequence. It is not to be done in a half-vast manner. Or if it is, such dickering about should not be a matter of pride, a litmus test of sensibility, or a means to disparage the adult athlete who thinks that limits are to be gauged from personal venture and that "extremes" are sometimes challenges with life-ennobling possibilities, as well as natural medications for the prevention of boredom and its cousin, mediocrity.

Now, let's turn the sword of freedom from the limp carcass of one dragon to another beast of infamy, namely, the evil monster that stole the term "Good Life" and uses it for nefarious purposes.

The "Good Life" dragon often seems to pick on the doctors and medical writers, who seem to worship at the claws of the creature by making statements that are variations of the following:

"The 'Good Life' is killing us." Always there is a recitation of elements of the good life, such as a mechanized society that allows limited movement, a preponderance of alcohol, fatty food, reckless use of drugs and tobacco, stressful living, and so on.

All right, you dastardly beast. Take that! And that! Such a view of the "Good Life" is kaakaa nonsense. Self-abuse is not the "Good

Life." The good life is great for you. That is why there is an entire wellness movement dedicated to its promotion and realization.

Well, the battle is over. I can't be sure I really dispatched these creatures of darkness forever but at least you should be safe for a while. Keep your eyes and ears alert for their return in one guise or another. And keep active in wellness—there are still bigger/meaner/ and uglier creatures out there waiting to pounce.

PART TWO

The Five Dimensions of High Level Wellness

Introduction: The Old Model

In 1976, I saw self-responsibility as the key to wellness, and nutrition, fitness, stress management, and environmental sensitivity as the other major components. In part two of the first edition, each of these dimensions warranted its own chapter. Every chapter focused on a set of principles for each dimension, followed by a review of applications and relationships among the dimensions.

This model worked very nicely for me for nearly ten years. I found that every issue of consequence could be fitted logically and without strain into one of the five areas.

Here is a drawing of the five dimensions as originally written.

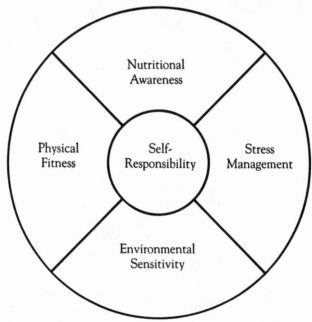

DIMENSIONS OF WELLNESS
1977–1986

Lately I've Been Thinking About . . .

A Realignment of the Five Dimensions

Despite the longevity of the original scheme, I have decided to reorganize the five dimensions. The new arrangement highlights other aspects that are too consequential to be subordinated to narratives within a dimension. The following diagram shows the nature of the changes.

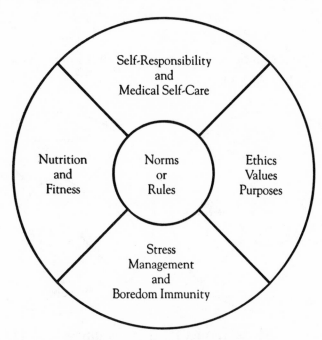

DIMENSIONS OF WELLNESS

When I reflect on my old and new dimensions and then compare the two with other models I realize that it really does not matter so much how the circle is divided or titled.

The following chart contrasts each of the two models I have offered with those of my friends Bill Hettler and John Travis. The color codes indicate the areas of obvious commonality amongst the four models. No doubt four other equally plausible ways of organizing the substance of wellness could be and probably will be drawn by others to come. Let's hope so.

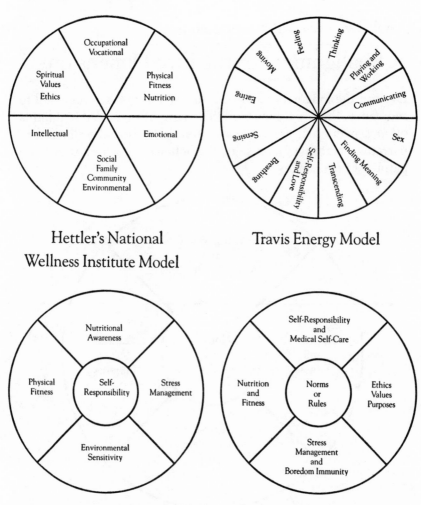

Hettler's National
Wellness Institute Model

Travis Energy Model

1977 Wellness Model (Ardell)   1986 Wellness Model (Ardell)

WELLNESS DIMENSIONS:
COMMONALITIES IN FOUR MODELS

What does matter very much is the explanation given by any model inventor to the dimensions he or she favors. In the remainder of this Part Two, I want to summarize why I think modifications to my own original model are in order.

The first modification you might notice is that everything has changed; the next is that nothing has changed, but each dimension has been altered. That second impression is what I intended. My ten years of lecturing and writing on wellness issues have provided an extraordinary continuing education, in the richest sense of that term. Week after week, I have had one occasion after another to learn more deeply the nature of a topic that is far more complex than I realized at the start of this career in 1976.

The first chapter in Part Two was self-responsibility. Because I viewed it as the core of the concept, I put it in the middle of the diagram and used it as the introductory chapter for the "Five Dimensions." My sense of the power of self-responsibility remains unchanged. In shifting it to one of the four quadrants in the circle, I mean to acknowledge two aspects that were neglected in the earlier edition: the role of "the rules" (an even more powerful variable), and the association between responsibility in general and medical self-care in particular. A commentary about each seems in order, followed by a brief look at each of the other dimensions, then and now.

Lately I've Been Thinking About . . .

Recognizing the Power of Rules or Norms

What makes people live or not live wellness lifestyles consistent with the principles of the five dimensions? I am now persuaded that the crucial variable is not knowledge, information availability, virtue, or will power; I think it is the nature of the rules people learned as children and obey as adults. Another word for rules is norms, a term popularized by Robert F. Allen in his book, *Lifegain.* Rules or norms are the codes—usually undefined and not even part of our conscious processes—that define what is normal and expected. Rules that are reinforced by the family and other groups shape lifestyles more than most of us realize. To live wellness lifestyles, therefore, we need to recognize the power of the rules that prevail, especially if they are unfriendly to wellness. Then we need to identify and join with others to rewrite the rules in favor of wellness, and practice them.

The first edition of *High Level Wellness* situated norms (without labeling them as such) in the dimension of environmental sensitivity. Now I think it belongs in the center of the circle as the core dimension for those seeking a framework for wellness.

Rules define what is expected. If your family reinforces poor food choices, sedentary living, negative behaviors, and blame/distrust/and other negative expectations, your prospects for even being open to wellness are diminished. However, if your early years were just the reverse—if wellness (whether called that or not) was the rule or norm—you will be not only open to but often fulfilled by health-enhancement information and experiences. This helps explain why over the past ten years the audiences at my wellness seminars have consisted of the wellest of the well, the healthiest people in any given town. I preach to the "true believers, the choir" of the fit and fulfilled because these people want more of what they already know is a good thing. The greatest wellness challenge ahead is to create the conditions, at the workplace and elsewhere, that will attract the masses who grew up with rules inimical to healthy living; people who think that such material, programming, and efforts are inapplicable or impossible for them.

Reflections on . . .

Self-Responsibility and Medical Self-Care

pages 94–112 This was, and remains, a super chapter, in my opinion. I could add stuff to it, but I would change none of the nine principles or even what was tacked on under "Further Perspectives on Self-Responsibility." I am including medical self-care to emphasize the

pages 102–104 importance of becoming a wise and informed consumer of medical services or resources, which really means knowing when and how to use the medical system.

pages 104–112 It might have added some interest at the time to include a discussion of a few "Programs Fostering Self-Responsibility," but I would not do so today. These particular programs were of appeal to a limited number of people, mostly Californians, and were businesses out to make money, not institutions dedicated first and foremost to the promotion of personal responsibility. Nothing wrong with the profit motive, but the dimension of self-responsibility was and remains far too important to associate it with a few controversial applications that addressed many other goals not at all tied to self-responsibility.

You already know by this time how I feel about the personal accounts or testimonials, so I will omit the usual self-recriminations on this facet of the chapter.

One of my two favorite features in this chapter provided tips to safeguard the reader from inappropriately adopting any of these or other programs or "new modalities," as they were identified. I refer to the questions given in a "consumer guide for assessing the new modalities." Anyone who did or in the future does follow these guidelines should remain clear of harm's way. This page remains one of my favorite features in this chapter; the other is the concluding quote from my mentor at the time, Harry Browne. It is my favorite statement on self-responsibility in a wellness context. If there's a better one, I'd sure be grateful to learn about it.

pages 110–111

page 112

Reflections on . . .

Nutritional Awareness

Most of the material is as useful today as when it was written. (Of course, that's my opinion—but since I'm the one writing this, my opinion counts for something!) Naturally, time and nutritional evolution have dated many references, and so on. That should pose no problem—you can easily tell what's what. However, I originally included a few statements, tests, and other materials that I dearly wish I had not. Nonetheless, they are reproduced in this edition so that you can see the changes in my thinking since then, and in the development of the wellness concept.

pages 113–133

What would go in my "Oh, I wish I didn't write that!" category or my "Dear Lord, I must have taken leave of my senses to have thought that!" division? The already-noted-and-disavowed Holmes Life Change Index, as well as the other techniques listed in the "Measuring Your Wellness" chapter. Other than that, I'm quite satisfied with the material.

Except for many of the details in *this* chapter. The overall principles are pretty good; it's the fine print that sometimes borders on the ridiculous.

page
121
First, the good news. The principles are OK. (Except for principle number eleven, "Don't overlook Grandmom's homilies"—this depends entirely on what your Grandmom knew and did about nutrition.) But in general, there are too many flaky details and not enough solid guidelines. And, as you might sense from my shift in the five dimensions, I underemphasized the intricate association between nutrition and fitness. These days, I believe that the two areas are indivisible. I even invented a way to express this relationship that dramatizes the extraordinary linkage: *Nutrition and fitness are inextricably intertwined.* That's why they are together now in the revised five-dimensional model.

Rather than review all the good stuff, I'll just summarize what I would withdraw.

pages
113–115
First, all the stuff on diseases caused by poor food habits. Sure, it is probably true that eating glop like Slow Decay Snack Cakes (they "last longer than you will") and high fat/low fiber diets year after year will cause half a dozen different diseases. But this emphasis masks a larger, more important issue: poor food habits (as well as high-risk addictions like alcohol abuse or smoking) are primarily symptoms of deeper perturbations, upsets, or psychological imbalances in the person. Why make such a big deal about symptoms when the underlying imbalances need attention?

pages
115–116
It would have been better to have omitted the faddist claims for certain foods (apple cider vinegar, nutritional yeast, garlic, and so on). I wish I had lightened up on ice cream, since I eat enough of it. (Hey, if your diet is terrific most of the time, then departures once in a while from perfection are OK. Especially if you are fit and getting plenty of exercise, have no diseases aggravated by occasional pleasure binges, and don't get guilty about eating in ways not approved by uptight wellness promoters, like yours truly in 1976.) The fact is, I have a lengthy wish list as far as this chapter goes. In fact, here it is. I wish:

pages
126–127
●I had noted that, if given a choice between being fat and going up and down on the scales, being fat is the better choice. And even this is an awful and unreal choice, somewhat like being asked if you would rather be shot or hanged.

●I had written more about: personal attitudes and responses to food; the excitement of nutritious food patterns; the positive challenge of life-enhancing choices; the advantages of healthy eating versus the crutch of vitamin supplements; the value of low fat/high fiber/high complex carbohydrate food patterns; the importance of eating a variety of foods; and the associations between nutrition and exercise. Fortunately, I did all this in my following book, *14 Days To A Wellness Lifestyle* (Whatever Press, 1982), so there is no need to repeat it all here.

●I had not introduced flaky (though possibly true, but by coincidence only) medical claims for certain foods— garlic for reducing blood pressure, or apple cider vinegar as an "antiseptic" (as in mouthwash?) and "healing agent," and other dumb remarks about watermelons, nutritional yeast, and "nature's herbs," for God's sake! (Like what? Poison oak?) Frankly, I think the only way watermelons will heal anything is from the way they are used by the comedian Gallager to make people laugh.* Hard belly laughter in heavy doses will kill anything growing inside you that doesn't have any business being there—and that's a fact. At least until the next edition. (I have to have something to set straight later on; everything else in this edition is gospel.)

pages
115–116

●I had steered away from wild claims and the reckless use of overkill assertions to make my points. There are enough abuses in food-processing practices; it should not have been necessary to claim that 80 percent of the food value in 3,500 calories is lost. I could not even find the source for that item in my records. I think it came from a nightmare, which was neither documented nor

pages
117–118

---

*You may not have *any* idea what Gallager does with watermelons. That's OK, it does not mean you are not a good person. I won't give away the act, but if you have a chance to see this funny guy do his thing, go for it. But don't sit in the first ten rows unless you want to get soaked or splattered with sledgehammered watermelons.

subjected to a double-blind crossover trial. Another like sin for which I repent (is this getting too religious?) was the suggestion to use honey or molasses. I wrote that sugar metabolism causes a loss of B vitamins, ergo molasses or honey would be a wise alternative. This was real dumb—compared to granulated sugar, honey has an additional 18 calories per tablespoon and triggers an even more dramatic fluctuation of blood sugar levels. Further, honey has no significant amounts of nutrients and, because it's sticky, it will rot your teeth faster than sugar. Leave it for the bears.

pages
130–131
•I had never mentioned raw milk. That was really bad. Every time someone got poisoned in California, I felt guilty! (Just kidding; I never pushed it that much. I just said I drink a glass now and then, which I stopped doing after writing this chapter—and before I got salmonellosis, brucellosis, diphtheria, streptococcus or tuberculosis, or other contaminant that is erased with simple pasteurization.)

pages
123–125
•I had not written about my own diet at the time, which gives me a stomachache to think about today. What particularly bothers me about the old diet in print is that I am not nearly so virtuous today. (I drink two cups of coffee daily, I eat sweets, do not take supplements, never fast, dislike herbal teas, and rarely eat granola). Does this mean I have gone downhill, lost all nutritional self-respect, and am addicted to fast foods, grease, and industrial chemicals? No. In fact, my diet is better today than in 1976, but it is free of rigidity and completely consistent with the dietary guidelines referenced in the first edition and updated regularly since that time.

page
119
•I did not promote herbal teas as an alternative to coffee and regular tea. Many such teas are fine, to be sure. But some brewed herbal teas have been shown to produce acids and toxins that build up in body tissues, according to a National Restaurant Association report recently cited in "Rethinking Nutrition," *USA Today* (October 16, 1985, p. 4D).

• Finally (I have worked myself over so severely I cannot continue this self-abuse or I shall cause hair to grow on my palms), a word about the readings. I should have mentioned *Jane Brody's Nutrition Book* (Bantam Books), Nancy Clark's *The Athlete's Kitchen* (Bantam Books), my friends Vicky Newman and Candy Cummins' *The Eater's Guide* (Spectrum) and colleague Covert Bailey's *Fit or Fat* series. I should have but I didn't. Of course, they had not been written yet. Nevertheless, no excuses are acceptable. After all, I could have waited. pages 242–257

Well, enough about nutrition. Frankly, I'm sick of the subject for now. Besides, it's time for dinner.

Henceforth, I will treat nutrition and fitness as an integrated issue—and I hope you will do the same.

Reflections on . . .

Physical Fitness

Fitness was my strong suit in 1976, and it remains so today. However, my appreciation for the significance of the other dimensions is far deeper than before. Still, repairs to the original chapter are in order, and would be even if the original fitness discussion had been written by a well-informed sportsmedicine physician or an exercise physiologist doing state-of-the-art research. Why? Because we know more now than we did then. And since the actual writer is but an ex-jock (well, let's say "adult athlete") and an "expert" only by self-study, experience, uncommon common sense, and divine inspiration (just kidding—I didn't have much experience), the need for filling in a pothole (if not a sinkhole) or two is clear and unmistakable. So I will. pages 145–161

First, the good news. As fitness jokes go, the opener wasn't bad. But these days I prefer shorter aerobic yuks. Like the account of the speedreader who just got out of the hospital. He was in an accident—he collided with a bookmark. (You see, if the joke is a bomb, at least an entire page has not been sacrificed.) page 145

I certainly did not overstate the benefits of regular exercise—or the hazards of sloth. The division of inner and outer joys works well, and I wouldn't change that, either. And the fitness pages 145–147 pages 147–150

pages
151–158 principles are still super—they will last another ten years, at least.

My modifications would not entail changes so much as different approaches. For instance, I would have a lot to write about the benefits of different exercise types; the value of the "sport of the eighties"—triathlons—which did not exist when *High Level Wellness* was written; the choice of characters for personal examples; and the nature of my own regimen, which has broadened and intensified.

page
152 But I *would* (and now will) correct the statements about how to compute maximum heart rate. The formula referenced in the fitness section (which appears in full in "Measuring Your Wellness," page 90) is simply not accurate, although it is still widely referenced and used. It may be useful for those age 40 and under, but even then it depends on certain variables associated with heredity and conditioning. A little background might help.

The formula for MHR was developed by Robinson in 1927 and promoted by the American Heart Association ever since. According to Dr. Mark Crookse, who has conducted more than 5,000 stress tests over a ten-year period, *very few patients** have maximal heart rates that correspond to the charts. Most of the 65-year-olds tested have heart rates between 160 and 172, not 150 to 160 as indicated on the charts. On the other hand, Dr. Ken Cooper's tables are quite accurate—he tested subjects with high motivation categorized by fitness levels, not just age.

For those who get romantic about formulas, here is a revised chart for determining (or even approximating) maximum heart rate (MHR). I have split it into two sections: one for the fit and one for the nonfit.

MAXIMUM HEART RATE (MHR)

ACTIVE** PEOPLE		INACTIVE PEOPLE
220 minus (age × .72)	——over 40——	220 minus (age × .90)
220 minus age	——under 40——	220 minus age

*Except for patients with disease.
**Active is defined as fifteen minutes of continuous endurance exercise two to three times per week for the three months previous to testing.

Thus, an active 50-year-old man might have a maximum heart rate of 184 beats per minute, whereas his inactive companion of like age would "max out" at 175. Why the difference? One likely reason is that the heart muscle (myocardium) of a trained, active person over 40 has greater compliance and is capable of greater stress. Paradoxically, at younger ages, the trained individual may have a *lower* maximum heart rate because catecholamine (adrenalin) response to maximal stress is less. Thus, there are two different curves for heart rate max with age. In an average inactive and an average active 65-year-old, a difference of about 15 beats may separate the two MHR values.

So much for the old "target zone" tables, particularly beyond the age of 50, if no allowance is made for fitness or its absence.

That may be more than you wanted to know about the matter, but I thought I would "make everything perfectly clear" for another decade or so.

Actually, it is a lot more than *I* care to know. I do not think tracking or plotting training heart rate is very interesting, necessary, or practical—certainly not after you have been "checked out" (assuming you feel the need to do that) or if you exercise regularly and are unconcerned with being "medical" about your exercise habits and routines.

So what *do* I care to know that gives me a sense of how hard to exercise on a given day? Jerry Gergley—a good friend, a remarkable athlete, and a highly regarded teacher who coordinates the University of Central Florida physiology laboratory—gave me a clue. Jerry, a top Hawaii "Ironman" triathlete in the Masters Division, insists that your "perceived level of exertion" is far more consequential and useful than some old-fashioned chart on maximal heart rate. To tune in to your perceived exertion level, you need "horse sense," not a chart or pulse counter. Factors that really count are such perceptions as temperature and/or humidity, attention to injuries or advent of soreness, awareness of the demands of the last or the next race, capability of your training partner(s), whether you are a morning or evening person, your morale at the time, how much rest you have had lately, and similar attunements to your own body and spirit on the move.

So pay more attention to yourself than to someone else's formulas. They may not have a wellness advocate in mind. But you—being one—will.

Reflections on . . .

Stress Management

pages
134–144 You already know how my thoughts about stress management have changed over the years from reading the Ardell Wellness Index in Part One. Stress is overrated. As with poor nutritional patterns and a lack of regular, enjoyable, and strenuous exercise regimens, stress-induced problems and hassles are just symptoms of larger, deeper difficulties.

I believe that if you are clear about your life purposes and principles; if you take pride in being physically fit; if you are well nourished and believe in accepting responsibility for as much as possible; and if, in short, you are excited and positive about each day of your life—then you have managed stress very well indeed.

Too much attention has been focused on deep breathing, muscle relaxation, visualization, and other remedial techniques for reducing stress, and too little on organizing one's overall lifestyle so that stress reduction is rarely needed in the first place. My feelings on this subject are so strong that I fear I may compose an interminable sentence, since I'm too excited and passionate on this issue to give myself the forced pause of a comma or, heaven forbid, a momentary halt with a period. Thus, I will make my point in verse. That way I don't have to slow down for as much punctuation—and you can read right through my excited prose.

> If you are having a great time most of the time,
> if you really like the people around you
> and those to whom you return each evening,
> if you have one or more projects that
> you deem worthy of you
> that you can do as well or better than anyone else,
> if, in short, you care deeply
> or feel enthusiastically about
> some things or people much of the time,
> then *you do not need to give a lot of priority*
> *to "creative visualization" or*
> *"biofeedback dots" or*
> *other gimmicks for noticing and managing stress.*
> *You are covered. Enjoy.*

Don't you agree?

Naturally, this is not to disparage stress management if it is kept in its place. Of course, stress is a factor in depression, disease, death, and dozens of other unpleasant situations, just as fever is a factor in meningitis and malaria. But fever is a symptom in these maladies, just as stress is a symptom in the myriad of problems attributed to it. It is not an independent cause.

Thus, stress *is* important; it remains one of the key dimensions of a high level wellness lifestyle. It just needs to be kept in perspective. Stress, well managed, should be one of the benefits of living near the heights of your potentials; stress management should not be used to string together a number of remedies for repairing structural (i.e., lifestyle) defects.

The word "stress" has been subject to a lot of misunderstanding, in part because of its usage by popularizers and in part because of all the programs, products, and services that are sold to cure ailments it is said to bring about. Stress, as you know, is a neutral word, neither good nor bad. But in the general press and in the literature up until the past couple of years, it has been portrayed as the scourge of the times.

I certainly was guilty of muddying the waters in the first edition. While I did provide eleven truly useful, sensible principles pages 138–143 for stress management, I also perpetuated the notions popular then (as now) by rambling on about diseases caused by stress, as well as about boring and relatively inconsequential stuff of limited use to the lay person (e.g., cycles of electrical activity in the pages 136–137 brain, flight or fight, and the adaptation syndrome). As the Ardell Wellness Index emphasized, stress doesn't *cause* anything; but the way you *respond* might cause all kinds of situations, for better or worse, over time. Finally, the way you respond is largely a condition of the way you live.

I promised not to continue to bemoan the presence of testimonials, so I will write no more about this. Except to "fess up" that what I reported doing then (i.e., progressive relaxation) is not pages 143–144 something I continued to do for many years after *High Level Wellness* was published. I do almost none of that now. Instead, I manage stress with vigorous daily exercise, a lot of good times as often as possible (lately it has been so often that the phrase "goofing around" comes to mind), involvement in work that I greatly enjoy and, as frequently as I remember to do it, taking deep breaths and giving thanks that the Earth is so green/the air so pure/I am so blessed, healthy, free, and alive. It's a lot more satisfying than standing on my head chanting Ohmmmmmm. Or employing other less drastic techniques after I got frazzled from neglecting my lifestyle.

In summary, techniques for stress management are all fine and dandy if kept in reserve, used when other positive strategies have momentarily broken down, or employed as a means to reach "higher states" of awareness, such as through meditation. As with vitamin supplements, they should not be perceived or used as alternatives to the real thing—namely, real food or, in this case, having a wellness lifestyle that works wonders for you nearly every day.

Lately I've Been Thinking About . . .

BOREDOM IMMUNITY

One wellness objective we all need is to find work and play that will keep us challenged and make our moments as valued as possible. Boredom is the archenemy of wellness. It is the leading cause of low level worseness and all its maladies, including smoking, drug and alcohol abuse, and a failure to take the positive initiatives associated with potent lifestyles.

Your score on the Ardell Wellness Index will tell you a lot about how you are doing in this regard. If it is way up there, you have no fear of boredom and its likely adverse consequences. You are immunized. But you are an exception: Those who need to hear or reflect on this message have an unfortunate habit of not reading wellness books.

The issue of boredom immunity is so important and closely tied to one's prospects for being open to and succeeding at wellness that I have decided to link it with stress management in the five-dimensional model.

How does one become immunized against boredom? Naturally, no pill or injection will work. You can't send away for it. You have to earn it, the old-fashioned way, as with anything else that is worthwhile in life.

You have to develop over time a wellness lifestyle, test it out, revise and expand it, and keep going through that process for years, deriving as much pleasure and satisfaction from the learning experience as possible.

You also need to recognize the hazard that boredom represents if you are not actively working to counter it. Schopenhauer wrote that mankind is apparently doomed to vacillate "eternally" between the two extremes of boredom and distress. But, with all due respect to this titan (in contrast to my pygmyism) in matters of existential philosophy, *I don't believe it.* If we have a wellness lifestyle going for us, we are not necessarily "doomed" between stress and boredom—neither "eternally" nor in the short run.

Psychiatrist Victor Frankel found that boredom brings more patients to psychiatrists than do stress or distress occasioned by any other single event or circumstance. In short, not knowing what to do with an abundance of free time can "do you in." Hans Selye knew this, too; he often quipped that there is nothing wrong with retirement so long as it does not interfere with one's (life) work.

Where do you start? One way is to become a wild and crazy guy, like Steve Martin. Another is to try *positive risk taking for wellness*, like my friend Mark Crookse.

Mark's story is an adventure story. It also illustrates one uncommon approach to boredom immunization, and provides valuable insights about boredom in the process.

MARK CROOKSE, RISK TAKER FOR WELLNESS

Like you and me, Dr. Mark Crookse of Kansas City is a risk taker. But he is more involved in the art *and science* of risk taking than most of us. Far as I can tell, he just may be the world's first *risk taker for wellness*.

Mark is a health educator. He does not often race into phone booths to dress for emergency services to his fellow man and woman. He has functioned in traditional health-promotion roles for many years, and is credited with the design of several midwest corporate wellness programs. He worked a couple of years at Baptist Medical Center in Kansas City—until his risk-taking notoriety made some of the institution's leaders uncomfortable. You see, Mark lived like a stuntman for a time to overcome boredom and to study risk taking. He did things like leap off a high bridge, swim across a dangerous river, scale a skyscraper, jump a car at high speed into a lake, skydive (with a parachute), and so on. He once swam and body-floated 350 miles down the Missouri river. He calls these heroic acts "wellness experiments," since he succeeded by using wellness tools such as physical fitness, visualization, and fear desensitization, along with conscious food choices and his strong belief in God. He describes these exploits and his research into boredom and risk taking in his book, *Wellness Through Risk Taking*. I suspect you will enjoy it if:

A. You are a Walter Mitty type;

B. You want to explore the relationship between boredom and disease;

C. You have a capacity to respect and enjoy creative approaches to living and teaching health concepts and applications; and/or

D. You are crazy enough to contemplate doing something bizarre, dangerous, outlandish, and/or "off-the-wall" either for wellness or for the hell of it.

Mark believes that boredom is synonymous with low level lifestyles that are plagued by smoking, alcohol abuse, drugs, lack of exercise, junk food addiction, and/or other self-destructive *vitality vitiators*. His work addresses all aspects of boredom as a wellness hazard. Mark's materials help the reader understand the connections between boredom and workplace problems, boredom and disease states, and boredom and societal disorders.

I should emphasize that wellness risk taking, Crookse-style, has not been restricted to physical stunts of derring-do. Believing strongly that psychological or emotional wellness is the key to true health, Mark has also discovered a *spiritual* aspect, not limited to physical risk taking. And the greatest spiritual rewards might await those who take risks relating to *social* spheres of life.

For example:

If, in the coming months, you find yourself at the Bristol Restaurant on Country Club Plaza—one of Kansas City's finer establishments—don't be surprised if you have occasion to meet Mark, as the *Wellness Caveman*.

Picture the scene. In comes the Wellness Caveman, briefcase in one hand and spear in the other. What do you say to a guy who destroys a relatively well-established norm that's hostile to cave attire in fashionable dining establishments?

Women in this restaurant often inquire about his distinctive attire. Mark offers a number of explanations:

"It relaxes me."

"Doing this periodically reassures me that I am not intimidated by the mores and social restrictions of society."

"It alleviates boredom."

"My wife divorced me, got the house and all my money, and now I've decided to get back to basics and simplify my life."

"I'm an animal."

"Well, you see, it's like this . . . I had a tough day at the office."

Men, on the other hand, rarely inquire—unless one is the manager of the establishment. *Then*, he asks. At first, tensely: "What is this? What is this about?"

Our man of steel, unblinking, replies: "Oh, just hanging loose."

To which the usual follow-up is: "Are you one of those telegram people?"

"Yes," replies Mark, "but I have already delivered my singing message and was too thirsty for a beer to go home and change."

A sigh of relief sets in ("At least the guy's not an uncontrollable wacko" is one likely thought), and a comment like "Well, OK, that's OK, then" usually follows. Mark believes that this exchange enables the manager to place him in some socially defined standard of deviancy, and judge him (more or less) as "safe to admit."

You may wonder, what does a caveman drink? Coconut milk. Money is seldom requested, which some of you may find reason enough to consider emulating the good Dr. Crookse. Entertainers don't have to pay.

When asked "Why the spear, the briefcase, the tie and white collar?" Mark responds along these lines:

"The spear represents man's aggressive nature, the briefcase is a symbol of modern man's carefully synchronized 9-to-5 schedule, and the collar and tie means status. It also means I must be high up in the tribe. Someday I may even be its leader."

"Does it bother you that people think you're weird?"

"No, it bothers me more if I fit in too well. Many things and people that originally seemed a bizarre aberration ended up as treasures or items of great interest. For example, the Edsel, Thoreau, Elvis, the Leaning Tower of Pisa, to name a few. By that,

I'm not saying I'll be a treasure or item of great interest someday, just that when I fit in, when I must appear normal, then I'm not quite as relaxed."

Men may be interested to know that there is one unanticipated phenomenon occasioned by this simple experiment in social risk taking. It seems that a considerable percentage of the establishment patrons of the gender opposite to Mark's respond in a somewhat primitive manner, demanding that he seize them firmly by their hair and remove them roughly from the grounds. (To do so would, of course, be rather at odds with Mark's character.)

Questioned about this reaction, one area psychiatrist speculated that Mark's appearance had touched some deeply ingrained primeval instinct in these women. At last report, a grant was pending to the local NOW chapter to further explore the situation—and make recommendations to area restaurateurs on how best to deal with disturbed female patrons.

If you would like to order a copy of Mark's book on wellness risk taking, invite him for a lecture or seminar on the topic, or just have him along to spice up your next dinner outing, write or call him as follows:

Mark Crookse, Ph. D., Director
Wellness Resources
Metabolic Research Laboratories, Inc.
9521 Mission Road, Overland Park, KS 66206
(816) 444-9521

Reflections on . . .

Environmental Sensitivity

pages
162–177

This was, in my opinion, the most creative of the five dimensions. The idea of organizing environmental issues into physical, social, and personal categories appeals to me still, and the focus on "personal space" seems sensible and useful. As usual, the best part of this chapter was the overall principles. In this case, principles were given for both the physical/social aspect of environmental sensitivity and personal aspects of the dimension. I am pleased to

pages
165–173

report, after examination of all these principles, that each seems even more significant now than it was ten years ago.

That's the good news.

There's really no "bad" news, but this chapter could have addressed and emphasized two areas that have received a great deal of attention over the years: *norms or rules* (now the hub of the "wellness wheel") and *spirituality*.

Lately I've Been Thinking About . . .

SPIRITUALITY

Spirituality means different things to people of varying religions, denominations, or factions within a denomination, as well as to people of varying cultures and nationalities. What is spirituality to Jerry Falwell would not seem so to Ayatollah Khomeini. This is a difficult area to address, given the potency and negativity that comes with dogma, creeds, and strong beliefs in what some perceive as moral absolutes. When one person's dogmas, creeds, and moral absolutes bump up against those of someone with a different set, the climate for thoughtful and considerate dialogue usually turns for the worse.

Yet despite the difficulty of addressing this ill-defined, arguable, and complex matter, it is clear that something about the "human spirit" belongs in a wellness model. It certainly deserves a lot more focus than I provided in the first edition, for example. Spirituality is the elusive issue that lies at the heart of a well-managed and examined wellness lifestyle. Rather than call it spirituality and invite all the misunderstandings attendant on the subject, I decided to address the matter in another context—namely, "ethics, values, and purposes."

ETHICS, VALUES, AND PURPOSES

I never met anyone who claimed that wellness was limited to being fit, responsible, happy, full of good humor, able to manage stressful events and circumstances, and otherwise being physically and psychologically healthy. Whether individuals profess belief in a deity or not ("religious" or otherwise), they have great concern about the meaning at the center—the proverbial "bottom line" of wellness. A tight definition of this essence of wellness is likely to remain elusive, but we can nonetheless appreciate the spirit of it all. Without it, fulfillment and perspective are harder to come by.

A secular philosophy works every bit as well as a total commitment of faith, and vice versa. In either case, a conscious awareness of and commitment to a personally workable set of well-defined, applicable ethics, values, and/or purposes seems to serve the individual who is in search of a rewarding and satisfying existence. This kind of framework permits one to live life to the full under varying circumstances and fluctuating health levels throughout a lifetime. Unfortunately, it is harder to *achieve* such a framework than to define what it looks like or consists of. I possess no formula, quick or otherwise, about how to do so.

Ethics, values, and purposes in life—or, if you prefer, a sense of spirituality—are less needed in good times than in bad, less vital when you are at the heights of well being than when you are ill or dying. In moments of peak performance, spirituality is less noticeably absent than in times of crisis or mourning. When the crowd is cheering and honoring your worth, beauty, and nobility, you may not miss an integrative belief system concerning "what it's all about." But if you are without such an emotional/intellectual anchor sometime when you are alone, hurt, and left to cope with incomplete resources, you will be sorely disadvantaged without some such system.

Nietzsche put it thusly: "He who has a *why* to live can bear with almost any *how*." But there is more to be gained from spirituality than merely a buffer that enables you "to bear" any burden and otherwise deal with the down side of life. It also makes life richer in good times. In short, it makes the peaks higher as well as the valleys comprehensible.

By cultivating a curiosity about and a life-long quest for your own truths about spirituality—in whatever context that satisfies, appeals, or "speaks" to you—you will be strengthening an integral, underlying component of wellness. You will be focusing on matters that fit the dimension of ethics, values, and purposes. Thus you will benefit by having all the following capacities:

●The ability to transcend difficulties and "explain" (to and for yourself) apparent tragedies and injustices.

•The ability to integrate different aspects of your existence, safeguarding the primacy of inner directions while being attuned to external signals and forces.

•The ability to be aware of what, to you, are worthy purposes in life, and an attendant sense of responsibility for acting accordingly.

•The ability to reach out to serve others (which also serves you and those around you about whom you care deeply).

•The ability to sense genuine inner achievements in the face of circumstances that, to others, would represent failures.

•The ability to find affirmations of your values, ethics, and purposes in creative work and fulfillment in the realms of beauty, art, and nature.

•The ability to realize that there are always choices— and that heartfelt and secure convictions give you the strength and serenity to live with your choices.

•The ability to know confidently that you, more than anyone or anything else, will decide what shall become of you, physically and emotionally.

•The ability to seize the opportunity to be all that you can be—and all without having to join the Army!

If all this is so, why haven't I placed ethics, values, and purposes in the center of the wellness circle? Because *there is no center*, in the sense of a rank order. At varying times in our lives, each dimension is more important than the others. But in the grand scheme of things, all are equally important. Neglect any one of the dimensions for a period of time and it will become the most important area for you—for a time.

Unfortunately, there are no guarantees that being aware of the importance of this dimension will, in itself, bring about all that I have sketched here. The many paths to peace of mind, fulfullment, strength to overcome/endure, and all the rest have been pondered by wise men and women for many centuries, and by philosophers, priests, rabbis, shamans, and just plain thoughtful folks in our own time. Of these, many have failed, and continue to fail! Why? I don't know. Maybe it goes back to the rules and early conditioning. Maybe it has to do with the support people do or do not get at critical times. More likely, it has to do with something else.

However, I do know that many individuals go through great travail trying to discover or to live with their ethics, values, and/or purposes in life. Most of us have known ministers, priests, psychiatrists or others in renowned professions who are alcoholics, who suffer depression or inner torment, and who simply cannot seem to achieve a faith in themselves or their own abilities to cope, let alone transcend. All the words and concepts count for little when there is no center that binds and holds it all together, however sincere, informed, and contemplative one may be. Spirituality is more mysterious than we sometimes acknowledge.

Yet there seems to be no feasible alternative to the search for meaning. There is so much to be discovered in the quest for new levels of understanding and satisfaction—and wellness lifestyles seem a promising framework for this ultimate purpose. It almost surely can be a rewarding pursuit for you. And for those who promote wellness to others, myself included, it is best not to interpret this dimension as being "for" or "against" any religious perspective, particular philosophical school, cultural group, or class of people. It is available to anybody and has equal potential value for all.

I hope you experience wellness as a valuable tool for finding satisfaction and consequence in your life. I hope you always interpret everything about wellness comfortably, in a manner that makes your time on Earth as rich as possible.

PART THREE

Toward a Healthier Nation

Introduction: Reflections on Upstream/Downstream

This fable was the most often-reproduced feature of the original book. The moral—that it pays to focus on underlying causes (upstream) rather than on symptoms (downstream)—still applies. Regrettably, the problem of downstream versus upstream is even greater today than when I wrote this parody of the health care system.

pages 179–180

Dividing Part Three into those actions you can take alone versus those best done in concert with others was an effective way of organizing matters, it seems to me. It allowed a breakdown of topics in that broad and vital area of "political wellness," or issues that affect your wellness prospects that lie outside the five dimensions and the jurisdiction of your own lifestyle.

Reflections on . . .
Practicing the Artful Complaint

I love this section. Back in '76 I felt it was of major importance. Now I think it is even more important.

pages 181–206

I wouldn't change a word—so I won't. But I will *add* a few. My favorite method of "artfully complaining" has been to write letters to celebrities or infamous persons. (Sometimes a single letter takes care of both!) For example, I have written to Sylvester Stallone, a sleazebag publisher or two, John Madden, and George Steinbrenner—there is no shortage of juicy candidates. The purpose in writing is to do just what I encouraged in 1976: to raise consciousness about wellness issues and thereby contribute to the growth of a constituency for healthy change in one realm or another. My way of raising consciousness was to share these letters with the public, wellness promoters, and others interested in positive health practices and healthier cultures. I reached the public by writing a weekly column, "The Ardell Wellness Letters: Going for the Real Gusto," in a local California newspaper; I reached wellness promoters, etc., by publishing some of the letters (and responses) in the *Wellness Report*.

Curious as to the recipients of Ardell Wellness Letters? Here is the list, plus a brief indication of the wellness issue raised—in a somewhat artful manner, I hope. (Of course, one man's art can be another's graffiti.)

If I left someone out who you believe needs or warrants a Wellness Letter, let me know and I'll put one out. Better yet, write one yourself. It's fun and good for your health. And maybe, someone out there will take you seriously and do something about whatever it is that needs rectifying.

THE ARDELL WELLNESS LETTERS

For about a year, I have been practicing the "artful complaint" on the following people (this list is not complete):

- The president of Arthur Anderson & Company, regarding what is missing in annual audits.

- Howard Cosell, regarding his doing an interview at a mythical hospital, Mt. Do-It-Yourself Medical Center.

- Mary Decker on self-responsibility, or dealing with the Zola Budds in life.

- The chairman of the board of Smith Barney, regarding ad copy for John ("Earn It") Housemann.

- Jerry Falwell, regarding the need to be aware that many do not realize he is just kidding.

- Bob Guccione at *Penthouse* magazine, regarding advice on a new way to sell a sleazy magazine.

- The manager of a California restaurant that served me deep fried whole wheat French toast. Unbelievable but true.

●Lazlo Toth, a master of the artful complaint, who gave me the idea to write wellness letters.

●John Madden, regarding fame, beer ads, MADD, and the presidency.

●The pope, regarding the problem with being pope— and what to do about it.

●The Proctor and Gamble Company, regarding how they can get Satan off their back.

●R. J. Reynolds Tobacco Company, regarding a proposed wellness program for the smoke pushers.

●The authors of *The Yuppie Handbook*, regarding an idea for a new best-seller they could call *The YIALAPW Handbook* (Youthful If Aging Lifestyle Artist Practicing Wellness)!

●Jack La Lanne, regarding how to use wellness to get attention.

●Percy Ross, the philanthropist columnist, regarding how to best distribute one million dollars.

●Pepsi Marketing leaders, regarding a better spokesman than M. Jackson or L. Ritchie.

●Roscoe Egger, Jr., the head of the IRS, regarding how to make paying taxes a joy—sort of.

●Jane Fonda, regarding the *true* meaning of "go for the burn."

●William F. Buckley, Jr., regarding his poor health habits.

●Newton Becker, regarding how to improve the qualifications of CPAs.

- Garrison Keillor, regarding wellness in Lake Woebegon.

- C. Everett Koop, M.D., regarding the surgeon general's role in wiping out worseness.

- Thomas Peters and Robert Waterman, regarding something they left out of their "search for excellence."

- Several letters to John and Jane Q. Public, regarding ads that seek to trick them and related matters that affect public opinion and consumer judgments.

- James Beggs, the administrator of NASA, regarding why I should be shot into space.

- Mikhail Gorbachev at the Kremlin, regarding why I (and others) should be allowed to jog in Moscow.

- Dr. Michael DeVries at Humana Hospital, regarding why we need a public forum more than another artificial heart transplant.

- George Burns, regarding a role for God in the matter of funds for retirees' health insurance.

- Hugh Hefner, regarding a few needed changes in the *Playboy* philosophy.

- Jimmy and Rosalyn Carter, regarding the value of their participation in the wellness movement.

- Peter Ueberroth, regarding the best way to solve baseball's problems.

- Clint Eastwood, regarding the line to use on smokers who annoy.

- George Steinbrenner, regarding a strategy to help the Yankees and their coach become happier people.

● President Reagan, regarding passage of his desired tax-reform program.

● The Reverend Peter Conley, regarding having my books banned in Boston.

● Sylvester Stallone, regarding a few problems inherent in his Rambo Rocky fantasies.

● The new president of the AMA, who owns a tobacco farm, regarding what he should do to reform the health habits of doctors.

Just to get you in the spirit, should you wish to do likewise, here are a few examples of Ardell Wellness Letters, or attempts at the artful complaint.

John Madden, Former Coaching Genius
Current Media Star and Beer Personality
% CBS Sports
51 W. 52nd Street
New York, New York 10019

Dear Coach:

You are some kind of guy! In a way, you're a reverse Cosell: nobody can get enough of you, and everybody either likes you, loves you, or is amused by you. It's a pretty enviable situation, but, as suggested in the preceding sentence, since it's you, there's no envy. You just can't lose.

But there is one tiny smudge on this splendid tapestry, and I would be grateful if you would bear with me while I respectfully mention it for your consideration. After all, your John Madden act (genuine as can be) is an art form—and thus subject to close scrutiny by admirers as well as detractors (of which there may be none in your case).

It's about those ads, Coach. Now I have *some* sense of humor and I certainly want to think that I can appreciate the value of having a few beers with your buddies and clowning around a bit in the process. No harm in that, I say.

But—read the papers (not just the sports or entertainment sections). Listen to the news, watch a few documentaries. There's a crisis out there—and your fans are the ones getting hurt (and hurting others). Sure it's fun to drink and act crazy—but drunk driving kills. In addition to the All-American good guys and other normals of our species, there are quite a few young and impressionable folks out there watching your example. And there are, to be sure, also vast numbers (millions?) of grown-up superjerks watching and imitating the superjocks in your beer ads. The message seems pretty clear: drink a lot, be loud, and you'll have lots of laughs and things will work out. You will be just like your sports heroes—including lovable John Madden.

Now don't get guilty or defensive about all this, John. I have a plan. It will do you no harm and in fact will add to your popularity, if that's possible. Actually, it is possible; there's one group that I don't think has climbed aboard the Madden bandwagon. In fact, I suspect this group probably thinks you are a public menace. With my plan, you can win them over, too! I'm thinking about MADD—Mothers (and Fathers and everybody else) Against Drunk Driving. Hell, you follow my plan, Coach, and it could be "Madden for President" in 1988.*

Are you Republican or Democrat? It matters not—you'll win either way.

Ready for my plan? Hope so, 'cause here it is.

Offer your services, for free, to MADD—and make your beer company pay for public service TV spots in support of a variety of safe driving messages (wearing seat belts, no drinking and driving, elimination of "happy hours" which promote abusive consumption as a "bargain," the buddy system for parties, and so on). Invite your ex-jock drinking pals to participate, also. See if you can get Danger-field to help out. It's the *only* way that guy will ever get any respect. And make sure the spots appear in prime time during big games; otherwise they might air on Sunday mornings between preachers and cartoons.

Well, that's it. Sure hope you like my plan and go for it. If you do, it will make all of us less afraid of the dark! (Most of us can handle a light going out on a train ride—it's the drive home at night that scares us. You never know when a fun-loving guy trying to be like Coach Madden may be coming around the corner or across the divider.)

Be well—and continued success and happiness.

*I'm sure you have not thought a lot about your cabinet yet—and I don't want to be premature. But, if you get stuck and can't think of anyone for secretary of defense, I might be interested. Or, if Butkas or one of the other linebackers seems a natural for this post, how about ambassador to England, or France, Sweden, New Zealand, Australia, Switzerland, or Canada? Liechtenstein?

James Beggs, Administrator
Space Flight Participant Program—NASA
400 Maryland Avenue
Washington, DC 20546

Dear Mr. Beggs:

I was delighted to read in a recent issue of *Life* magazine that NASA
will deliver "the ultimate payload of a consumer society" into space
sometime in 1985, namely, a "tourist" or citizen. Specifically, a
teacher, to be nominated in early 1985 by peers on the basis of a six-
to eight-page application, with selection set for May.

Well, in all modesty, I think I have just the candidate with all
the "Right Stuff" for you. C'est moi!

I know I should save this for the six- to eight-page application I
would like you to speed my way, but you are probably dying to know
why I think I'm your man—so I'll highlight a few of the strong points
of my candidacy.

● For starters, I'm in fabulous shape. I run marathons, do
triathlons, cross country ski, shoot rapids (backwards), pump iron,
and always take the stairs. Of course, I do fall asleep before 8:00 pm
every night and cannot rise before 10:00 am, but this should not be
a big problem if you do not expect the tourist to do any work on
board, anyway.

● I'm great company—and as a teacher of wellness lifestyles I
would be superb for purposes of the crew's morale and continuing
education. I mean, face it, you don't want to bring along just *any*
teacher. What would a first grade teacher do—read to the astronauts? ("Look Jane. See it go. See it go up. Up, up.") You have to
admit—that would get old *real* fast. Then you have a morale problem. Or, suppose you get a biology teacher. You want somebody cutting up frogs on the Space Shuttle? And so it goes—all the traditional
teachers, while lovely people and deserving of rides on future
flights, are not ideally suited for the *first* endeavor of this genre. By
contrast, imagine the benefits of bringing a wellness promoter. I
have this dynamite slide show with two carousel projectors and a dis-
solve unit, and video tapes on the Planning for Wellness system used
to train seminar participants to sustain their good lifestyle intentions. (In this case, the astronauts on duty.) I can divide the crew into
small groups for experiential processes . . . maybe I should save this
for the application!

Suffice to note that I'll cover the key principles in nutrition the
first day, we'll focus on fitness the next, self-responsibility the next,
and the first time something goes wrong we'll delve into stress management. By the time we land, all crew members will be paragons
of wellness virtue.

And now the best part of my candidacy—the overall effect of the experience, when the cheering has died down and heart rates are back to normal, mine included.

I'm talking about the meaning of it all. Going beyond personal glorification. I'm talking about style, class, even panache. No beer commercials for this famous figure. Quite the contrary—the attention given to the wellness concept during the entire process of selection, the flight itself (especially my lectures from space), and the post-flight hoopla will draw the eyes and hearts of hundreds of millions of citizens all over the world to the attractions of wellness living. A lifestyle philosophy pioneered right here in the old U.S. of A. Get the flags out.

And I can tell little boys and girls everywhere that if they live a wellness lifestyle, maybe they will get shot into space someday, too.

I'm already looking forward to my Great Adventure in space. In the meantime, I have taken to hanging upside down a lot from my roof to simulate the effects of weightlessness. If you have other suggestions, please pass them along.

Harrison L. Rogers, M.D., President
American Medical Association
535 N. Dearborn Street
Chicago, IL 60610

Dear Dr. Rogers:

Greetings. Congratulations on the occasion of your election to the Presidency of the American Medical Association (AMA).

You will be relieved to know that I will not be at all critical about that farm you own on which tobacco is grown. I know you have received a lot of grief ever since the Chicago Sun-Times revealed this bit of compromising data. In my opinion, this firestorm of outrage is off the mark. Heck, if you were not growing tobacco on this land, someone else surely would be. Besides, how could you know that someday you would be "El Presidente" of the world's most powerful medical organization? M.D.'s do all kinds of things that seem to conflict with common sense—why make an example of you? As I see it, the real problem is the *appearance* of conflict. The very idea of a public figure doctor being involved in such an insidious activity for profit is just going to bother a lot of idealistic people—especially since the AMA is trying to repair its image as a "do-nothing" organization on the smoking issue. But, don't worry. At least I won't hold this against you.

I won't, that is, if you roar into action in support of a wild idea I have to prevent such embarrassments in the future and, more important, encourage doctors to become better role models for healthy living!

Support for this idea may not be so difficult to secure after all, because I have been reading that the AMA has come out for all kinds of good reforms on lifestyle matters. Take smoking, for instance. Goals and directions adopted at the last AMA convention urged varied efforts to "snuff out tobacco" by the Year 2000 (maybe you *should* sell that farm), action against fraudulent and just plain misleading tobacco company advertising, an end to Federal tobacco price supports, a stop to free cigarette samples, support for public protection from secondhand smoke, and even control of smoking by employees of the AMA.

My idea for doctors as wellness role models that I want you to spearhead is just a logical next step for the AMA. You should not have any trouble at all seeing it through the organization. And, best of all, I want you to take all the credit for the plan.

Consider me your secret advisor.

But the idea does require that the AMA take really bold action to convince the skeptical citizenry that the organization is *really* dead serious about reducing U.S. health care costs and improving the health status of the people.

So, assuming that you are ready to lead the AMA into a bold course of action, here is my plan. All you need to do is run with it.

Have the AMA determine that doctors who smoke, abuse alcohol, get fat through sedentary living, act stressed out and hostile, eat Twinkies and other junk foods in public and/or otherwise set a terrible lifestyle example for patients will henceforth be brought before AMA tribunals on a charge of medical malpractice!

Why not? Are such physicians not being derelict in their roles as teachers? Should doctors not show us by example how to live a healthful life? While it has been a few years since the infamous ads that "more doctors recommend Chesterfields than any other brand," it is not necessary to look back to the fifties to find doctors whose specialty you would think is modeling low level worseness. I say have the AMA put a screeching halt to this sorry situation, and thereby move us closer to the goal of a smokeless and well society by the year 2000!

But, is it practical, you are probably wondering? Who would be the persons with the responsibility or moral authority to challenge the doctors on their awful lifestyle habits, unconditioned physical appearances, stressed out/hostile personalities, or spiritually void/joylessly dull personal lives, to name but a few malpractice possibilities under the new system?

Patients would, of course! Pharmacists would also be valued tipsters. So would nurses, receptionists and particularly bankers, who see doctors more than most of us.

This plan has rich possibilities. In cases of disputes, there could be televised wellness trials with great educational potentials. You could hire Judge Wapner to preside over a People's (Medical) Court. Or, on a more positive note, elect the Wellest of physicians in each community to the "Doctor Bowl" or other celebratory local event. How about a contest for the doctors with the healthiest lifestyles, with divisions for both sexes and varied age categories? What fun it would be to invent new criteria for scoring.

I do hope you go into action immediately with my plan, which I offer to you at no charge.

Good luck. Call if I can be more helpful than I have been already.

By the way, are *you* fit? Happy? Do you practice stress management techniques? How's your diet? Don't smoke any of that stuff you grow, do you?

Be well. Send quarterly reports on how the plan is going, if it's not too much trouble.

Clint Eastwood, Tough Hombre
Star of Clint Eastwood Movies
Box 125
Pebble Beach, CA 93953

Dear Clint:

Howdy. Of all the lessons subtly conveyed in your silver-screen morality plays, the one I like best is that a man cannot be too careful in the choice of his enemies. Yes, that's the "reality" I got out of all those punch-em-out, hunt-em-down, run-em-over, shoot-em-up shows you produced and acted out—and I sure do hope I did not miss the point. Of course, "reality" is a pretty subjective thing and we should not be limited by the way others construe it. As that great philosopher Lily Tomlin has observed: "What is reality but a collective hunch?"

Thinking of which brings me to the point: I have a hunch about the reality of America's greatest health hazard. If I am right about this hunch, then I think you can apply my idea in your next movie through your choice of the right enemies—and help a lot of people in the process. Interested so far?

It's about smoking. Despite all the warnings, posters, research, articles, and so on, about 30 percent of adults still smoke. (I know you don't, thank God.) One reason (there are many) is that very few authorities and public figures take the problem seriously enough. They pussyfoot and dance around the smoking monster like a bunch of do-gooder pansies. Not like the way you would handle the problem, Clint. Take the Surgeons General, for example.

For years, all they did was put a sissy-like warning on the side of cigarette packs with inane messages like: "Warning: the U.S. Surgeon General has determined that smoking may be (recently updated to *is*) hazardous to your health." Big deal: Smokers already know that. Can you imagine a smoker reading that just before he/she lights up and thinking: "Wow, is that so? Sure glad I was warned. I'll just throw these away." Of course not.

It's time to get "Clint Eastwood tough" on smoking! Let's make it a capital offense—at least for repeat offenders. Let's lock-em-up and throw away the key. Let's punch-em-out, hunt-em-down, run-em-over, and shoot-em-down! That's the reality we have to go with if we really want to stop this craziness.

Of course, smokers in Congress, smoking sympathizers, and bleeding-heart-do-gooders would never allow such a get-tough stand. That's where you and movie escapist-propaganda come in. You can make smokers your enemies in future scripts. Have them commit assorted mayhem with their obnoxious weeds. For example, show them lighting up in elevators, airplane rest rooms, theatres, gas stations, health clubs, or anywhere else where non-smokers are breathing. Then do your Clint Eastwood routine. Walk up real close, glare white heat into their watery eyeballs, and invite them to put it out now or die! If they give you even the slightest resistance, let them know in no uncertain terms that they either stop smoking (for life) or else. Try to express this choice in a memorable way. For your convenience and use, I have invented a great line you could use as a warning if a smoker looks like he or she might take just one last puff. Here it is:

"Go ahead—make my day!"

Be well.

George Steinbrenner III, Owner/Tyrant
New York Yankees—Yankee Stadium
New York, NY

Dear George:

Well, Billy's back—but you and I know he's not going to last long. If he doesn't punch out some marshmallow salesperson, kick an umpire, pass secrets to the Orioles, lose ball games, or otherwise self-destruct, then you will have to fire him for personal reasons—such as failure to genuflect, grovel, or grunt graciously in your presence.

You need a backup manager ready to go—when Billy gets the old heave-ho. Not Yogi, Ralph, or some other retread. A fresh face— someone unknown to the fans and to the game itself who can bring a dramatic new look and emphasis not just to the Yankees but to all of baseball.

Guess who, George? Moi!

Hire me now and I will turn the Yankees into a fun bunch of happy holistic warriors by Labor Day. I will immediately put players and coaches on an "eat to win" diet. Those with an excess percentage of body fat will go on a Dick Gregory special (no food!). Everyone will be trained to meditate before going to bat. No one will blame anyone else—self-responsibility will be our motto. Every player will be cross-trained in distance swimming, biking, and running for greater endurance, stamina, and flexibility. Classes will be held before all home games in transformation, breakthrough performance, high self-esteem, affirmations, the Zen of winning, energy balancing, body work therapies, accelerated learning and hair restoration. Before road games, we will practice firewalking, prosperity consciousness, megavitamins for baserunning, creative pet care, and Bach flower remedies for slumps and slide burns. I will not neglect the applications of astrology, herbology, hypnosis, or craniology to sore arms, drug abuse, burnout, greed, smoking, groupie overload, and other occupational hazards of the game.

All players will be trained in advanced hugging by Leo Buscaglia. My tenure will be a time of very exciting personal growth for players and their spouses. Please don't fire me before my "New Age" management style has had a chance to rub off on the fans. They need more help than the players.

I do not promise or predict that the Yankees will win more games under my management, nor, to tell the certain truth, do I *care* a great deal about this limited perspective. (It's *how* the game is played that counts, George.) But I can tell you this, given that your team is near the bottom: We won't be any worse than the Yanks are now! And we'll be a hell of a lot healthier and have a lot of laughs. Good luck and be well. My best to Billy.

Ronald Reagan
President of the United States
The White House
Washington, DC

Dear Mr. President:

Greetings. I do not want to see your tax reform initiative delayed, so I thought I should write you at once. It is evident that every special interest group in the Nation is seeking to have its turf treated favorably, and I would not want you to hold up the program waiting for wellness promoters to declare what we want out of reform.

As you well know, these are turbulent times in the 400-billion-dollar health services industry. The provision and financing of medical care are undergoing revolutionary changes. The methods of reimbursement, the dynamics of competition, the great pressures of deregulation, and the emergence of citizen skepticism about high technology treatment all constitute conditions for a revolution in the way Americans view health and obtain medical care.

At a later date, I could give you a complete plan as to how you could shape a much better health system. For now (I'm very busy) I will just tell you what to do about Medicare, which accounts for the lion's share of the federal deficit.

Make Medicare a vehicle for wellness and a part of your tax reform program.

Institute a 469th diagnostic-related group (DRG) for which the government will reimburse medical providers and institutions. This DRG number 469 would be for incipient worseness and would enable a medical institution to admit individuals (on an outpatient basis) for some form of wellness training *before* they qualify for one of the other 468 DRG categories! This DRG would, of course, be the least expensive of all the DRG categories: a very modest sum, say, $100 per person per year, should suffice for counseling and training patients who smoke, are sedentary, bored, or just stressed out, a little depressed, mired in low self-esteem, or who otherwise seem to be excellent candidates for a lifestyle refresher and "picker-upper."

At a cost of a mere billion or two, you will be able to assist mega-numbers of our citizens to give themselves the ultimate tax credit—a healthy lifestyle that is satisfying, effective, and life sustaining.

Don't worry about the details. Have one of your cabinet officers give me a call and I'll explain how to do it. Or, if I'm in the area I'll be glad to come over for dinner with you and Nancy. Be well.

The Rev. Peter Conley, Spokesman
Archdiocese of Boston
2121 Commonwealth Avenue
Boston, MA 02135

Dear Father Conley:

The purpose of this letter is to solicit your aid in a conspiracy. Inasmuch as you manage publicity for an institution that seeks to do good and serve the interests of both mankind and the Lord, I just know you are going to love my conspiracy idea.

A little background is in order. I got the idea for this conspiracy in reading about your promotional talents in a variety of newspapers and magazines in recent weeks. It seems the ex-nun authors of the risque new book entitled *Lesbian Nuns: Breaking Silence* and their publishers at Naiad press are crediting you with the fact that their book has gone from absolute "nowhere anonymity" to the best-seller list. One of the co-editors, Nancy Manahan, is quoted as saying you were "marvelous," and promises to send you a bouquet.

I'm sure that modesty constrains you from taking full credit for this book's commercial success. But the fact is you did it, Father Conley. What's more—and here is where my conspiracy plan comes in—I think you can do it again. Let's review your tactics for a moment.

When you read that the ex-nuns were to appear on a local NBC TV show to promote their expose of hanky-panky in the nunnery, you protested to the Boston station on the grounds that "public discussion of this book would offend decency." What's more, you succeeded—the station cancelled the interview!

Anyone in San Francisco (or anywhere outside of Boston) could have predicted what would happen next when word of a book's being "banned in Boston" got out. Notoriety ensued, the authors became overnight celebrities, and sales took off. As of last week, *Lesbian Nuns* was fifth on the Bay Area non-fiction charts, excerpts are running in the sleazy sex tabloid *Forum* magazine, and ex-nun Manahan and her co-editor Rosemary Curb are about to take off for London to launch the British edition of their book.

As to your role in making *Lesbian Nuns* a hit, I think Ms. Manahan summed it up best when she said: "You can't buy that kind of publicity."

And that's where you fit into my conspiracy. Actually, it will be *our* conspiracy if you consent to my plan. You see, Father, I can't buy "that kind of publicity" either. And I need it for a cause I know you support, namely good health, self-responsibility, sound diet, strenuous (not moderate) exercise, stress management, and all that sort of thing. I know the Church has nothing against any of this, but here is my idea.

I want you to come out against the publication, reading, discussion, sale, or existence of my new book entitled *The History and Future of Wellness* (Kendall Hunt, Dubuque, IA, 2nd ed., 1985)! Make up some ridiculous reason why it should be suppressed by Catholics and other proper thinkers far and wide, but especially in your area. Yes, my goal here is nothing less than to have this book *banned in Boston*.

I can think of nothing else that will do as much to insure its success.

On what basis would you object to a wellness book? Here are a few possibilities:

● People would get so wholesome that they would have nothing left to confess.

● People would get so fit they would become narcissistic about their bodies.

● People would demand whole wheat wafers at Communion— and what would the Church do with its supply of non-nutritious white wafer bread?

● People might expect all priests and nuns to participate in active sports despite their age—and physical condition—and it won't be easy keeping up with the likes of Sister Marion Irvine.

● Women who pursue wellness to exercise extremes will experience amenorrhea, a sneaky form of birth control—and we all know the Church's position on that!

Well, you get the idea. It doesn't matter if the reasons are sensible or not—it's the magic of censorship that counts.

If you join me in this conspiracy, check your mailbox. There will be another bouquet on the way.

Be well.

Sylvester "Rambo Rocky" Stallone
9665 Wilshire Blvd., #200
Beverly Hills, CA 90212

Dear Mr. Stallone:

Greetings. I write on behalf of wellness practitioners and promoters everywhere. (No, they did not ask me to write on their behalf, but, what the hell, where would you be if you waited for somebody to tell you to invent "Rocky"? There are some things a guy just knows he has to do, if you know what I mean.)

First of all, congratulations on the success of "Rambo." One hundred million dollars in five weeks is pretty good box office action—and your fee of twelve million for doing the movie is not bad, either. That's more than I've made in years.

I have to tell you straight out that this is not exactly a fan letter. Oh, I reluctantly enjoyed a few Rocky episodes before tiring of the genre after, let's see, I think it was Rocky 212. That was the one where Rocky's second son's daughter wins the women's heavyweight title from the Commie amazon from Transylvania. In a comeback, of course. The Rambo thing sounded awful from the reviews, even though a large segment of the public obviously ate it up. Naturally, the public can be wrong, as witness Richard Nixon, rich punk rockers, Jerry Lewis, Muzak, and much more.

Nevertheless, I decided to see Rambo only after encountering four bits of information:

1. Somewhere I read that you work out five hours a day, burning about 12,000 calories. Anybody with the discipline to do that can't be all bad. I exercise two hours daily—and I thought I was committed. *You* are committed—I'm a dilettante. And, I respect what you have done with your body. I once wrote a book based upon research as to the superb health implications of such practices (termed "heroic acts"). Anyway, I'm impressed.

2. Somewhere else I learned that you want to stay "uncivilized" and that you profess "a desire to stay on the edge of madness" because this "allows for creative leaps."

3. On a talk show I heard that you believe in reincarnation, that you were once a monkey or toad or something in Central America as well as a nobleman who lost his head on the guillotine during the French Revolution. You certainly must have an interesting resume.

4. What made Rambo must viewing was a comment by our president, Ronald Reagan. It was at the end of the hostage crisis in Lebanon, and he had just seen your movie. He said: "After seeing Rambo, I know what to do the next time."

All this aroused my interest, so off I went to the local bijou (past the stores selling no less than 30 different Rambo products) and saw your movie.

After watching you single-handedly (well, with a little help from a pretty girl) wipe out about a third of the Vietnamese and Soviet armies and probably all Mekong Delta pirates (but you spared the snake), I decided I'd better write you.

Now look here, Sylvester "Rambo Rocky" Stallone! You have got to get yourself under control. In the first place, don't worry about staying uncivilized or on the edge of madness. You're covered. Secondly, while you have every right to make any kind of fantasy movie you want for wimps, psychos, deviants, and just plain folks overcome with a sense of powerlessness who enjoy such escapist nonsense, you must for the sake of the Earth and us wellness types exercise some caution if our President is going to base his foreign policy on this kind of "Rambomaniacal" silliness.

I do not think it is a good idea to make movies which encourage our President to function "on the edge of madness," even if his looniness is creative. He has bigger guns than Rambo and Rocky together—and some innocent people could get hurt if he does "next time" in the real world what you did last time in a film.

Sylvester, Sir, there *are* alternatives to reliance upon violence, hatred, grudges, revenge, and monosyllable grunts for problem solving/conflict resolution purposes, not to mention stress management. Try deep breathing when the urge to decimate arises. Eat regular, nutritious meals. Listen to classical music. You ought to sleep more. Take some time off. Work on your relationships. Read some poetry. Build a more positive self-concept. Attend a wellness seminar. If you want more advice, just call anytime—no charge. Follow my suggestions and you will get to win next time, even if the U.S.A. doesn't invade Vietnam.

You may, sans the gore and carnage, lose a million or two at the box office, but look at it this way: you don't really *need* the money and we will all be better able to sleep at night knowing you are setting a better—and safer—example for our President.

Be well.

And here are a few replies:

Dear Mr. Ardell:

Thanks for inquiring. I try to do twenty or thirty minutes of bicycling indoors three times a week, and once a year I go to one of those health places (in Mexico, Rancho La Puerta). The doctors seem to think I am in moderately good shape. You were very kind to inquire.

Yours faithfully,

Wm. F. Buckley, Jr.

Dear Mr. Ardell:

Thank you for writing and telling me that you enjoyed reading my autobiography.

I'm glad you found my story so satisfying. It shows the truth of the lesson I learned very early on—that hard work and perseverance will pay off, and that people working together can move mountains.

I appreciate your sending me the Ardell Wellness test to take. I took the test and scored in the highest category.

Thank you for your support.

Best wishes.

Sincerely,

Lee Iacocca

Dear Doctor Ardell:

Thank you very much for your letter of 8/8/85 and I appreciate your support. A.M.A. certainly supports and is an active advocate of a healthy lifestyle for all Americans and we welcome your encouragement of this for all of our citizens.

I've tried very hard to practice what I preach and have succeeded reasonably well. I'll have to admit that I would be a little nervous about having my colleagues try me for "malpractice" if I went over my "alotted" weight! Active encouragement is great but mandatory recriminations might have an adverse effect.

Thanks again for your support.

Sincerely,

Harrison L. Rogers, Jr., M.D.

363

You are probably thinking: "Why does he write these letters? What a crank!" Well, I have good reasons. Here are a few of them:

- Writing these letters is a very enjoyable and creative challenge.

- Thinking of the likely reactions has been enjoyable so far, in all cases.

- Receiving an occasional response is a big thrill—in most cases.

- Writing a letter to whomever you choose to address is a valued privilege possible only in a free and tolerant society. Besides, it's cheap!

- Wellness is too important to be presented grimly—and these letters are not grim. (This point cannot be repeated too often.)

- The lessons of the evolving wellness philosophy should be translated to events and behaviors in the "real world."

- Public figures are role models (unfortunately so, in some cases). Therefore, a few letters from wellness-conscious observers might encourage a few of them to reflect a bit and maybe even shape up to become better models. More likely, the letters will be ignored—but no harm in trying.

Wait, I just thought of another justification.

Ever get the feeling that you are looking for wellness in all the wrong places, searching for interest in too many faces that are simply turned elsewhere? Of course you do—and that is perhaps the best reason for wellness letters to big shots. Those who most need to hear about wellness are not ready to listen—the topic has little appeal. That's precisely why they ought to be exposed to a wellness outlook, because they have spent years ignoring its precepts and rewards. But if you identify a wellness issue with, or at least relate it in some manner to, a big star, hero, heroine, or miscreant whom they recognize—then you have captured their attention.

Reflections on **.** **.** **.**

INFLUENCING THE MODEL
FOR NATIONAL HEALTH INSURANCE

In 1976, I challenged the idea of national health insurance with a commentary about all the disincentives that such federal entitlements would bring. Ten years later, I feel the same way, except that now I am against nearly *any* form of health insurance, save perhaps catastrophic coverage. pages 193–194

The problem with health insurance is that not many programs are set up with healthy people in mind. For this reason, if you have an interest in wellness lifestyles, you may want to look carefully at the value of health insurance policies. I personally consider them a relatively poor investment. (A bit of a digression is in order before this gets too heavy. Of course, *health* insurance is a misnomer. What is called health insurance is in fact a *sickness payment plan*. You receive no benefits if you do not get sick. Ever tried "calling in well"? Try it tomorrow. Call the boss in the morning and say something like this: "Hiya, Chief. I just read *High Level Wellness* and I'm feeling great. And it's a beautiful day. Yes, sir—I'm on top of the world. No way would I come to work today." See how much enthusiasm you get for that. Maybe, someday, employers will permit time off for "extreme wellness.")

Since sick insurance is a "free" fringe benefit for about 90 percent of U.S. employees, concern about its value is of interest mostly to the self-employed or others not covered at their workplace or eligible for public assistance via Medicare or Medicaid. Or is it? Are there reasons for the 90 percent to be concerned?

Well, one reason could be the twelve-billion-dollar tax loss diverted from the U.S. Treasury, due to health insurance deductions by corporate insurors.

While the U.S. Treasury may not have profited from the fact that I haven't bought insurance for over ten years (although I had coverage during a time of association with a hospital), I personally have saved a bundle. I reasoned, "Why spend all that money if I am not likely to get sick, based on the lifestyle I enjoy?" After all, I don't smoke, use drugs, abuse alcohol, or otherwise depart from the straight and narrow path of righteousness most days of the week (well, at least I exercise vigorously, manage stress well, eat wisely and in accordance with established wellness guidelines, enjoy my work, have a super support system, and so on). This policy saves me a lot, although it *is* a risk. (In fact, with all the money I saved, I could get me one of those mechanical hearts and still be financially ahead.)

The key question is: Just how risky is it to forego a sickness-protection plan of some kind? Is this what Dr. Crookse calls "positive risk taking?" Or might I be the health-system equivalent of an uninsured motorist—a threat to my solvency as well as the fiscal security of anyone with whom I collide (e.g., those depending on or affected by me)? How will the hard-core ill who are not on public assistance be protected at reasonable cost if the healthy do not subsidize the system? And yet, is it reasonable to require or expect the prudent to pay in order to cover not only their own risks but also those whose lifestyles almost guarantee dependence on the system?

I wondered about these questions recently when I paid a bill in California for a few hours of care by physical therapists for a sports-related neck and shoulder problem. The receptionist told me the "normal" charge would be over $175, but, given my situation of no insurance, I would be charged only a third that amount. Of course I was delighted, but later I had to wonder: What if this single transaction were repeated regularly throughout the nation? Would all health services cost a third less if the recipient had no health insurance? Applying this kind of thinking to just 10 percent of medical transactions, imagine the inflation factor caused by health insurance!

A glance at the big picture may be of use here.

Private health insurance grew rapidly between 1945 and 1960. During this span, the number of people with coverage rose from 32 million to 122 million. In the same period, physician expense protection costs leaped from $5 million to $83 million. The numbers took off a second time in 1965, when Medicare and Medicaid were enacted, giving substantial coverage to those who needed it the most—the elderly and poor. All this contributed mightily to the explosion of health-care costs. Now every company wants to stop the increases, and a proliferation of strategies are being developed to restrain the costs of doing business under the present arrangements. But more is at stake than the high cost to individuals, companies, and institutions: When a system biased toward sickness services fails to discourage or even *warn* against sickness-causing behaviors, then what we have on our hands is a disaster.

Health insurance *should* pay for services that help people to stay well. It *should* pay for classes for wellness education. It *should* allow for self-care training and support.

Some of the people who think this way are against the very idea of health coverage as now constituted. Physician Robert Mendelsohn, for example, believes that treatment often causes more harm than comfort or healing, except in limited cases (e.g., emergency care for shock, trauma, broken bones, and so on).

Of course, this is not a popular outlook. Nevertheless, when a system does not deliver your money's worth *unless* you get sick, something is out of whack. (It's a fact that in today's medical system, you can't "win" without losing.) I wonder why rebates are not a part of all policies.

Wellness promoters claim that the only way to cut costs in a significant and nondraconian sense is to help people stay well in the first place.

But maybe there is also another way—reduce or eliminate the buffer of health insurance, at least as it is now designed. Why subsidize smokers and alcoholics, the sedentary, and others who expend too little effort to stay out of the system?

Analysts such as Victor Fuchs, John Knowles, Robert Rodale, and countless others have been saying the same thing for a long time. As Fuchs writes in *Who Shall Live?* "When consumers pay for health care (or any goods and services) directly, they tend to more carefully weigh the costs of the purchase against the benefits."

It seems common sense to reward healthy behavior, and irrational to subsidize self-destructive lifestyles with government and private health-insurance entitlements. Government does it, but you do not have to. Of course, if you are employed and sick insurance is part of the fringe-benefit perks—congratulations. Just do not use those "benefits" more than necessary. Also, ask your personnel or benefits department manager whether the coverage could be optional, with the "option" being dropping you from the plan and directly giving you the amount of money that has been earmarked for your health insurance. Many workers do not realize that insurance is not really "free"—they pay for it with a lower wage.

If you do not have health insurance at work, consider whether buying it on your own is worth your while. You will want to insure your auto, home, and maybe your life (though that's a bargain with the Devil if there ever was one), but perhaps health-insurance money for occasional doctor and other professional medical services might better be used for other purposes.

Someday, when a wellness consciousness has been adopted by a significant number of people, it may be possible to strike a better deal with Blue Cross or Blue Shield or the other operations that manage this business. Until then, start with the idea that insurance should be a way to plan for a positive outcome—and, incidentally, to help pay when illness treatment is required. While no one should be discouraged on the basis of disability, heredity, age, or, of course, the usuals (gender, race, etc.), there may well be a need for other lifestyle considerations.

Since, during all the years of illness consciousness, there has been no interest in such a program it will first be necessary to work out a system for defining, then assessing, what kinds of lifestyles would affect eligibility for affordable wellness insurance.

To whom could society entrust such a task?

No problem. Elect me Czar of Wellness, and I'll have the system ready in a fortnight or 14 days, whichever comes first.

In the meantime, try to remember that a healthy lifestyle is your best insurance policy—in the first, middle, and last analysis.

Reflections on . . .

Helping to Create
a New Kind of Planning System

Lately I've Been Thinking About . . .

THE DEMISE OF HEALTH PLANNING
AND THE RISE OF
ALTERNATIVE PROMOTERS

Health planning was the most promising agent for leading a wellness revolution, or so I thought in 1976. Several planning agencies did innovative work for a few years, but federal and local support for health planning itself was largely discontinued by the
early 1980s, and the role of wellness advocacy fell to other institutions, such as hospitals and business corporations. (For a full review of these developments, you may want to see my recent
book, *The History and Future of Wellness*.)

pages 207–213

Most people are familiar with wellness programming in the
corporate or hospital sectors, but what about on a college or university campus? College campuses are a major force for wellness
promotion. At the University of Wisconsin–Stevens Point in July
1985, approximately 30 campus-based wellness promoters gath-
ered to compare notes. The meeting was not far along before it
became evident that the campus was virgin turf. Only 14 of those
in attendance represented schools with existing programs—but
all were preparing either to get under way or expand. Naturally,
other programs from across the country could have been reviewed had their schools been represented. But little is known
about the range of models for promoting wellness lifestyles on
campus. Here is a quick sketch of one approach, by a relatively
small school in Florida. (Remember, this is an example; not *the*
way.) One reason for being connected with organizations like the
new National Wellness Association, Healthy America, and the
National Center for Health Promotion is so that you can, with
minimal fuss or expense, obtain information about creative pro-

grams.* Enough background—here is a summary of the process and structure at the University of Central Florida, Orlando.

Just under way, wellness programming is focused at a new Campus Wellness Center located next door to the Student Health Service (SHS). The entire operation is under the control of the SHS, which is run by a physician, in this case one dedicated to the wellness concept (John Langdon, formerly of Sioux Falls, SD). The wellness program itself, however, is managed and led in nearly all important ways by a committee of about 15 students from diverse areas of influence on campus. The Student Wellness Advocate Team (SWAT), coached by yours truly and many others, is the heart and soul of the program. UCF has approximately 16,000 students. The SHS is funded by a health-service fee of $24 per student. These funds support an extensive medical service, open 24 hours a day (12 on Saturday; tough luck if you get a cold or VD on Sunday), as well as the wellness program.

The SWAT has identified a series of skill areas of value and interest to the students, including such basics as fitness, nutrition, stress management, medical self-care, and a series of practical topics including conflict resolution, healthy sexuality, and leadership training. The SWAT is now organizing a series of training sessions for other students in each of these areas. A peer-education approach will be used to bring student trainers to dorms, fraternities, sororities, and elsewhere on and off campus, as requested by interested organizations.

Other aspects of the SWAT's work include setting up facilities throughout the campus to make wellness activities convenient. The idea is to seize whatever "teachable moments" come about via interactive videos, software programs, and easy-to-use computers installed at sites most frequented by the students.

Plans are under way to ensure the availability of healthy choices in the dining and cafeteria areas; a smoke-free campus is considered by many on the SWAT as a prime target goal (removing all cigarette machines is on the agenda). Naturally, the Campus Wellness Center is a resource for video tapes and books about the many health topics promoted in the program. Visiting lectur-

*For example, if you have an interest in finding a job in wellness, you might benefit by examining a free pamphlet from The National Center for Health Promotion on that subject. Write them at 3772 Plaza Drive, Suite 5, Ann Arbor, MI 48104.

ers are another part of the SWAT's agenda. In the first months of the year, such notables as Drs. Ruth (sex), Robert Willix (fitness), John Travis (energy/spirituality), and Earl Ubell (intimacy) were in residence on campus.

Dr. Langdon, approaching the leadership at UCF, justified the focus on wellness as part of a quality higher education:

> We seek to supplement the valued "unity of knowledge, ethical concern and social responsibility" that are cherished dimensions of the educational ethic at UCF. We propose an action expressly designed to provide our students with an awareness of another dimension integral to a comprehension of reality and a rounded education. We ask nothing less than curricula modifications that will provide a built-in opportunity to put to a judicious test the student's powers of intellect and judgment in support of living a whole, examined, and fulfilling lifestyle.
>
> We owe wellness education to every young man and woman who comes to UCF. Wellness educations *should* have been provided in the homes since infancy; such training *should* have been given in the elementary and secondary schools since adolescence; and wellness awareness and options for varied mastery of its fundamentals *should* have been part of everyone's cultural and social inheritance. Unhappily, this cherished consummation has not been the fortune of most of our charges. We can go along with the normative neglect that exists, rightfully noting that wellness is not an expressed element of the educational contract between the student and this University— or we can act to support our sense of the larger mandate of a great institution to highest ideals and larger purposes. Our request begs the latter initiative.
>
> Students here and elsewhere in America are *not* getting the idea that their attitudes, habits, behaviors, and lifestyle commitments and values have immense and all-encompassing consequence for their futures—as much so in fact as their ability to recall formulae and dates, to reason critically, and to master today's state-of-the-art content and axioms in diverse disciplines. But the mastery of a healthy and self-reinforcing, evolving lifestyle has extrinsic value beyond the student's capacity to minimize exposure to disease and mediocrity. It will render our graduates more employable! The evidence for a growing interest by such firms as Tenneco, ETNA Life and Casualty, Texas Instruments, and a long list of other major corporations in healthy job candidates is too evident to overlook. Tenneco, for example, has demonstrated after years of experimentation with employee wellness programming that the participants in such activities are the same employees who earn the highest performance ratings. As a result, company policy is to motivate a greater percentage of their work force to engage in wellness lifestyles—*and to focus future hires on those who already practice healthy living.*

The goals for the program are as follows:

1. In one year's time, to create an awareness of and a favorable attitude toward wellness among a majority of the on-campus students at the university.

2. In one year's time, to have in place a comprehensive peer-learning process under the auspices of SWAT. The SWAT will also prepare and publish a *Campus Wellness Report*, which will be distributed throughout the campus.

For more on campus wellness, write the unofficial but generally acknowledged coordinator for programs on the topic, Connie Kunda, Ph.D., Director of Wellness, Muhlenberg College, Allentown, PA 18104.

Lately I've Been Thinking About . . .

SOMETHING WORTH COMPLAINING ABOUT, ARTFULLY OR OTHERWISE

Writing letters is one thing, being wary about "health" insurance another, and having an interest in wellness programming on campus and elsewhere yet another; but there are some anti-wellness matters so profound that you have to be on the alert nearly all the time to safeguard yourself against them. Unfortunately, doing so is extremely difficult. These forces can creep up on you when you least expect them. I have in mind such "biggies" as famine and drought, hurricanes and cyclones, nuclear fission, wind shear, bubonic plague, and cigarette smoke.

I had strong feelings about smoking when I wrote *High Level Wellness*. I am no less concerned about this wretched habit today.

A *USA Today* survey in September 1985 showed that cigarette smoking is the number one factor in eliciting a *turnoff* response in someone of the other sex. By contrast, people seem almost tolerant of other well-established and time-tested yuks and vices, such as obesity, unkempt appearance, loudness, too much aftershave, sour disposition, a preoccupation with looks, appearing conceited, or too much makeup. So, better to be an overweight, conceited slob with a big mouth and heavy makeup, excessive aftershave and a Nazi personality than to be a smoker. In fact, if you smoke, I suspect there's no hope for any social life whatsoever unless you can find another smoker to socialize with.

If militant anti-smokers like yours truly have their way, that might be even more of a hassle in the years ahead. Here is a summary of a few recent developments that may be of interest.

On the legal front: Product-liability suits from a small army of characters who smoked their fool heads off for years and now want to make the manufacturers responsible for their behavior actually constitute a genuine threat to the $57-billion-a-year tobacco industry. This is a classic case of litigants who deserve each other. Pending are 35 cases. The reason for the renewed hopes for the "breakthrough" victory is that there have been changes in the law that now penalize manufacturers in tort cases for making a product that is inherently unsafe, regardless of extenuating circumstances. This twist is a result of something lawyers call "strict liability" theory from product cases in the late 70s. What it really represents is a chance to blame someone for the dumb things you did. It may be OK when the one being sued is a tobacco company, but it's not such a wise alternative to personal responsibility for your own current life situation and future options.

On the economic front: Some universities are into divestiture, not only against South Africa but in protest against a blight far worse than apartheid, namely cigarette manufacturers. Reports that such stalwart institutions of high learning as Harvard are preparing to unload tobacco company stocks has investors running scared. Naturally, this affects the value of tobacco stocks. One analyst is quoted as saying, "There are 35 opportunities for lawyers to strike gold. They would have to be real idiots not to get *one* of these suits right. And once the first suit is lost, tobacco stocks will collapse."

Richard Daynard, a prominent law professor, writes that 700,000 actions a year could be taken against the tobacco purveyors, based on current morbidity and mortality data linked to smoking!

On the cancer-training front: Domestic consumption is down! Only 595,000,000,000 (that's *billion*) of the yellow-brown scum sticks were consumed this year, versus 600 billion last year. There has been a 4 percent drop in cigarette use in the past three years. (Why don't I feel cheered by this statistic?) That's the good news.

Before continuing, a parable seems in order. Are you ready for this?

Doctor phones patient: "Hortense, I have some very bad— and some *very, very* bad news for you. Which do you want first?"

Hortense: "Hey, Doctor, you need work on your bedside manner. Ease it to me, will ya? Don't be so blunt. You want to scare an old girl to death? Give me the simple bad news first."

Doctor: "Hortense, my dear. It's awful. You have 24 hours, max—if you are lucky."

Hortense: "My God! What could be worse than that? What's the *very, very* bad news?"

Doctor: "I was supposed to call you yesterday."

So here is the *very, very, very* bad news: On the world scene, smoking is rising dramatically, especially in poor nations where ad marketing is targeted and where antismoking campaigns practically don't exist. According to the *AMA News* (October 4, 1985), in China and India one third of the male population is addicted to cigarettes by the time they are 20 years old.

On the political front: At least 50 more local governments have adopted anti-smoking provisions, and 57 are pending. The federal tax of $.16 a pack was passed by the Senate Finance Committee; some had tried to raise this to $.40. Next time, maybe. One Ann Arbor study showed that an increase to $.32 would lead 3.5 million Americans to quit or decide not to start, which in turn would prevent 875 million premature deaths.

The AMA is coming on strong against smoking—and it is about time! It probably senses the rise in public intolerance for the existing norm permitting this truly foul and repulsive practice in otherwise civilized places. AMA members recently adopted a resolution calling for a total ban on all tobacco advertising. In coordinated action on Senator John Chafee's (R, R.I.) bill to raise the tax, 43 groups joined forces into a coalition representing no less than 30 million antismokers. A Boston research specialist, Dr. Michael Charney, urges his fellow physicians to attack cigarette makers through lawsuits. He believes that by referring cancer-stricken patients to attorneys, doctors help drive up the cost of the product, thereby protecting the young, who are most sensitive and resistant to increases in the cost of smoking. In the September 20 issue of the *AMA News*, Dr. Charney recalls that family doctors used to warn patients away from mosquito-plagued areas because of the diseases known to be transmitted by mosquito-borne infections—and he suggests that the same principle is in play now. Suits against the tobacco pushers make sense because the cigarette makers "are the mosquitoes of the 20th Century."

On the research front: A Kentucky study just released suggests that pregnant smokers may be maiming their babies! How lowdown can they get? It has long been known that low birth weights were found in babies born to smokers; now, birth defects such as retardation, abnormal facial features, and heart defects have been linked to two-or-more-pack-a-day offenders. Most recently, a link between parental smoking and inner ear infections in young children has been demonstrated. Which raises the question: "Shouldn't a pregnant smoker be arrested for child abuse?" Also, where are the "Right to Lifers" when we need them?

You think I'm picking on (pregnant) women smokers? Check this: Another study at the University of Washington showed that male smokers have fewer sperm! What is more, what fewer, wimpy sperm they do have are not even regular in shape. How disgusting! And, as you might expect, they *move* less than the sperm of nonsmokers. Think of that—sedentary sperm. These are among the results of 12 studies with 4,000 men.

As cigarettes become less accessible, more costly, less acceptable, more dangerous, and more obvious as a cause of or contributor to millions of disorders and deaths, perhaps consumption in 1986 will *fall* a few billion more, and continue to do so for the coming decade—to the point where an historic last puff will be celebrated before the Year 2000.

Once this dragon is slain (current toll is 350,000 U.S. deaths annually and $40 billion in health-related costs), the forces of the wellness revolution can join in battle against megadragons of the Galaxy, like nuclear fission, bubonic plague, and creatures of that ilk.

P.S. One more front: Hot Flash from the as-yet-not-world-renowned *WAAKO Institute*: What do you think would happen if a scientist went to the media with proof of a link between smoking and AIDS? Recent research at the Wellness Attitude Adjusters and Kinesthetic Organizers (WAAKO) Institute shows that smoking is even worse than anyone ever would have guessed. Ready for this?

SMOKING CAUSES A.I.D.S.!

That's right. I saw the data. You can always trust the WAAKO Institute. In this historic study, which should appeal to all better publications (like the *National Enquirer*, for instance), smokers were shown to have *air-insufficient delivery systems*, or an AIDS syndrome, in comparison with nonsmokers.

Before concluding this diatribe, I should report something that may serve as a time capsule for the present, a sort of "sign of the times." *Time* magazine publisher John Meyers noted, in the October 7, 1985, issue, that Americans have clearly developed a new awareness about the way they look and feel—and that *Time* has responded to that interest with a new weekly section, "Health and Fitness." *This is good.* Not to be outdone, *Time*'s chief editor offered this: "A major change in modern life has been the increasing understanding of the benefits of fitness and preventive medicine. It is not a fad or craze. It is not a jog, it is here for the long run." *This too, is good,* particularly in view of the fact that *Time* distributes about 25 million copies of each issue.

It's possible that this little item in *Time* will prove more influential than *both* editions of *High Level Wellness*. Fine, I can handle it. Still, don't you wish they were not a year or two behind? Come on, *Time*, you should know better. The title, "Health and Fitness" is redundant: there is no genuine fitness without health—and "health" assumes a fit body. What the editors should be pushing is a *wellness* section—*and that's a very good thing.*

Maybe we should write to Anastasia Toufexis and Georgia Harbison, two fit and healthy young writer types pictured in full athletic glory to whom the boss men of *Time* have entrusted this cushy assignment. The sooner they learn about wellness (including "health and fitness" and a great deal more), the faster the movement will move toward levels of well-being as yet unimagined by those who see true health as something to be "moderate" about.

While you are at it, why not write John Meyers an "artful complaint"-type letter about all the ads that *Time* still features for products that don't promote fitness, health, and all other aspects of the wellness "boom"? I refer to the five pages of inane smoking ads that appear in the same issue as the health and fitness column!

If you want to see hypocrisy in action, examine *Time*'s so-called health and fitness supplement (October 14, 1985), and note how much it tells you about the hazards of smoking. I'll save

376

you the trouble: Not a word! Naturally, the ads are there, spread all through the magazine.

Oh well. There is always *gradual* change, if only a bit of patience can be mustered. Of course, if you cannot muster patience, you can always write the editors at *Time* an artful complaint. If readers cancelled or chose not to renew their subscriptions in protest against tobacco advertising and its attendant constraint on the quality of reporting, maybe change at *Time* would happen a little less gradually. What do you think?

Wellness Resource Guide
The Honor Roll of Books

Reflections on . . .

A Wellness Resource Guide
The High Level Wellness
Honor Roll of Books

pages
215–293 This was a useful section, if the feedback I received from readers represents how most people responded to the book. This selective annotated bibliography answers the (silent) question, "Where do you go after *High Level Wellness?*" My recommendations for further reading in the five dimensions of wellness still strike me as a good, solid way to educate yourself about wellness. Although many of these books are somewhat dated now, the majority are still worth examining, if you have not already done so. The best of the lot, still provocative and fresh, are those written by Harry Browne, A. H. Maslow, Ivan Illich, Marc Lalonde, and Halbert Dunn.

Of course, many worthwhile books on the subject of wellness have appeared since 1976—and a good thing, too! Rather than compiling an exhaustive listing of these publications, I'm adding a brief, unannotated, updated list at the back. Peruse at the risk of becoming more wellness conscious.

Though ten years have passed, I can not think of a better way to say goodbye to you, the reader who has honored me by reading all this copy, than to repeat the close I wrote for the first edition:

There is excitement, adventure, enjoyment, and fulfillment for us on this Earth. A wellness lifestyle will not guarantee or assure that you experience these states, but it will certainly bend the odds your way. At a minimum, you can expect that a healthy body, emotional equilibrium, and an alive mind will give you one hell of a good start.

Be well.

Lately I've Been Thinking About . . .

MORE BOOKS THAT ARE
GOOD FOR YOUR HEALTH

If knowledge is power, then knowledge about wellness is powerful healthy. Here's my list of books worth reading on the subject of wellness that have been published since the original edition of *High Level Wellness* came out.

Dimension of Norms or Rules:

Allen, Robert F. *Lifegain*. New York: Appleton-Century-Crofts, 1981.

Blanchard, Marjorie, and Tager, Mark. *Working Well*. New York: Simon and Schuster, 1985.

Irving, John. *Cider House Rules*. New York: William Morrow, 1985.

Dimension of Self-Responsibility and Medical Self-Care:

Greening, Tom, and Hobson, Dick. *Instant Relief: The Encyclopedia of Self-Help*. Wideview Books, 1979.

Kemper, Donald, et al. *Pathways*. Boise, ID: Healthwise, 1985.

The New Holistic Handbook: Living Well in a New Age. Lexington, MA: Stephen Greene Press/Penguin Books, 1985.

Roberts, Toni M., Tinker, Kathleen, and Kemper, Donald W. *Healthwise Handbook: A Guide to Responsible Health Care*. Garden City, NY: Doubleday, 1979.

Sobel, David S., and Ferguson, Tom. *The People's Book of Medical Tests*. New York: Summit Books, 1985.

Sobel, David Stuart, and Hornbacher, Faith Louise. *An Everyday Guide to Your Health*. New York: Grossman, 1973.

Vickery, Donald M. *Lifeplan for Your Health*. Reading, MA: Addison-Wesley, 1978.

Wildavsky, Aaron. "Doing Better and Feeling Worse: Health in the United States." *Daedalus: Journal of the American Academy of Arts and Sciences* (Winter 1977).

Dimension of Nutrition and Fitness:

Bailey, Covert. *Fit or Fat*. Boston, MA: Houghton-Mifflin, 1978.

Bailey, Covert. *Target Diet*. Boston, MA: Houghton-Mifflin, 1984.

Brody, Jane. *Jane Brody's Nutrition Book*. New York: Bantam, 1982.

Burger, Robert E. *Jogger's Catalog*. New York: M. Evans and Co., 1978.

Clark, Nancy. *The Athlete's Kitchen*. New York: CBI Publishing Co., 1981.

Devries, Herbert A. *Health Science: A Positive Approach*. Santa Monica, CA: Goodyear, 1979.

Eisenberg, Arlene, and Eisenberg, Howard. *Alive and Well: Decisions in Health*. New York: McGraw-Hill, 1979.

Farquhar, John W. *The American Way of Life Need Not Be Hazardous to Your Health*. New York: Norton, 1978.

Fixx, James F. *The Complete Book of Running*. New York: Random House, 1977.

Kuntzleman, Charles T. *Activetics*. New York: Wyden, 1978.

McCoy, Kathy, and Wibbelsman, Charles. *The Teenage Body Book*. New York: Pocket Books, 1978.

Newman, Vicky, and Cummins, Candy. *The Eater's Guide*. Englewood Cliffs, N.J.: Prentice-Hall, 1981.

Osman, Jack D. *Thin from Within*. Washington, DC: Review and Herald Publishing Association, 1981.

Piscatella, Joseph C., and Piscatella, Bernie. *Don't Eat Your Heart Out Cookbook*. New York: Workman Publishing Co., 1983.

Smith, David. *The East/West Exercise Book*. New York: McGraw-Hill, 1976.

Dimension of Stress Management and Boredom Immunity:

Carney, Richard (Ed.). *Risk Taking: Implications for the Behavioral Sciences*. St. Louis: Mosby, 1979.

Crookse, Mark. *Wellness Through Risk Taking.* Pompano Beach, FL: Exposition Press, 1985.

Davis, Martha, et al. *The Relaxation and Stress Reduction Workbook.* Richmond, CA: New Harbinger Publications, 1980.

Gawain, Shakti. *Creative Visualization.* Mill Valley, CA: Whatever Publishing, 1978.

Pelletier, Kenneth R. *Mind As Healer, Mind As Slayer: A Holistic Approach to Preventing Stress Disorders.* New York: Delta, 1977.

Schafer, Walt. *Stress, Distress and Growth.* Davis, CA: International Dialogue Press, 1978.

Tanner, Ogden. *Stress.* New York: Time-Life Books, 1976.

Zuckerman, Marvin. *Sensation Seeking: Beyond the Optimal Level of Arousal.* Hillsdale, NJ: Lawrence Erlbaum Assoc., Inc., 1979.

Dimension of Ethics, Values, and Purposes

Allen, Robert F. (with Charlotte Kraft). *Beat the System: A Way to Create More Human Environments.* New York: McGraw-Hill, 1980.

Ardell, Donald B. *The History and Future of Wellness.* Dubuque, IA: Kendall/Hunt Publishing Co., 1986.

————, and Tager, Mark. *Planning for Wellness: A Guidebook for Achieving Optimal Health.* Dubuque, IA: Kendall/Hunt Publishing Co., 1982.

Brilliant, Ashley. *I May Not Be Totally Perfect, But Parts of Me Are Excellent.* Santa Barbara, CA: Woodbridge, 1979.

Dyer, Wayne W. *Your Erroneous Zones.* New York: Avon, 1976.

Ryan, Regina Sara, and Travis, John W. *Wellness Workbook.* Berkeley, CA: Ten Speed Press, 1981.

Shanor, Karen. *The Shanor Study: The Sexual Sensitivity of the American Male.* New York: The Dial Press, 1978.

Index

Book reviews are in italics.

A

Absenteeism, and wellness, 315
Active, definition of, 334n.
Acupuncture, 29
Additives, food, 117
Add Years to Your Life and Life to Your Years (Gore), 274–75
Advertising, tobacco, 374
Age, and fitness, 335
Aging, 57–58
    and exercise, 146
Aikman, Ann, 263
Airola, Paavo, 243
Alcohol, 95–96, 100, 119
    suggested legislation on, 196
Allen, Robert F., 327
AMA News, 374
Ardell Wellness-at-the-Workplace Test, 317–20
Ardell Wellness Culture Test, 312–15
Ardell Wellness Stress Test, 309–12
Are You Confused? (Airola), 243–46
ARICA, 107
Arteriosclerosis, exercise and, 146
Assertiveness, 142
Athlete's Kitchen, The (Clark), 333

B

Bailey, Covert, 333
Beggs, James, wellness letter to, 353–54
Bennett, Hal Z., 266
Benson, Herbert, 258
Be Well (Samuels and Bennett), 266–68
Bioenergetics, 107
    for stress control, 14
Blood pressure, garlic for, 116
Blue Cross Association, 222
Books, on wellness, 215–92
    recently published, 378–81
Boredom:
    books on immunity from, 380–81
    effects of, 339
    immunity from, 338–42
Born to Win (James and Jongeward), 219–21
Boston Women's Health Collective, 225

Brain, 57
    cycles of activity of, 136–37
Bran, for digestion, 116
Breakfast, need for, 122
Breathing techniques, importance of, during exercise, 155–56
Brewer's yeast, as source of Vitamin B, 132
Brody, Jane, 333
Browne, Harry, 216
Buckley, William F., 349, 363
Buddy system, for pursuit of wellness, 62
Business, role of, in wellness, 186–88

C

Cafeterias, junk food in, 199
Caffeine, effect of, on the body, 119
Calisthenics, for exercise, 156
Cancer, and smoking, 373–74
Carbohydrates, 118, 132
Carlson, Rick, 227
Centering, 34–35
Cereals, sugar-coated, suggested legislation for, 196
Children:
    decision to have, 168
    illness in, 176
Cigarettes, addiction to, 374. *See also* Smoking
Clark, Nancy, 333
Coffee. *See* Caffeine
Colleges, wellness programs at, 369–72
Communities, international, 289–99
Community action, 209–12
Competition, as stress, 152
Complaint, reflections on the artful, 347–65
Computer video, interactive, 301
Conley, Peter, wellness letter to, 359–61
Cooking, of fruit and vegetables, 120
Crookse, Dr. Mark, 339–42
    address of, 342
Culture, and wellness, 312–13, 328. *See also* Norms
Cummins, Candy, 333

D

Danyard, Richard, 373
Davis, Adelle, 246
Death, 6–7
Decision making, 101
Dieting. *See* Weight control
Diet for a Small Planet (Lappé), 286–88
Digestion, 115, 166
    fiber and, 120–21
    sugar and, 118
Divestiture, of tobacco stocks, 373
Downing, George, 261
Dreams, 37
Drinking. *See* Alcohol
Dunn, Dr. Halbert L., 283, 300

E

East West Academy of Healing Arts, 41–42
Eastwood, Clint, wellness letter to, 356–57
Eater's Guide, The (Newman and Cummins), 333
Eating, mood during, 121, 122, 166–67
Education, in health field, 97
End of Medicine, The (Carlson), 227–28
Erhard Seminars Training (EST), 105–106
Esalen Institute, 42–47, 297
Ethics, 343–46
    books on, 381
Excellence, 316, 320
Exercise (*See also* Physical fitness), 333–34
    benefits of, 146–48
    isometric, 156–67
    isotonic, 157
Exertion, perceived level of, 335

F

Fasting, 36, 128–29
Fats, 132
Fiber, 116, 118, 120–21, 132
Fight or flight response, to stress, 137
Fit or Fat (Bailey), 333
Fitness:
    approaches to, 334
    books on, 380
    reflections on physical, 333–35
Flour, white, 118
Folk Medicine (Jarvis), 248–49

Food:
    attitudes toward, 331
    processed, 117–18, 167
    reflections on fads about, 330–32
Food chain:
    and diet, 166
    eating on, 166–67
Food habits, as symptoms, 330
Food processing, 331–32
14 Days to a Wellness Lifestyle (Ardell), 331
Frankel, Victor, 339
Fringe benefits, and wellness, 367–68
Fuchs, Victor R., 229, 367

G

Garlic, 115–16
Gergley, Jerry, 335
Glasser, William, 270
Gomez, Joan, 272
Gore, Irene, 274
Gross, Leonard, 277

H

Happiness, 98–99, 100–101, 171
Hay fever, exercise and, 147
Headaches, biofeedback for, 14
Healing: A Doctor in Search of a Miracle (Nolen), 237–41
Health:
    definitions of, 64–66
    holistic, definition of, 5, 55
Health centers, 7
    hospitals as, 191–93
    need for, 47–48
Health Hazard Appraisal, 307
Health insurance, 193
    reflections on, 365–68
Health planning:
    reflections on, 369–72
    role of, 207–208
Health Systems Agencies (HSA), 208–12
Healthy America, 369
Heart rate (pulse rate), determining, 89–91, 152, 334–35
Herbs, in cooking, 130
High Level Wellness (Dunn), 283–86
History and Future of Wellness (Ardell), 369
Holmes Life Change Index (LCI):
    applicability of, 311
    reflections on, 307–309
    stress management and, 85–87
Honey, 116, 332
Hospitals, as health centers, 191–93

How I Found Freedom in an Unfree World (Browne), 216–19
How Not to Die Young (Gomez), 272–74
HSA. *See* Health Systems Agencies
Human Life Styling: Keeping Whole in the Twentieth Century (McCamy and Presley, 288–92
Hypertension, garlic for, 116

I

Iacocca, Lee, 363
Iatrogenesis, 4, 193
Illich, Ivan, 231
Illness:
    in children, 176
    meaning of, 56
Illness-Wellness Continuum, 298
Insomnia, biofeedback for, 14
Intramural sports, need for, 148
Inventory, of personal wellness, 66–82

J

James, Muriel, 219
Jane Brody's Nutrition Book (Brody), 333
Job, in wellness, 370n.
Jogging, 6, 36
Jongeward, Dorothy, 219
Journal, keeping of, 15–16

K

Kunda, Connie, address of, 371

L

LaLonde, Marc, 233
Langdon, John, 370–71
Lappé, Frances Moore, 286
Lawsuits, product-liability, and tobacco, 373, 374
Legislation, needed for wellness, 194–97
Leonard, George, 275
Let's Eat Right to Keep Fit (Davis), 246–47
Letters, wellness, 348–63
Life Change Index. *See* Holmes Life Change Index
Lifegain (Allen), 327

M

McGuire, Thomas, 249
McQuade, Walter, 263
Madden, John, wellness letter to, 351–52
Massage, 44

Massage Book, The (Downing), 261–63
Maximum Heart Rate Test Profile, 307
Meadowlark Wellness Center, 20–24, 297
Medical Nemesis (Illich), 231–33
Medication, need for, 53
Medicine:
    books on, 221–22
    changing, to wellness, 183–85
    cost of, 3–4
    modern, 18, 50
Meditation, 5, 6
    effect of, on the body, 140
Megavitamin therapy, 130
Mendelsohn, Robert, 367
MHR (maximum heart rate). *See* Heart rate, determining
Milk, raw, 130–31, 332
Model:
    Ardell's, of the dimensions of wellness, revised, 324–27
    Hettler's National Wellness Institute, 326
    Travis Energy, 326
Moderation, considerations on, 321–22
Morehouse, Lawrence E., 277

N

National Center for Health Promotion, 369, 370n.
National Wellness Association, 369
Nature, as a healer, 51
New England Center, 25–27
Newman, Vicky, 333
New Perspective on the Health of Canadians (LaLonde), 233–37
Nietzsche, Friedrich William, 344
Nitrates, 117
Nolen, William A., 237
Norms (rules):
    and attitudes toward wellness, 327–28
    books on, 379
Nutrition, 113–33
    books on, 242, 333, 380
    at Meadowlark, 21–22
    principles of, 115–22
    reflections on awareness of, 329
    at San Andreas Health Council, 35–36
    at Wellness Resource Center, 16–17, 131–33
    at Wholistic Health and Nutrition Institute, 29

Nutrition Against Disease (Williams), 255–57
Nutrition and Health: An Evaluation of Nutritional Surveillance in the United States (U.S. Senate), 253–55

O

Our Bodies, Ourselves: A Book by and for Women (Boston Women's Health Collective), 225–27
Overeating, 35
Overweight. *See* Weight control

P

Performance, breakthrough, 316
Personal expectations, 168–73
Physical fitness, 145–61
    books on, 270
    principles of, 151–58
    at San Andreas Health Council, 36–37
    at Wellness Resource Center, 17
Podiatry, 29
Polarity balancing, 106–107
Positive Addiction (Glasser), 270–72
Proceedings of the Conference on Future Directions in Health Care (Blue Cross Association, et al.), 222–25
Productivity, and wellness, 316
Protein, need for, 119–20, 131
Proverbs, Chinese, 321
Proxmire, William, 280
Psychosynthesis, 15, 106
Pulse rate. *See* Heart rate
Purpose, need for, in life, 99. *See also* Ethics

Q

Questionnaire:
    Health Hazard Appraisal, 87–88
    Holmes Life Change Index, 85–87
    Nutrition, Health, and Activity Profile, 88–89
    Voice Stress Analysis, 82–85
    from Wellness Resource Center, 11–14

R

Reagan, Ronald, wellness letter to, 358–59
Relaxation Response, The (Benson), 258–61
Research, on the effects of smoking, 375
Reuben, David, 252

Risk taking, social, 340–41
Rockefeller Foundation, 222
Rogers, Harrison L., wellness letter to, 354–56, 363
Rules. *See* Norms
Ryan, Regina, 298

S

Samuels, Mike, 266
San Andreas Health Council, 33–40
Save Your Life Diet, The (Reuben), 252–53
Self-care. *See* Self-responsibility
Self-responsibility, 49–51, 94–112
    books on, 216, 221–22, 379
    at Esalen Institute, 43
    principles of, 98–101
    reflections on, 327, 328–29
    at San Andreas Health Council, 34
    at Wellness Resource Center, 8, 12–13, 15–16
Selye, Hans, 268–69, 339
Sensitivity, environmental, 162–77
    book list, 283
    principles of, 165–73
    reflections on, 342–46
    at San Andreas Health Councils, 37–38
    space shaping, 173–76
Silva mind control, 107–108
Small business, support for wellness in, 315
Smoking, 95, 100, 166
    provisions against, 374–75
    reflections on, 372–77
    suggested legislation on, 195, 196
    and the worseness-oriented, 303–304
Soybeans, 115
Space-shaping, 168–76
Spirituality, 343
Stallone, Sylvester, wellness letter to, 361–62
Steinbrenner, George, wellness letter to, 357–58
Stress:
    competition and, 152
    reactions to, 137, 309, 311–12, 336–37
Stress (McQuade and Aikman), 263–66
Stress management, 134–44, 175–76
    books on, 258, 380–81
    exercise for, 60

Holmes Life Change Index and, 85–87
principles of, 138–43
reflections on, 336–38
at San Andreas Health Council, 37
voice stress analysis and, 82–85
at Wellness Resource Center, 12, 14–15
Stress Without Distress (Selye), 268–69
"Strokes," 54–55, 95
Sugar, effect of, on the body, 118
Sunflower seeds, 116
Supplements, need for, 128

T

Tax credit, for wellness activities, 189–90
Tea, herbal, 332. *See also* Caffeine
Teeth, sugar and, 118
Test: Ardell Wellness Stress, 309–12
Ardell Wellness Culture, 312–15
of wellness in the workplace, 315–20
Testimonials, reflections on value of, 305
Tests, revised, for measuring wellness, 306–23
Time magazine, on fitness, 376–77
Tooth Trip: An Oral Experience (McGuire), 249–52
Total Fitness: In 30 Minutes a Week (Morehouse and Gross), 277–80
Transactional Analysis (TA), 15, 54–55, 95, 108, 219
Transcendental Meditation (TM), 139, 143
Travis, Dr. John, 296–302
address of, 302

U

Ultimate Athlete, The (Leonard), 275–77
University of California, Health Policy Program, 222
University of Central Florida, wellness program at, 370–71
U.S. Senate, 253

V

Values. *See* Ethics
Vegetarianism, 125–26
Vending machines, suggestions for, 195
Vinegar, apple cider, 116, 331
Vision, 14–15

Vitamin A, 133
Vitamin B complex, 132–33
Vitamin C, 130–32
Vitamin D, 133
Vitamin E, 132

W

Water, types of, 127–28
Watermelon, 116, 331
Weight control, 126–27, 149
reflections on, 330
"Well Medicine/Traditional Medicine Continuum," 297–98
Wellness:
consciousness of, 347
dimensions of high level, 324–46
principles of, 49–54, 302–303
reflections on measuring, 306–23
social possibilities of, 205–6
Wellness centers, reflections on, 296–97
"Wellness Community Newsletter" (Travis and Travis), 299
Wellness ethic, reflections on, 302–305
Wellness Report, 299–301
letters in, 348
Wellness Resource Center, 6, 8–19, 131–33
Wellness Through Risk Taking, (Crookse), 340
Wellness Workbook for Helping Professionals (Travis), 298
Wellness/Worseness Continuum, 306
Wheat germ, 116
Wholistic Health and Nutrition Institute (WHN), 6, 27–33
Who Shall Live? Health, Economics, and Social Choice (Fuchs), 229–31
Williams, Roger J., 255
Workplace, as wellness center, 185–88

Y

Yeast, nutritional, 116
YMCA:
exercise programs, 154
fitness evaluations, 89–90
Yoga, 36, 40, 139, 156
Yoghurt, 115
You Can Do It! Senator Proxmire's Exercise, Diet and Relaxation Plan, 280–82